Biotechnological Approaches in Waste Management

Waste generation from industrial and domestic sectors is imposing a very challenging environment and the intervention of biotechnology offers a viable solution for their effective management. This book deals with the employment of biotechnological aspects for waste treatment including the basic concepts, biochemical processes, and various technologies for pollutant reduction and production of value-added products for a cleaner environment. It covers different aspects of biotechnology in the conservation of environment dealing with the sustainable management of waste through the concept of waste-to-economy along with the management of environmental pollutants and natural resource conservation.

- Focuses on ecological approaches i.e., the use of biocatalysts and biotechnological approaches for waste management
- Explores the different biotechnology-based solutions for the removal of environmental pollutants
- Covers various microbiological routes, technological options for waste to energy, removal of contaminants, and the production of value-added products
- Reviews the bioremediation potential of microbial strains and enzymes
- Explores the significant routes of biotechnological means of obtaining eco-friendly products substituting the hazardous chemical-based products

This volume is aimed at researchers and professionals in environmental, biotechnology, and chemical engineering.

Novel Biotechnological Applications for Waste to Value Conversion

Series Editors:

Neha Srivastava, IIT BHU Varanasi, Uttar Pradesh, India and
Manish Srivastava, IIT BHU Varanasi, Uttar Pradesh, India

Solid waste and its sustainable management is considered as one of the major global issues due to industrialization and economic growth. Effective solid waste management (SWM) is a major challenge in the areas with high population density, and despite significant development in social, economic and environmental areas, SWM systems are still increasing the environmental pollution day by day. Thus, there is an urgent need to attend to this issue for green & sustainable environment. Therefore, the proposed book series is a sustainable attempt to cover waste management and their conversion into value-added products.

Nanobiotechnology for Safe Bioactive Nanobiomaterials
Poushpi Dwivedi, Shahid S. Narvi, Ravi Prakash Tewari and Dhanesh Tiwary

Sustainable Microbial Technologies for Valorization of Agro-Industrial Wastes
Jitendra Kumar Saini, Surender Singh and Lata Nain

Enzymes in Valorization of Waste
Enzymatic Pre-treatment of Waste for Development of Enzyme based Biorefinery (Vol I)
Pradeep Verma

Enzymes in Valorization of Waste
Enzymatic Hydrolysis of Waste for Development of Value-added Products (Vol II)
Pradeep Verma

Enzymes in Valorization of Waste
Next-Gen Technological Advances for Sustainable Development of Enzyme based Biorefinery (Vol III)
Pradeep Verma

Biotechnological Approaches in Waste Management
Rangabhashiyam S, Ponnusami V and Pardeep Singh

Agricultural and Kitchen Waste
Energy and Environmental Aspects
Dan Bahadur Pal and Amit Kumar Tiwari

For more information about this series, please visit: www.routledge.com/Novel-Biotechnological-Applications-for-Waste-to-Value-Conversion/book-series/NVAWVC

Biotechnological Approaches in Waste Management

Edited by

Rangabhashiyam S, Ponnusami V and Pardeep Singh

CRC Press
Taylor & Francis Group
Boca Raton London New York

CRC Press is an imprint of the
Taylor & Francis Group, an **informa** business

First edition published 2023
by CRC Press
6000 Broken Sound Parkway NW, Suite 300, Boca Raton, FL 33487-2742

and by CRC Press
4 Park Square, Milton Park, Abingdon, Oxon, OX14 4RN

CRC Press is an imprint of Taylor & Francis Group, LLC

ISBN: 9781032036298 (hbk)
ISBN: 9781032036342 (pbk)
ISBN: 9781003188292 (ebk)

DOI: 10.1201/9781003188292

Typeset in Times
by codeMantra

Contents

Editors

Rangabhashiyam S. is an assistant professor in the School of Chemical and Biotechnology, SASTRA Deemed University, India. He received his Doctor of Philosophy degree from the National Institute of Technology, Calicut, India. He has received Post-Doctoral Fellowship from Max Planck Institute for Dynamics of Complex Technical Systems, Germany, received National-Post Doctoral Fellowship from SERB-DST, India, selected as Young Scientist by DST, India, for the BRICS Conclave held in Durban, South Africa, and received Hiyoshi Young Leaf Award from Hiyoshi Ecological Services, Hiyoshi Corporation, Japan. His major research interests are bioremediation and wastewater treatment. He is an Editorial Board Member in *Scientific Reports, Biomass Conversion and Biorefinery,* Associate Editor in *International Journal of Environmental Science and Technology, IET Nanobiotechnology, Frontiers in Environmental Chemistry,* Academic Editor of *Adsorption Science and Technology* and Editorial Board of *Scientific Reports.* He has published more than 90 papers and also contributed several book chapters including editing books from Elsevier and Wiley. He is listed in the World's Top 2% Scientist published by Elsevier, Stanford.

Ponnusami V. is Associate Dean in the School of Chemical & amp; Biotechnology, SASTRA Deemed University, India. He graduated from A. C. Tech., Anna University, and did his doctoral research in SASTRA Deemed University, India. He has rich industrial and academic experience. His research interests include domestic and industrial wastewater treatment, bioconversion of lignocellulose, and bioprocessing. His group is working on photocatalysis, production of renewable fuels, and microbial polysaccharides. He had published over 50 research papers in international journals.

Pardeep Singh is an assistant professor in the Department of Environmental Study, PGDAV College, University of Delhi, New Delhi, India. He obtained his doctorate from the Indian Institute of Technology (Banaras Hindu University), Varanasi. He was also selected as Young Scientist by DST, India, for the BRICS Conclave held in Durban, South Africa. His research interests include waste management, wastewater treatment, water scarcity, and global climate change. He has published more than 75 research/review papers in international journals in the fields of waste and wastewater treatment/management. He has also edited more than 40 books with various international publishers like CRC Press, Elsevier, Springer Nature, Wiley, and IGI.

Contributors

Sanjida Aktar
Department of Environmental Sciences
Patuakhali Science and Technology University
Patuakhali, Bangladesh

Ayesa Akter Suhi
Department of Agronomy
Patuakhali Science and Technology University
Patuakhali, Bangladesh

Sam Aldrin Chandran
School of Chemical and Biotechnology
SASTRA Deemed to be University
Thanjavur, India

V. Anbuganesan
Department of Environmental Sciences
Bharathiar University
Coimbatore, India

A. S. Archana
Department of Environmental Sciences
Bharathiar University
Coimbatore, India

Nur Izyan Wan Azelee
School of Chemical and Energy Engineering, Faculty of Engineering
Universiti Teknologi Malaysia (UTM)
Skudai, Malaysia
Institute of Bioproduct Development (IBD)
Universiti Teknologi Malaysia (UTM)
Skudai, Malaysia

Ganesh Babu Malli Mohan
School of Chemical and Biotechnology
SASTRA Deemed to be University
Thanjavur, India

Nur Afiqah Badli
Department of Chemistry, Faculty of Science
Universiti Teknologi Malaysia
Johor Bahru

Nurul Nabila Huda Baharudin
Department of Chemical Engineering, College of Engineering
Universiti Malaysia Pahang
Gambang, Malaysia

L. Benedict Bruno
Department of Environmental Sciences
Bharathiar University
Coimbatore, India

Muhammad Abd Hadi Bunyamin
Faculty of Social Sciences and Humanities
Universiti Teknologi Malaysia UTM
Skudai, Malaysia

Rohaida Che Man
Department of Chemical Engineering, College of Engineering
Universiti Malaysia Pahang
Gambang, Malaysia

Aayush Kumar Choudhary
Department of Chemical Engineering
National Institute of Technology
Tiruchirappalli, India

Daniel Joe Dailin
School of Chemical and Energy Engineering, Faculty of Engineering
Universiti Teknologi Malaysia (UTM)
Skudai, Malaysia
Institute of Bioproduct Development (IBD)
Universiti Teknologi Malaysia (UTM)
Skudai, Malaysia

Hesham Ali El Enshasy
School of Chemical and Energy Engineering, Faculty of Engineering
Universiti Teknologi Malaysia (UTM)
Skudai, Malaysia
Institute of Bioproduct Development (IBD)
Universiti Teknologi Malaysia (UTM)
Skudai, Malaysia
City of Scientific Research and Technology Applications (SRTA)
New Burg Al Arab, Egypt

Vinodini Elango
Department of Chemical Engineering,
National Institute of Technology
Tiruchirappalli, India

Farah Shahirah Mohd Fairuz
School of Health Sciences
Universiti Sains Malaysia
Kubang Kerian, Malaysia

Siti Fatimah Zaharah Mohd Fuzi
Department of Technology & Natural Resources, Faculty of Applied Science & Technology
UTHM
Panchor, Johor

Godwin Glivin
Department of Energy and Environment
National Institute of Technology
Tiruchirappalli, India

N. Kalaiselvan
Department of Energy and Environment
National Institute of Technology
Tiruchirappalli, India

H. Hareesh Krishnan
Department of Energy and Environment
National Institute of Technology
Tiruchirappalli, India

A. Ayush Kumar
Department of Chemical Engineering,
National Institute of Technology
Tiruchirappalli, India

P. Suresh Kumar
Indian Council of Agricultural Research- National Research Centre for Banana
Trichy, India

Luo Zaini Mohd Izwan Low
School of Chemical and Energy Engineering, Faculty of Engineering
Universiti Teknologi Malaysia (UTM)
Skudai, Malaysia
Institute of Bioproduct Development (IBD)
Universiti Teknologi Malaysia (UTM)
Skudai, Malaysia

Alaa El Din Mahmoud
Environmental Sciences Department, Faculty of Science
Alexandria University
Alexandria, Egypt
Green Technology Group, Faculty of Science
Alexandria University
Alexandria, Egypt

Tomoyuki Makino
Graduate School of Agricultural Science
Tohoku University
Sendai, Japan

Nor Hasmaliana Abdul Manas
School of Chemical and Energy Engineering, Faculty of Engineering
Universiti Teknologi Malaysia (UTM)
Skudai, Malaysia
Institute of Bioproduct Development (IBD)
Universiti Teknologi Malaysia (UTM)
Skudai, Malaysia

V. Mariappan
Department of Mechanical Engineering
National Institute of Technology
Tiruchirappalli, India

Nasratun Masngut
Department of Chemical Engineering, College of Engineering
Universiti Malaysia Pahang
Gambang, Malaysia

Shamim Mia
Department of Agronomy
Patuakhali Science and Technology University
Patuakhali, Bangladesh

Md. Mehedi Hasan Mithu
Department of Agronomy
Patuakhali Science and Technology University
Patuakhali, Bangladesh

Wan Nur Aini Wan Mokhtar
Department of Chemical Sciences, Faculty of Science and Technology
Universiti Kebangsaan Malaysia
Bangi, Malaysia

Mohd Akmali Mokhter
Department of Chemistry, Faculty of Science
Universiti Teknologi Malaysia (UTM)
Skudai, Malaysia
Advanced Membrane Technology Research Centre (AMTEC), School of Chemical and Energy Engineering, Faculty of Engineering
Universiti Teknologi Malaysia
Johor Bahru, Malaysia

Muhammad Hilman Abdul Mustapa
Department of Chemical Sciences, Faculty of Science and Technology
Universiti Kebangsaan Malaysia
Bangi, Malaysia

Sheeba Narayanan
Department of Chemical Engineering
National Institute of Technology
Tiruchirappalli, India

Vasantha M. Nayagam
School of Chemical and Energy Engineering, Faculty of Engineering
Universiti Teknologi Malaysia (UTM)
Skudai, Malaysia
Institute of Bioproduct Development (IBD)
Universiti Teknologi Malaysia (UTM)
Skudai, Malaysia

Nurul Zahidah Nordin
School of Chemical and Energy Engineering, Faculty of Engineering
Universiti Teknologi Malaysia (UTM)
Skudai, Malaysia
Institute of Bioproduct Development (IBD)
Universiti Teknologi Malaysia (UTM)
Skudai, Malaysia

Ojshwi Prakash
Department of Chemical Engineering
National Institute of Technology
Tiruchirappalli, India

M. Premalatha
Department of Energy and Environment,
National Institute of Technology
Tiruchirappalli, India

Nurul Elia Aqila Abu Rahim
School of Chemical and Energy Engineering, Faculty of Engineering
Universiti Teknologi Malaysia (UTM)
Skudai, Malaysia

M. Rajkumar
Department of Environmental Sciences
Bharathiar University
Coimbatore, India

Nurrulhidayah Salamun
Department of Chemistry, Faculty of Science
Universiti Teknologi Malaysia (UTM)
Skudai, Malaysia

Nur Fatien Muhamad Salleh
School of Health Sciences
Universiti Sains Malaysia
Kubang Kerian, Malaysia

Miguel Angel Sanchez-Monedero
Department of Soil and Water Conservation and Organic Waste Management
CEBAS-CSIC
Murcia, Spain

Joseph Sekhar Santhappan
Mechanical Section, Department of Engineering, Shinas College of Technology
University of Technology and Applied Sciences
Shinas, Oman

Joseph Sekhar
Department of Engineering
University of Technology and Applied Sciences
Shinas, Oman

Shanmugaprakasham Selvamani
School of Chemical and Energy Engineering, Faculty of Engineering
Universiti Teknologi Malaysia (UTM)
Skudai, Malaysia
Institute of Bioproduct Development (IBD)
Universiti Teknologi Malaysia (UTM)
Skudai, Malaysia

Nurasmat Mohd Shukri
School of Health Sciences
Universiti Sains Malaysia
Kubang Kerian, Malaysia

Ashim Sikdar
Department of Agroforestry & Environmental Science
Sylhet Agricultural University
Sylhet, Bangladesh

S. Soundarya
Department of Environmental Sciences
Bharathiar University
Coimbatore, India

Alok Tripathi
Department of Chemical and Biochemical Engineering, School of Engineering
Indrashil University
Rajpur, India

R. Vishnupradeep
Department of Environmental Sciences
Bharathiar University
Coimbatore, India

Dayang Norulfairuz Abang Zaidel
School of Chemical and Energy Engineering, Faculty of Engineering
Universiti Teknologi Malaysia (UTM)
Skudai, Malaysia
Institute of Bioproduct Development (IBD)
Universiti Teknologi Malaysia (UTM)
Skudai, Malaysia

Nur Nadia Binti Mohd Zakaria
Department of Chemical Engineering, College of Engineering
Universiti Malaysia Pahang
Gambang, Malaysia

Preface

With the growing issues of the major environmental problem, appropriate technology is required to overcome the pollution problem routed from domestic and industrial sectors. The biotechnological approach to environmental protection is a greener and more economical to combat environmental pollution. The book is framed with chapters covering different aspects of biotechnology in conserving the environment. The book offers possible solutions for different environmental issues caused by modernization and increasing population worldwide through suitable biological methods and sustainable biotechnological-based environment-friendly approaches.

Environmental biotechnology involves the different technological applications based on living/non-living organisms and/or enzymes for the environmental problems addressing diverse pollutants, including emerging contaminants, with the merits of efficient and hazard-free practice. The book covers different biotechnology-based solutions for the removal of environmental pollutants; provides information pertinent to the removal of contaminants, characteristic types of toxic chemicals, precious elements, and emerging contaminants; reviews the bioremediation potential of microbial strains and enzymes; introduces the technological aspects covering suitable bioreactor configurations in the treatment of wastewater; and explores the significant routes of biotechnological means of obtaining eco-friendly products substituting the hazardous chemical-based products.

Specifically, these aspects are covered in the below-mentioned chapters: 1. Bioreactors for Biomass Conversion – Solid State Fermentation, Slurry Reactors, Airlift reactors; 2. Immobilized Enzyme Technologies for Removing Water Pollutants and Toxic Contaminants; 3. Value-Added Products from Microalgae; 4. Clean-Up of Marine Oil Spills through Bioremediation Method; 5. Bioreactor Scale-Up Strategies; 6. Biotechnological Advancements in the Treatment of Plastic Wastes; 7. Production of Biopolymer from Waste Materials as the Suitable Alternative for Plastics; 8. Microbial Pigments Production Using Agricultural Biomass Residues; 9. Nanotechnology-Associated Bioremediation for the Elimination of Emerging Contaminants; 10. Phytoremediation Potential of Some Bioenergy Crops – A Review; 11. Sustainable Approach for Extracting Precious Metals from Electronic Waste Materials; 12. Conversion of Organic Waste to Economically Valuable Products: Recent Advancements with Challenges.

1 Bioreactors for Biomass Conversion

Solid-State Fermentation, Slurry Reactors, Airlift Reactors

Aayush Kumar Choudhary, Ayush Kumar A., Ojshwi Prakash, Godwin Glivin, N. Kalaiselvan, H. Hareesh Krishnan, M. Premalatha, and V. Mariappan
National Institute of Technology, Tiruchirappalli

Joseph Sekhar
University of Technology and Applied Sciences

CONTENTS

1.1 INTRODUCTION

Bioenergy harnessed from biomass has been used predominantly for the production of heat, electricity, and biofuels, which takes up the bio-electrochemical, biological, and physico-chemical routes for its efficient production (Liao et al., 2018). Cellulose, the primary component of lignocellulose biomass, has the potential to be **utilized** as a source for chemicals and for liberating energy. The annual production of biomass evaluated as 10^{11} **tons** has the prospective to sequester 2×10^{21} joule. Going by the

DOI: 10.1201/9781003188292-1

numbers, Earth's plants in a decade can utilize the energy stored as conventional crude oil as cellulose, lignin, and hemicellulose. The obstacle has always been for the scientists to generate fuels based as building blocks for civilization by accessing these polymers.

The hydrolysis of lignocellulosic biomass is assisted by the less hazardous cellulose solvents which are easy to manage and control. Salts that possess melting points near or below the ambient temperature have been used as a solvent for chemical derivatization. The biomass hydrolysis can be demonstrated by the dissolution of linen in sulfuric acid post water dissolution, on heating it is transformed into a fermentable sugar. Disrupting the inter- and intra-chain hydrogen networks, strong acids decrystallize the cellulose, making it accessible to reagents. Thus, catalyzing the hydrolysis of these bonds of glycosidic nature, strong acids can cleave the hemicellulose and cellulose into sugars (Binder & Raines, 2010; Binder & Raines, 2010).

The use of crops has popped up as an alternative to fossil fuels as renewable resources to override the glaring issues of feedstock shortage. This solution brought problems hand in hand creating turbulences in the agricultural market consuming land which instead could be used for food production, ultimately leading to a state of rising global food prices. The most obvious path has been trodden to solve this queued problem where marginal lands not suitable for the growth of food crops are in turn being utilized for the cultivation of energy crops (Knápek et al., 2021).

Microalgae cultivation is one of the most promising undertakings within this technology. Terrestrial crops like sunflower and soybean lack by a tenth factor in their lipid productivity when compared to microalgae. Growth abilities in non-arable patches utilizing the wastewater nutrients and significantly higher photosynthetic efficiency are other advantages of microalgae cultivation (Zhang et al., 2018). Temperature and operating pH are also rated influential parameters in the microbial composition for the anaerobic type digesters. The feeding sludge, the key source of microbial seeds, is regarded as one of the main environmental factors for anaerobic bioreactors/digesters.

Mixotrophic, heterotrophic, and photoautotrophic are the various categories of microalgae cultivation, depending on the energy and carbon source adopted for the process. In case of cultivation by photoautotrophic cultivation, photosynthesis is used to convert the inorganic carbons in bicarbonate, carbon dioxide and light into a valuable organic matter. Microalgae utilize the organic carbon sources in heterotrophic cultivation, from the glucose or acetic acid present in the culture media to synthesize the carbohydrates, chlorophyll, and proteins in the absence of light energy. Mixotrophic cultivation offers the liberty for microalgae cells to reproduce under photo- and heterotrophic conditions, capable of using both organic and inorganic carbons as the energy threshold for their growth (Zhang et al., 2018). The operating complexity puts mixotrophic cultivation at disadvantage in spite of its ability to reduce the photo-limitation effect present in the photoautotrophic cultivation and any sort of bacterial contamination, which is a potential risk present in the cultivation by heterotrophic routes.

Solid-state fermentation (SSF) has been viewed as a potential technology to aid the production of food, pharmaceutical products, and chemicals classed as microbial products. Biopulping, bioremediation, biobeneficiation, and bioleaching are the effective routes, where the microbial processes can be utilized. As the name indicates, SSF is observed in the absence of any free flowing liquid. The substrates that need to support the growth and metabolism of the microorganism need to possess enough moisture. The environment-friendly behavior backed up by lower energy requirements and lower wastewater production makes SSF an opportunistic technology in the processing of agro-industrial residues (Pandey, 2003).

Bioreactors are one of the critical units in any conversion process involving microbes, considering their ability to host a stable environment to catalyze the metabolism. The microbial conversion is impacted by the heat and mass transfer characteristics in the bioreactors.

1.1.1 Process Type

There are several different processes for conversion of biomass into usable energy. They can be broadly classified into Thermal, Biological, and Physical methods. Thermal methods of biomass conversion include combustion, gasification, and pyrolysis of different biomass feedstock. This can be used to produce a variety of fuel gases and hydrogen depending on the composition of the air in which the process is carried out. Physical methods are hydrolysis, liquefaction, crushing, pelletizing, etc. The biological methods include anaerobic digestion and fermentation.

1.1.2 Fermentation

Fermentation is the most used process in industries to produce a wide range of products from antibiotics to enzymes and other organic products (Xia et al., 2021). Biomass can also be converted into biofuels using fermentation. Individual microbial strains and the feedstock used characterize the production levels from a fermentation process. The production capability can then impact the interactions between the momentum transfer fields developed inside a bioreactor depending on the scale of operation. The key parameters that impact the fermentation include aeration, pH, stirrer speed, liquid and gas flow rates, DOT (Dissolved Oxygen Tension), pressure, exhaust oxygen and CO_2 levels, and temperature. The production of the metabolites and the growth of the microbes are critically dependent on the oxygen being supplied in submerged fermentation (Liu & Wilkins, 2020).

Fermentation is an anaerobic process used to break the polysaccharide molecules of biomass feedstock. A biological process that involves the conversion of complex substrates into lower-level simple components, which are beneficial to people and various applications on the industrial scale, is observed as fermentation. The secondary metabolites like enzymes and antibiotics are liberated during this process. Alcohol and acids of organic origin are labeled as the primary products of fermentation. The productivity is inherently dependent on the nature of the substrate as the rate of consumption of nutrients varies for each of the substrates. Wheat bran, rice straw, vegetable waste, and paper pulp are some commonly used substrates (Kuila & Sharma, 2018).

The benefits of the fermentation process are the moderate operating conditions and sustainability characteristics. The design of bioreactors for fermentation

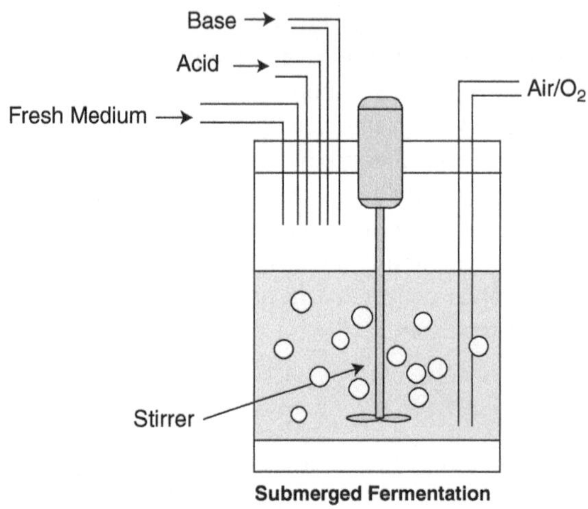

FIGURE 1.1 Submerged fermentation reactor.

applications is dependent on the fermentation environment, the natural conditions of the chosen fungi, yield/efficiency desired, product quality, and other process parameters. Fermentation can either be SSF or submerged fermentation (SMF) (Arora et al., 2018). Figure 1.1 shows the setup of a SMF reactor.

Microorganisms need to be controlled in the atmosphere for effective production of superior quality end products attaining high yields and optimum productivity levels in submerged production. The SSF is comparatively slower which raises the residence time of the substrates for effective completion of the process. SSF is effective in a low moisture environment so it is best suited for fungi and microorganisms.

The optimization of the design principles and the simple applicability make stirred tank reactors the go-to approach for fermentation operation on the industrial scale. The flow field generated requires a detailed and intricate study to cover the large range from laminar to turbulent regimes through the transient state.

1.1.3 Hydrolysis

Hydrolysis is one of the widely adopted techniques for conversion of high solid concentrations. Hydrolysis takes place through the breaking of polysaccharides in the feed biomass in an aqueous solution. Typically using enzymes as catalysts, hydrolysis promises high efficiency and economic operating conditions. The mild operating conditions, low energy requirements, and higher efficiency favor enzymatic hydrolysis over saccharification down the chemical route.

The low inhibitors generated during enzymatic fermentation add to the advantages of their application. Conventional distillation processes require high solid feed concentrations typically over 15% on dry basis. These processes are not economical because of the viscosity preventing efficient transport processes. Hence, the economics of solid-state processes should be improved by studying novel techniques. Simultaneous saccharification and fermentation is another technique to improve the overall hydrolysis efficiency (Nieves et al., 2016). Compared to a 56.3 yield at 21%, a 75.3% yield was obtained at 15% of the solid loading which increases the efficiency significantly.

The design of bioreactors for hydrolysis should consider several factors like the configuration, mode of operation, enzyme and substrate, reaction mechanism, operating conditions, the yield required, etc. The most common types of bioreactors used are stirred tank reactors and membrane reactors (Pino et al., 2018). Stirred tank bioreactor, filled up to 70%–80% of the medium, is the common type of bioreactor used in industries. It essentially comprises a number of agitators connected to an external motor in a cylindrical vessel. The time of mixing and energy consumption is regarded as important metrics to estimate the mixing time efficiency. To further restrain the power consumption, the impeller can be varied in the stirred tank. Membrane bioreactors are instrumental for the hydrolysis by the enzymatic approach where the polysaccharides like cellulose are used. The small size components like glucose are liberated in the process which possesses inhibitory behavior; however, they are easily detached by membranes. Membrane bioreactors reduce the loss in enzymatic activity by reducing the applicable shear force (Shokrkar et al., 2018).

1.1.4 Anaerobic Digestion

Anaerobic digestion (AD) is a sustainable technique of conversion of biomass feedstock into biofuels. Several other value-added products apart from biogas are produced from AD process which makes this process more desirable than conventional methods. But the economics of this process should be studied and made viable for large-scale industrial applications. Hydrogen, fatty acids, and other carbon-based products are obtained during the bio-gasification process via digestion (Qin et al., 2021). Hydrolysis, acidogenesis, acetogenesis, and methanogenesis are the stages that must be accomplished to complete any reaction down the AD path. The biogas production is observed from methanogens which grow at inherently low redox potential. Methane and carbon dioxide are the principal components of the produced biogas, which is the desired product (Zhang et al., 2016). AD has been instrumental in reducing the sludge volume generated during wastewater treatment which is regarded as expensive to incinerate or deposit in fills. The renewable energy can be recovered from the microbial decomposition of the organic section of the sludge which further cuts down the expenditure on treating wastewater.

The anaerobic digesters under application include the standard rate digesters which have the liquid layers segregated and a high rate digester which involves mixing, uniform feed loading, and heating facilities. Digesters arranged with chambers in series provide the required buffering capacity and a stable operation of the AD reactions for varied microbial population.

1.1.5 Reactor Types

There are many different kinds of bioreactors that are used for different biological and biochemical processes. Some of them are stirred tank reactors, rocker reactors, airlift reactors, slurry reactors, fixed bed reactors, fluidized bed reactors, etc. The selection of these reactor types depends on the application and feedstock type. The process conditions in some reactors do not support the life of cell cultures of some species and so this must be considered before selecting the reactor. In this work. SSF reactors, slurry reactors, and airlift reactors will be discussed in detail.

1.1.5.1 Solid-State Fermentation

SSF is a sustainable process with very low environmental effects and is also economic in terms of large-scale implementation. SSF has a higher production rate of enzymes thus producing significantly better yields when compared to conventional processes. Under conditions of varying pH and temperature, SSF produced more stable enzymes than SMF. The thermostability and resistance against acidic and basic environment make the enzymes viable for industrial application.

The setup of an SSF reactor is shown in Figure 1.2. It consumes less energy and gives a shorter fermentation time. Also, the production of by-products is less, thereby minimizing the risk of bacterial contamination. But there are several process inconsistencies to be studied to improve the transport processes and other operational parameters. The study of kinetics of the process is difficult due to the tough measurement of biomass for microbial growth.

SSF is utilized under the conditions that the solid surface is moist, providing significantly higher end product concentrations, higher stability of the liberated products, improved efficiency of fermentation, and cultivation of substrates that are inherently insoluble in water. The easier preservation and monitoring regulations make SSF a suitable process in various industrial applications involving sporulation. The various

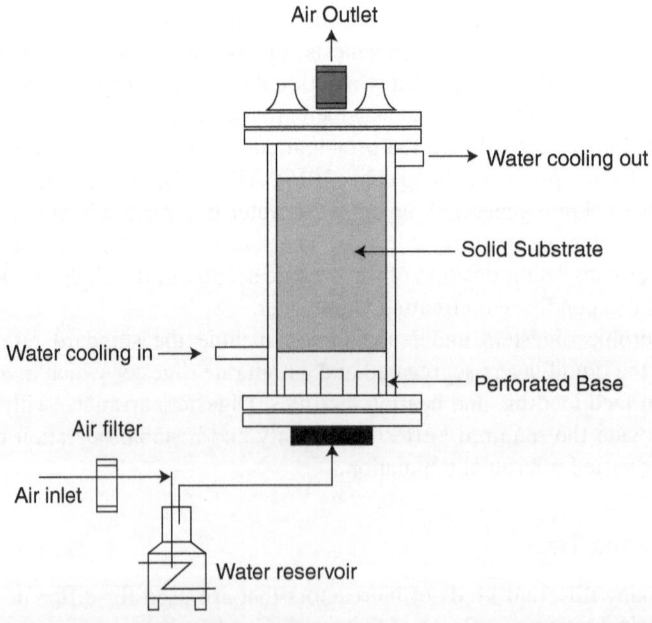

FIGURE 1.2 Solid-state fermentation reactor.

advantages offered by the SSF process are outweighed by the problems in scaling up enzyme production. The parameters moisture, oxygen gradients, pH, and temperature inside the bioreactor pose major hindrance in the scale-up operations. The agitation of the solid substrates presents a separate challenge, which is ultimately responsible for the generation of the compositional gradients in the operational environment. Agitation significantly increases the rates of heat and mass transfer and also plays an important role in the formation of aggregates (Chilakamarry et al., 2022).

pH is regarded as an essential factor varying due to the metabolism as metabolic rates decrease considerably with a lowering of pH. Organic acids like citric, gluconic, and lactic acids are secreted during fermentation which is considered the most likely reason for the drop in pH levels. Temperature impacts the efficiency of SSF due to the temperature sensitivity of enzymes and metabolite growth and development. The development of fungi is most effective in the 20°C–55°C range of temperature. Optimum moisture levels need to be maintained as the diffusion of nutrients and growth of microorganisms drop steadily under reduced moisture environments. On the other hand, high humidity levels restrict the transmission of gases and bacterial competition, leading to particle agglomeration. The water requirements of microorganisms are recognized as water activity instead of the solid substrate water content. The inert matrix for enhanced adsorption of carbon and energy resources is labeled as a fundamental macromolecule structure. Particle size is regarded instrumental in the ability of substrate to interchange with the microorganism's growth, mass, and heat transfer in SSF.

SSF reactors are mainly of four categories: rotary drum bioreactors, tray reactors, packed bed bioreactors, and fluidized bed reactors. Rotary drum reactors are constantly agitated with circulation of air. The main components include the drum, pump, electric motor, and the mechanical parts like gearbox. They may or may not have a paddle but the air is circulated near the reactor headspace and not the bed. Packed bed bioreactors have a stationary bed where the fluid is forced through the bed. Fluidized beds are continuously agitated with a forced circulation of air. Tray reactors are totally stationary and air is not forced through the bed but is circulated around it (Leite et al., 2021).

The tray type offers a key advantage of easier scale-up possibility of the generated results, making them reproducible on the industrial scale. The tray reactor design characteristics that allow the variation in the number of trays while maintaining the same tower height aid the scale-up and reproducibility abilities. The air diffusion and heat transfer limitations affect the scale up from bench to the pilot scale in case of the packed bed bioreactors.

1.1.5.2 Slurry Reactor

Slurry reactors are an important type of gas–liquid–solid multiphase reactors. They provide several added advantages over conventional reactors such as more efficient mixing, better heat and mass transfer characteristics, and overall cost reduction owing to better mixing in the reactors. The working of slurry reactors is similar to fluidized bed reactors where a solid particle is suspended in a fluid medium, and the gas is passed through the reactor vessel. These solid particles are usually catalysts that are very fine in nature and help in carrying out the reaction between a gas and a

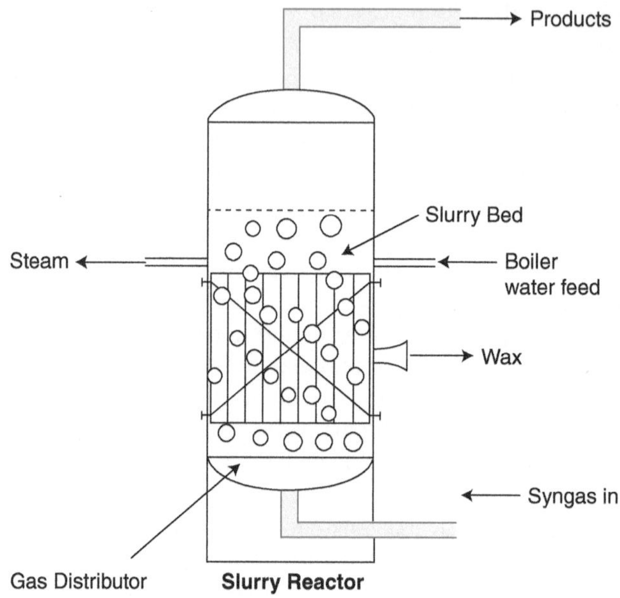

FIGURE 1.3 Slurry reactor.

liquid. The main distinction between fluidized bed and slurry reactors is that in fluidized bed reactors, the suspending medium is generally the reacting gas, but a fluid is used in slurry reactors (Yang et al., 2021).

As shown in Figure 1.3, slurry reactors have a slurry bed with solid catalyst particles suspended in a liquid bed through which the gas is pushed via the syngas inlet. A water feed is provided, and a gas distributor is present in the reactor. The products come out of the product outlet present near the top of the reactor. Slurry reactors have important biochemical applications like the separation of pharmaceutical components from water for wastewater treatment (Janssens et al., 2017), industrial biochemical reactions like hydrogenation, oxidation, etc. There are several challenges in slurry reactors like the effects of solid particles present in the mixture, gas sparger performance, and complex flow regime characteristics. To overcome these challenges, a solid catalyst return system is used. Slurry reactors are beneficial for catalyzed systems because of the well-defined liquid flow (Yang et al., 2021). High level of liquid back mixing in slurry reactors impacts the overall conversion of the reactant drastically and hence, perforated plates should be used to reduce the liquid axial dispersion (Geng et al., 2021). In bioremediation problems, slurry bioreactors are used for controlling conventional issues like inefficient mixing, low microbial population, etc.

Several advantages of slurry reactors include the high heat capacity in the case of exothermic reactors which yield a temperature stability leading to efficient heat recovery and transfer characteristics. In case the catalyst gets deactivated, it can be replaced easily as they are small particles. Another advantage of particle size is a very low intra-particle diffusion resistance leading to an efficiency nearing 100%.

The overall mass transfer coefficients in slurry reactors are high as compared to packed bed reactors. Moreover, the internal temperature gradient values can be neglected due to the presence of a near-uniform temperature throughout the reactor. Membrane slurry reactors are used to minimize the energy required for the pumping of solid particles and minimize catalyst hold-up. Hence, the volume of the reactor is reduced and, hence, the contact time decreases. This leads to high production efficiency as unwanted side reactions are not present in slurry reactors.

1.1.5.3 Airlift Reactor

Airlift bioreactors are used mainly for shear-resistant microorganisms. Pneumatically agitated systems are used to circulate the broth in these reactors providing efficient transport characteristics leading to highly energy-efficient systems (Zhang et al., 2019). The transport of oxygen is efficient in slurry-type reactors as the flow is vertically circulating and the design is made to promote the mass transfer characteristics. They are widely used in fermentation, wastewater treatment, and other biological applications due to the reduced contamination risk and simplicity of construction. They are compatible with denser solutions where the mixing characteristics are better than traditional bubble cap trays. As shown in Figure 1.4, airlift reactors consist of a gas flow inlet and an outlet with a gas distributor present inside the reactor.

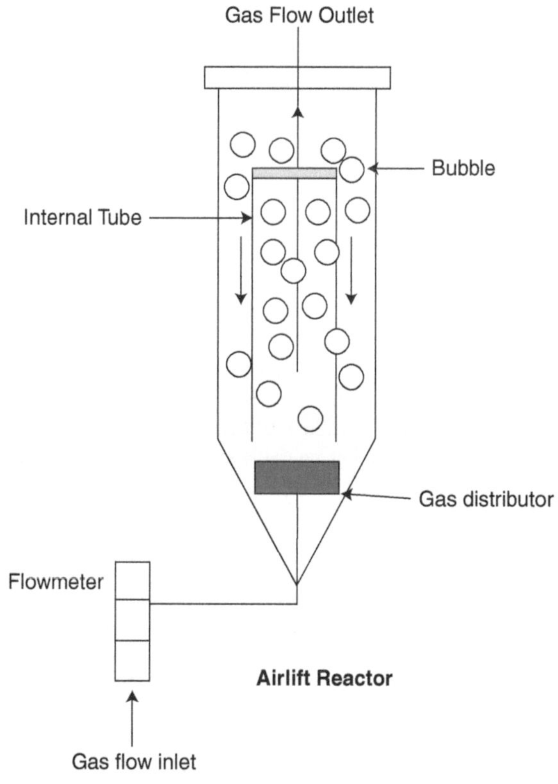

FIGURE 1.4 Airlift reactor.

The image used has been generated by authors using draw.io software.

Even in low-cost applications like wastewater treatment, these reactors are highly efficient because of better flow characteristics and better driving forces. The main criterion for the design of airlift reactors is the fluidization of the bioreactor. The lowest circulation velocity required in the riser for the least shear force between the carriers should also be calculated in order to design a suitable reactor. It should be made sure that the surface area available for the reaction is the highest with a sufficiently long retention time (Pelivanoski et al., 2020).

1.2 CONCLUSION

Bioreactors are essentially specialized reactors for biological reactions like fermentation, AD, biological synthesis, etc. Finding applications in almost all industries ranging from food to pharmaceuticals, bioreactors are high performance instruments fundamental to any biochemical process. In this chapter, they have been categorized based on the process type and reactor design type. Important processes that have industrial applications like fermentation, hydrolysis, and AD are dealt with in this chapter. Several reactor types like stirred tank reactors, slurry reactors, SSF reactors, and multiphase reactors like slurry and airlift reactors are described in this chapter. Design challenges and process intensification possibilities are discussed with the latest advancements in the field leading to an all-round description on bioreactors. Novel bioreactors like slurry and airlift reactors can be readily offered as replacements to the traditional packed bed reactors and trickle bed reactors suited for biochemical reactions with various mechanical and chemical stimuli. The future possibilities include studies in process intensification and scaling up of bioreactors from lab scale to high scale industrial reactors. Several studies related to modeling and simulation can be carried out for a better understanding of bioreactors improving the efficiency and yield leading to sustainable applications in several industrial processes.

REFERENCES

Arora, S., Rani, R., & Ghosh, S. (2018). Bioreactors in solid state fermentation technology: Design, applications and engineering aspects. *Journal of Biotechnology*, *269*, 16–34. https://doi.org/10.1016/J.JBIOTEC.2018.01.010

Binder, J. B., & Raines, R. T. (2010). Fermentable sugars by chemical hydrolysis of biomass. *Proceedings of the National Academy of Sciences*, *107*(10), 4516–4521. https://doi.org/10.1073/PNAS.0912073107

Chilakamarry, C. R., Mimi Sakinah, A. M., Zularisam, A. W., Sirohi, R., Khilji, I. A., Ahmad, N., & Pandey, A. (2022). Advances in solid-state fermentation for bioconversion of agricultural wastes to value-added products: Opportunities and challenges. *Bioresource Technology*, *343*, 126065. https://doi.org/10.1016/J.BIORTECH.2021.126065

Geng, S., Mao, Z. S., Huang, Q., & Yang, C. (2021). Process intensification in pneumatically agitated slurry reactors. *Engineering*, *7*(3), 304–325. https://doi.org/10.1016/J.ENG.2021.03.002

Janssens, R., Mandal, M. K., Dubey, K. K., & Luis, P. (2017). Slurry photocatalytic membrane reactor technology for removal of pharmaceutical compounds from wastewater: Towards cytostatic drug elimination. *Science of the Total Environment*, *599–600*, 612–626. https://doi.org/10.1016/J.SCITOTENV.2017.03.253

Knápek, J., Králík, T., Vávrová, K., Valentová, M., Horák, M., & Outrata, D. (2021). Policy implications of competition between conventional and energy crops. *Renewable and Sustainable Energy Reviews, 151*, 111618. https://doi.org/10.1016/J.RSER.2021.111618

Kuila, A., & Sharma, V. (Eds.). (2018). *Principles and Applications of Fermentation Technology*. https://doi.org/10.1002/9781119460381

Leite, P., Sousa, D., Fernandes, H., Ferreira, M., Costa, A. R., Filipe, D., Gonçalves, M., Peres, H., Belo, I., & Salgado, J. M. (2021). Recent advances in production of lignocellulolytic enzymes by solid-state fermentation of agro-industrial wastes. *Current Opinion in Green and Sustainable Chemistry, 27*, 100407. https://doi.org/10.1016/J.COGSC.2020.100407

Liao, Q., Chang, J., Herrmann, C., & Xia, A. (Eds.). (2018). *Bioreactors for Microbial Biomass and Energy Conversion*. https://doi.org/10.1007/978-981-10-7677-0

Liu, E., & Wilkins, M. R. (2020). Process optimization and scale-up production of fungal aryl alcohol oxidase from genetically modified *Aspergillus nidulans* in stirred-tank bioreactor. *Bioresource Technology, 315*, 123792. https://doi.org/10.1016/J.BIORTECH.2020.123792

Nieves, D. C., Ruiz, H. A., de Cárdenas, L. Z., Alvarez, G. M., Aguilar, C. N., Ilyina, A., & Martínez Hernández, J. L. (2016). Enzymatic hydrolysis of chemically pretreated mango stem bark residues at high solid loading. *Industrial Crops and Products, 83*, 500–508. https://doi.org/10.1016/J.INDCROP.2015.12.079

Pandey, A. (2003). Solid-state fermentation. *Biochemical Engineering Journal, 13*(2–3), 81–84. https://doi.org/10.1016/S1369-703X(02)00121-3

Pelivanoski, B., Detmann, B., Ooms, K., Winkler, M., Vasyukova, E., & Denecke, M. (2020). Design of a 1000L pilot-scale airlift bioreactor for nitrification with application of a three-phase hydrodynamic mathematical model and prediction of a low liquid circulation velocity. *Chemical Engineering Research and Design, 153*, 257–262. https://doi.org/10.1016/J.CHERD.2019.10.018

Pino, M. S., Rodríguez-Jasso, R. M., Michelin, M., Flores-Gallegos, A. C., Morales-Rodriguez, R., Teixeira, J. A., & Ruiz, H. A. (2018). Bioreactor design for enzymatic hydrolysis of biomass under the biorefinery concept. *Chemical Engineering Journal, 347*, 119–136. https://doi.org/10.1016/J.CEJ.2018.04.057

Qin, S., Wainaina, S., Liu, H., Soufiani, A. M., Pandey, A., Zhang, Z., Awasthi, M. K., & Taherzadeh, M. J. (2021). Microbial dynamics during anaerobic digestion of sewage sludge combined with food waste at high organic loading rates in immersed membrane bioreactors. *Fuel, 303*, 121276. https://doi.org/10.1016/J.FUEL.2021.121276

Shokrkar, H., Ebrahimi, S., & Zamani, M. (2018). A review of bioreactor technology used for enzymatic hydrolysis of cellulosic materials. *Cellulose, 25*(11), 6279–6304. https://doi.org/10.1007/S10570-018-2028-4

Xia, J., Wang, G., Fan, M., Chen, M., Wang, Z., & Zhuang, Y. (2021). Understanding the scale-up of fermentation processes from the viewpoint of the flow field in bioreactors and the physiological response of strains. *Chinese Journal of Chemical Engineering, 30*, 178–184. https://doi.org/10.1016/J.CJCHE.2020.12.004

Yang, T., Geng, S., Gao, F., He, T., Cheng, J., Huang, Q., & Yang, C. (2021). Investigation of hydrodynamics and mass transfer in an internal loop airlift slurry reactor integrating mixing and separation. *Separation and Purification Technology, 259*, 118209. https://doi.org/10.1016/J.SEPPUR.2020.118209

Zhang, L., Zhang, B., Zhu, X., Chang, H., Ou, S., & Wang, H. (2018). Role of bioreactors in microbial biomass and energy conversion. In: Liao, Q., Chang, J. S., Herrmann, C., & Xia, A. (Eds.). *Bioreactors for Microbial Biomass and Energy Conversion*. Green Energy and Technology. Springer, Singapore. https://doi.org/10.1007/978-981-10-7677-0_2

Zhang, Q., Hu, J., & Lee, D. J. (2016). Biogas from anaerobic digestion processes: Research updates. *Renewable Energy, 98*, 108–119. https://doi.org/10.1016/J.RENENE.2016.02.029

Zhang, T., Wei, C., Feng, C., Ren, Y., Wu, H., & Preis, S. (2019). Advances in characteristics analysis, measurement methods and modelling of flow dynamics in airlift reactors. *Chemical Engineering and Processing-Process Intensification, 144*, 107633. https://doi.org/10.1016/J.CEP.2019.107633

2 Immobilised Enzyme Technologies for the Removal of Water Pollutants and Toxic Contaminants

Nur Izyan Wan Azelee, Nor Hasmaliana Abdul Manas, Nurrulhidayah Salamun, Mohd Akmali Mokhter, Muhammad Abd Hadi Bunyamin, and Nurul Elia Aqila Abu Rahim
Universiti Teknologi Malaysia (UTM)

Siti Fatimah Zaharah Mohd Fuzi
UTHM

Nasratun Masngut
Universiti Malaysia Pahang

CONTENTS

DOI: 10.1201/9781003188292-2

2.1 INTRODUCTION

The world energy consumption is projected to increase by 50% between 2018 and 2050 (EIA, 2019). Therefore, this increase is expected to give rise to undue burden on natural resources and creating challenges on energy conservation and sustainability, environmental consequences, and quality of life (Temesgen et al., 2021). In addition to energy, resource consumption per capita continues to increase because of the growth of global population as well as the rise of consumer aspirations. Nowadays, with the expeditious pace of industrialisation and rising consumer demands, such augmentation will inevitably imply significant anthropogenic impact on the ecosystems. The biggest concern is disposal of effluents from industries and municipal sources poses threats and is giving adverse effects on the environment (Chowdhary et al., 2020). Significantly, the composition of industrial effluents varies substantially depending on the different fields and industries, technology features in industrial sectors, population density, climate, and even cultural and social practices in different areas (Han et al., 2018).

Pollutant is a substance or energy introduced into the environment because of the human activity which is the source of contaminants. Whilst micropollutants (MPs) refer to anthropogenic chemicals which occur in aquatic environment over (potential) natural background level, but the concentrations persist at trace levels (which can be μg/L range). The MPs in the environment has becoming a problem of major relevance, especially in heavily urbanised areas (Rodrigo-Comino et al., 2020). The MPs are categorised by their anthropogenic origin and their occurrence at low concentrations. Bioaccumulation, toxicity, and resistance to degradation are reasons for potential risks of emerging MPs. There are broad sources for production of MPs, ranging from agriculture, traffic networks, households, or industries which would then enter waterways through diverse routes. MPs can be transferred via run-off or leaching process from farming or as different site pollution, for which wastewater treatment plants are important examples (Nematollahi et al., 2022).

Wastewater comprises of several microorganisms, natural and synthetic MPs such as biodegradable organic components, nutrients, organic and inorganic materials (for example detergents, pesticides, acids, and bases), heavy metals, radionuclides, pharmaceuticals, personal care, and nanotechnology products. All these find their way to surface water resources. This could give rise to inevitable damage to the aquatic ecosystem and to humans as water's aesthetic value is compromised. Statistically, it was revealed that approximately half of the total chemicals production is represented by hazardous constituents whereby nearly 20% of them had significant acute effects and environmental degradation (EUROSTAT, 2016).

According to the United Nation report, only 20% of wastewater flows back into the ecosystem being treated or reused. According to WHO, approximately 2 billion people use drinking water source contaminated with faeces leaving them at risk of health hazard. Some examples are discussed here such as pharmaceutical contaminants, preservatives, biocides, and pesticides, dyes, polycyclic aromatic contaminants, and dyes-containing hazardous substances, as well as dioxins and polychlorinated biphenyls-based pollutants.

The pharmaceutical constituents are of significant attention due to their relative stability and recalcitrant nature. It was found that over 3,000 substances are utilised as pharmaceutical ingredients such as painkiller, beta-blockers, impotence drugs, antidepressant, antidiabetics, antibiotics, X-ray contrast media, lipids regulators, etc. (Lambert and Skelly, 2016; McGrane, 2016). Pharmaceutical contaminants can happen via agriculture run-off, landfill leachates, human and animal feeding operations, as well as urban run-off.

As for preservatives, various contaminants are derived from household good and personal care products including parabens, disinfectant, fragrances (musk), antifungal agents, insect repellents hormones, shampoos, steroids, sunscreen, cosmetics as well as analgesics materials (Pal et al., 2014). On the other hand, pesticides are chemicals utilised for controlling crops while biocides are mainly used for the non-rural environment. There are various categories of biocides such as penicillin, cephalosporin, tetracycline, etc. Biocides are substances used to control weed, bituminous waterproofing, and grass management (Margot et al., 2015). Nowadays, the number of fertilisers, biocides, and pesticides are increasing with the increasing demand for agricultural crops leading to increased biocides and pesticides contamination and eutrophication of groundwater and surface water.

Another significant MPs is organic contaminant called polycyclic aromatic contaminants (PACs). PACs are hydrophobic, relatively stable, and semi-volatile in the environment. The main sources of PACs are pyrolysis process and incomplete combustion coal, petroleum, and biomasses (Abdel-Shafy & Mansour, 2016). Moreover, because of its good volatile properties, PACs can easily combine with soil, sediments, air, water, and food (Beriro et al., 2016; Ma & Harrad, 2015; Nielsen et al., 2015). Bilal et al. (2018) claimed that predominantly industrial sector preoccupies a great amount of diverse arrangement of synthetic dyes including diazo, azo, basic, acidic, disperse, reactive, metal-complex, etc. These dyes are mostly toxic, teratogenic, or carcinogenic compounds. Unrestricted discharge of dyes and/or their decay by-products pose a severe threat to public health and environment when they enter the water bodies (Bilal et al., 2017a, b; Chatha et al., 2017).

Apart from that, incineration of certain types of health-care waste, smelting of metals, soils and sediments, fossil fuel combustion and emission of gasoline/diesel vehicles could generate countless environmental contaminants. Sany et al. (2015) reported that there are contaminants that present in suspended solid form such as polychlorinated biphenyls (PCBs), polychloro-dibenzo-p-dioxins (PCDDs) and polychloro-dibenzofurans (PCDFs). This is because they are less soluble, have low vapour pressure and have high n-octanol/water coefficient. With the emergence of consciousness at multiple levels, the expansion of pollution control technologies and to a more diligent legislation on management of waste has risen to mitigate the environmental impact of wastewater treatment process.

For example, European legislation endorsed the development of local integrated and sustainable management plans, in order of preferences that comprise prevention, waste valorisation, and the use of landfill only for the disposal of refuses that are not able to recover. In some places such as Italian municipalities, the new legislation, the fast growth of solid waste production and the recurring landfill closings have stimulated the expansion of incineration and recycling/reuse programmes. Such programmes must envisage an integration of socio-economic, environmental, and technical considerations.

According to SWOT analysis reported by WHO, major strengths of the Association of Southeast Asian Nations (ASEAN) are natural resource base, socio-economic growth, resilient economy, poverty alleviation, basic policy, and regulatory framework for sustainable development. Nevertheless, the shortcomings include gaps in policy or regulatory, recycling/reuse programme and plan, or treatment and disposal infrastructure and institutional mechanism (Fiorucci et al., 2003). However, ASEAN countries offer major opportunity in all aspect of waste management based on 3Rs across the value chain. With certain intervention, ASEAN countries could face up the challenge of natural capital exhaustion, green growth transition and sustainable development. Traditionally, there have been various methods applied in the industries for the removal of environmental pollutants such as sedimentation (He et al., 2021), adsorption (Silva et al., 2021), ozonation (Li et al., 2021), chemical oxidation (Farzaneh et al., 2021), coagulation (Alibeigi-Beni et al., 2021) and many more. Unfortunately, majority of the methods have several disadvantages which include high processing cost, the use of toxic solvents and chemicals, the production of toxic by-products and the need for expensive and sophisticated equipment.

2.2 UTILISATION OF IMMOBILISED ENZYME TECHNOLOGY FOR BIOREMEDIATIONS

Enzyme technology has long time been used as one of the promising technologies for bioremediation especially due to its green, low energy input, non-toxic, reduced by-products generation, mitigating wastewater treatment, and environmentally friendly characteristics (Ivanov et al., 2019). However, as time passes by, huge concern has been put on the cost, recyclability, robustness, and stability of the enzymes when being used in their free form (free enzyme). The drawbacks of using free enzyme are becoming more apparent when being used at the industrial scale where most of the processes involve harsh process conditions. Hence, immobilised enzyme has caught the attention of having enhanced performances compared to the previous conventional free enzymes. Immobilised enzyme is a form of heterogeneous biocatalyst with improved characteristics. Figure 2.1 shows the benefits portrayed by immobilised enzymes as compared to the conventional technology, free enzymes and microbial technology. Huge investment has been done focusing on the development, optimisation, operation and implementation of the immobilised enzymes for various applications.

Due to all the mentioned constraints associated with suspended enzyme treatment, need for a better method is highly on demand and immobilised enzyme technology is foreseen to be able to overcome these limitations. The effectiveness of immobilised enzyme will strongly be dependent on the support material or carrier it is being attached or immobilised to. In most cases, organic and inorganic support has

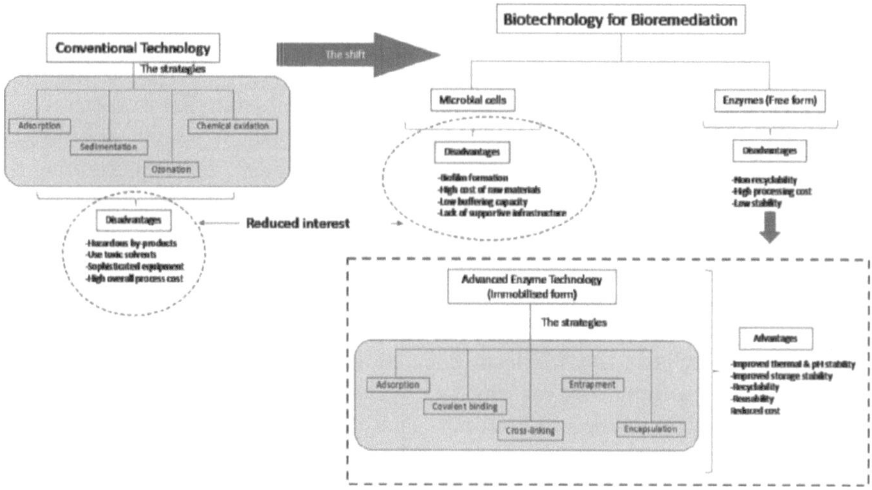

FIGURE 2.1 Advantages of immobilised enzyme technology for bioremediation.

been widely studied for the enzyme immobilisation as well as composite materials (hybrid materials) (Zdarta et al., 2021). Most importantly, the chosen support material must be biocompatible and having high affinity towards the enzyme. Screening and optimisation for the best carrier for enzyme immobilisation should provide enzyme with improved performance including having high stability as well as high mechanical and heat resistance. The applications of immobilised enzymes have been tested for various bioremediation purposes including biodegradation of hazardous dyes, phenolic compound, bisphenols and its derivatives, pharmaceuticals, and for heavy metals removal.

Besides the vast study on the immobilised enzyme, microbial remediation has also been widely researched. Immobilised enzyme is more preferable than immobilised microbes as microbes tend to have problems such as biofilm formation. There are a few methods of enzyme immobilisation which are adsorption (attached on the surface), cross-linking (requires a cross-linker), covalent bonding (bonding pairs between enzyme and carrier), entrapment (enzyme is entrapped inside the matrix), and encapsulation (enzyme is encapsulated inside a polymer). Among them, adsorption method is seen to be the most simple, easy, cost-effective, efficient for the removal of various pollutants, flexible design, and able to remove very low concentration of pollutants. Other advantages of utilising immobilised enzyme for bioremediations are improve recovery, environmentally friendly and having low maintenance cost as the enzyme can be regenerate. The characteristic of the support plays important role in enzyme immobilisation. Inert support with porous structure makes the enzyme to be well dispersed inside the matrix and does not interact with other chemicals which may affect enzyme performance. Immobilised enzymes have increased functional stability with pH and temperature tolerance compared to the free enzyme. The drawbacks of utilising free enzymes are instability, high production cost and problems with separation between the product, enzyme, and system (Ranjan et al., 2019).

2.3 IMMOBILISED ENZYME TECHNOLOGIES FOR DYES AND PHENOLIC COMPOUNDS REMOVAL

Dyes and phenolic compounds are among the recalcitrant industrial wastewater pollutants that are toxic and carcinogenic. Dyes and phenolic compounds are released into various water regions due to poor wastewater treatment, and they infiltrate the food chain (Lu et al., 2009; Zdarta et al., 2021). Enzymatic degradation is effective in removing these persistent pollutants from the water source by converting it into non-toxic substances (Akhtar et al., 2005). Enzymatic conversion attains high-efficiency rate, results in less hazardous production and can be readily removed from the post-reaction mixture. In fact, enzymes have been used for dye decolourisation from water solution (Lu et al., 2009, Zdarta et al., 2021), especially synthetic dyes that are hardly degraded such as azo dyes which are widely used in industry. Among various enzymes used, ligninolytic enzymes can catalyse ring cleavage of aromatic compounds. Oxidoreductase enzymes, such as laccase and peroxidase, can catalyse oxidation reaction for phenolic removal from wastewater. There is a need for an effective method of enzymatic degradation to remove those pollutants in large volumes as free enzymes endure low stability and limited reusability (Zdarta et al., 2021). In recent years, enzyme immobilisation that overcomes the limitations of free enzymes has also been developed for synthetic dyes and phenolic compounds removal. Especially in degradation of these persistent pollutants, immobilised enzymes are of a great technology used for its stability and reusability properties.

Table 2.1 shows various enzymes with different immobilisation approaches used for removal of dyes and phenolic compounds. The efficiency of enzymatic degradation depends on the enzyme origin, the kind of support material employed, the presence of any other substance in the solution, and the process condition and parameters. The physico-chemical characteristics and shape of the support material surface and type of enzyme used define the immobilisation approach (Ali Khan & Alzohairy, 2010). Enzymes are immobilised through adsorption, cross-linking, encapsulation, and covalent binding. Adsorption and encapsulation are the simplest and most basic approach of immobilisation based on weak bonds such as Van der Waal's forces. Meanwhile, immobilisation through covalent bond requires other cross-linking chemicals and it provides stronger enzyme binding.

The immobilisation of horseradish peroxidase (HRP) on cationic microporous starch (CMPS) has successfully removed 86% p-chlorophenol using the adsorption method. The study shows that synthesised CMPS successfully supports the enzyme during phenolic compound removal. The findings also highlighted that CMPS has many pores that increased the enzyme efficiency, and improved enzyme stability towards denaturation by pH solution, organic solvent, and temperature (El-Naggar et al., 2021). Encapsulation of HRP in phospholipid-templated titania exhibited thermal stability improvement, pH stability and high tolerance against inactive agents, thus improving the enzyme efficiency. The removal of phenol achieved was 92.99% and the immobilisation promotes a good capacity of enzyme reutilisation (Jiang et al., 2014). Immobilisation of laccase enzyme on magnetic nanoparticle for phenol degradation was performed using dialdehyde starch (Fe_3O_4-NIL-DAS) as a cross-linker. This research discovered that ionic liquid modification and cross-linking immobilisation

TABLE 2.1
Enzyme Immobilisation Strategies for Different Dyes and Phenolic Compounds Removal

Type of Enzyme	Immobilisation Strategy	Type of Carrier	Targeted Pollutants	Process Description	Removal Efficiency (%)	Reference
Soybean hull peroxidase	Adsorption and cross-linking by using glutaraldehyde	Chitosan beads	Phenolic compounds	pH optimum: 6.0 Temperature: 30°C Time: 90 min	Coffee Processing Wastewater = 32.69% phenolic removal Synthetic Phenolic Solution = 79.18% phenolic removal	Chagas et al. (2015)
Horseradish peroxidase	Adsorption	Cationic microporous starch	p-chlorophenol	100 mg of CMPS at pH = 6.0 and 100 units of enzyme	86% p-chlorophenol removal efficiency	El-Naggar et al. (2021)
Horseradish peroxidase	Encapsulation	Phospholipid-templated titania	Phenolic compound and dye	HRP content 130 U, H_2O_2 8 mM 50 mL	79.72%	Jiang et al. (2014)
Horseradish peroxidase	Covalent binding	Functionalised RGO-SiO_2 nanocomposite	Phenols and dyes	Temperature: 40°C Time: 90 min	100% phenol removal efficiency 100% decolourisation of most dyes 70% Reusability of the initial activity after ten cycles	Vineh et al. (2020)
Laccase	Cross-linking (dialdehyde starch as cross-linker (Fe_3O_4- NIL-DAS)) + covalent bonding	Magnetic nanoparticles modified by amino-functionalised ionic liquid	Phenolic compound	Temperature: 25°C pH: 7.0	85.8% phenolic compound removal	Qiu et al. (2020)

(Continued)

TABLE 2.1 (*Continued*)
Enzyme Immobilisation Strategies for Different Dyes and Phenolic Compounds Removal

Type of Enzyme	Immobilisation Strategy	Type of Carrier	Targeted Pollutants	Process Description	Removal Efficiency (%)	Reference
Polyphenol oxidase	Adsorption	Chitosan/montmorillonite (CTS/MMT) and chitosan-gold nano- particles/ montmorillonite (CTS-AuNPs/MMT) composites	Phenolic compound	Temperature: 30°C 50 mM, pH 7	94.3% removal phenol efficiencies	Wang et al. (2020)
Laccase	Covalent binding	Epoxy-functionalised silica	Phenolic compound	Enzyme loading on support: 30 mg/g optimum pH: 4.5 Time: 24 h	95% removal phenol efficiency	Mohammadi et al. (2018)
Laccase	Adsorption	Magnetic bimodal mesoporous carbon	Phenolic compound	Time: 30 min Temperature: 45°C	78% Phenol removal and 84% p-chlorophenol removal	Liu et al. (2012)
White rot fungus	Adsorption	Wood chips of Italian poplar	Phenolic compound	Temperature: 30°C, pH: 6.0	87.05% phenol removal 72.09% COD	Lu et al., (2009)
Peroxidases	Adsorption	Bitter gourd (*Momordica Charantia*)	Textile dyes	Temperature: 40°C, pH: 3.0–4.0	>90% dyes degradation	Akhtar et al. (2005)

are effective for phenolic compounds removal in wastewater (Qiu et al., 2020). In a study, immobilised HRP onto functionalised RGO-SiO_2 through covalent bonding promoted 100% decolourisation efficiencies for most dyes and achieved 100% phenol removal efficiency (2,500 mg/L). This study confidently shows that HRP could effectively be used as an enzyme for phenol and dye degradation from the aqueous solution, and RGO-SiO_2 was an efficient matrix for the immobilisation of RHP via covalent binding. These results reported that catalytic activity improved by RHP, and it was found that HRP was less sensitive towards pH changes. Covalent binding is effectively preserved against deactivation throughout the degradation of pollutants (Vineh et al., 2020).

Factors such as reaction time, contact time, solution pH, initial pollutant concentration, cross-linker agent and concentration affect the immobilised enzyme efficiency for dyes and phenolic compounds removal. Chagas et al. (2015) indicated that enzyme efficiency of immobilised soybean hull peroxidase is becoming more dependent on the temperature after immobilisation. They have also reported that there was a difference in phenolic removal efficiency between the coffee processing wastewater (CPW) and synthetic phenolic solutions (SPS) even the experiment was run at the same conditions and using the same enzyme and carrier. CPW achieved much lower removal efficiency than SPS, which were 32% and 79%, respectively, due to the high complexity of the coffee processing effluent (Chagas et al., 2015). The finding shows that the presence of other substances in the solution affects the enzyme efficiency. A study by Wang et al. (2020) revealed that the most influencing factors that affected the immobilised polyphenol oxidase to remove phenolic compounds are solution pH and temperature. Solution pH is a major factor affecting the enzyme ionisation state. With the increased temperature, the removal efficiency of the phenolic compound is also increased, and the optimal temperature was 30°C. However, the removal efficiency decreased at a temperature higher than optimal due to thermal deactivation when the temperature exceeds the enzyme tolerance level (Wang et al., 2020). An optimum enzyme/substrate ratio (E/S) is another crucial parameter to minimise enzyme consumption and to ensure the maximal efficiency of the enzymatic reaction. Wang et al. (2020) have found that increasing the E/S has no significant effect on the removal efficiency. On the other hand, lower optimal ratio significantly improved catalytic efficiency of the immobilised polyphenol oxidase (Wang et al., 2020).

2.4 IMMOBILISED ENZYME TECHNOLOGIES FOR PHARMACEUTICAL BY-PRODUCTS REMOVAL

Considering the active development of human and veterinary medicines, and growing expanse of antibiotics, drugs and hormones, sewage disposal of these pharmaceutical wastes into the environment (rivers, lakes and soil) is a serious issue of concern. Chlortetracycline, carbamazepine, diclofenac, oestrogen and ibuprofen are examples of hormones and drugs that are identified to influence aquatic life (Yusuf, 2020). Current waste treatment method does not completely remove trace amounts of these compounds. New and more efficient methods to remove them are required.

Researchers and industries have shown an escalating interest to efficiently remove these compounds, which may include the application of immobilised enzymes (Naghdi et al., 2017). Pharmaceutical active compounds in the wastewater were numerously reported to be successfully degraded by immobilised oxidoreductases (Becker et al., 2017; García-Delgado et al., 2018; Garcia et al., 2019; Lacerda et al., 2019; Naghdi et al., 2017; Simón Herrero et al., 2019; Taheran et al., 2017; Wen et al., 2019; Xu et al., 2015; Yusuf, 2020). Oxidoreductase enzymes are among the best candidates due to their capability to oxidise pollutant compounds (Yusuf, 2020). Laccase gained a great interest among other oxidoreductase enzymes, since it only needs a simple co-substrate which is oxygen (Yusuf, 2020). Therefore, laccase is suitable for wide applications as it has low specificity with the capability to use oxygen as the electron acceptor and high pollutant removal yield.

Previously, *Trametes versicolor* laccase was covalently immobilised onto biochar-polyacrylonitrile membrane to treat antibiotic (chlortetracycline), anti-inflammatory (diclofenac) and antidepressant (carbamazepine) residues in water (Taheran et al., 2017). Degradation of chlortetracycline, diclofenac and carbamazepine were at 63%, 72% and 48%, respectively. After 30 days, immobilised enzyme retains high activity (94%) from its initial activity at 4°C, compared to the free enzyme which left only with 32% from its initial activity. Immobilised enzyme showed better pH, storage and thermal stability than free laccase and after ten cycles, able to maintain about 20% from its initial activity. In a different study, immobilised biocatalyst graphene oxide supported laccase successfully degraded ibuprofen (Yusuf, 2020). Stages of carrier binding, cross-linking and physical adsorption were carried out to produce such biocatalyst. The biocatalyst action in the presence of vanillin as a mediator, successfully converted 100% ibuprofen into biodegradable compounds such as N-(2,6-dichlorophenyl) indolin-2-one, 2,6-dichloroaniline, 4-isobutylacetophenone and 2-(2,6-dichlorophenylamino)benzaldehyde (Yusuf, 2020).

Naghdi et al. (2017) reported carbamazepine removal using immobilised laccase on acid-treated nanobiochar. They reported a maximum of 86% removal from synthetic wastewater and secondary effluent that contain the drug. The immobilised enzyme activity decreased to 6% after seven cycles. Another study on carbamezapine removal using modified polyimide aerogels as a support for laccase was reported by Simón Herrero et al. (2019). In their study, immobilised laccase exhibited carbamazepine removal by 76% from synthetic wastewater and 74% from secondary effluent. In addition, the removal efficiency remained high after seven cycles (50% for synthetic wastewater and 65% for secondary effluent). Another study, mesoporous materials from bentonite-derived with laccase immobilised was used to degrade tetracycline (Wen et al., 2019). The degradation efficiency of tetracycline by immobilised laccase in the presence of 1-hydroxybenzotriazole (HBT) was reported more than 60% after 3 h of the treatment. After five cycles, the immobilised laccase retained over 30% from its initial activity as a result of enzyme leaching during washing stages. This was due to the degraded binding forces between the carrier and enzyme (Wen et al., 2019).

García-Delgado et al. (2018) reported the removal of sulfonamides and tetracycline by immobilised laccase onto stevensite and biochar. The immobilised laccase with the help of redox mediator (either ABTS or syringaldehyde) exhibited up to

100% removal of sulfonamides and tetratcyclines. ABTS was a better mediator than syringaldehyde in terms of detoxification, kinetics of removal and removal extents. HRP supported by Poly(acrylic acid)/poly(vinyl alcohol)/SiO_2 membrane was developed to degrade paracetamol from spiked water (Xu et al. 2015). The paracetamol degradation rate was over 80% and reduced to 40% after seven cycles. Although the degradation rates between free and immobilised HRPs are about the same at 84.4% and 83.5%, respectively, the immobilised enzyme has the possible reusability which certainly added to its benefit.

Enzymes can successfully degrade hormones, such as oestrogens. Becker et al. (2017) immobilised laccase from *Myceliophthora thermophila* and *Trametes versicolor* onto two supports; ceramic membranes and polymeric beads of IB-EC1 by adsorption, to remove oestrogen in real wastewater and spike water. After 24 h treatment, 91% of oestrogen activity was removed by the enzyme. Laccase entrapped on copper alginate–chitosan bead and calcium were reportedly used to remove another type of hormone, 17α-ethinylestradiol (EE2) (Garcia et al., 2019). Immobilised laccase is able to remove about 80% of EE2 at a temperature of 28°C and pH 5, after 24 h of treatment. Furthermore, the removal yield maintains high at 70%, after three cycles. The same hormone (oestrogen) also reportedly being treated using laccase immobilised on *Luffa cylindrica* fibre (Lacerda et al. 2019). After 8 h treatment, the maximum EE2 degradation was 75% than that of the free laccase which is 79%. Although exhibited lower yield than the free laccase, the immobilised laccase presented possible reusability while maintaining 25% of its removal efficiency after seven cycles. The removal efficiency and storage stabilities of immobilised enzyme on various support was reportedly enhanced than that the free enzyme as shown in Table 2.2. It should be noted that the immobilised oxidoreductases application in the treatment generally yielded in over 60% of pharmaceutical residues removal.

2.5 CRITICAL FACTORS INFLUENCING THE EFFICIENCY OF IMMOBILISED ENZYMES AND THEIR CHALLENGES

Enzymes have recently been used to degrade numerous resistant environmental pollutants. This method has been shown to be ecologically beneficial since the breakdown products are less hazardous than the starting pollutants. Moreover, even under moderate conditions, enzymes show high efficiency and selectivity when they catalyse complex chemical reactions (Kashefi et al., 2019). As generally known, enzymes can be used in the free or immobilised form. Free enzymes alone normally show high enzymatic activity. However, it is not suitable for continuous process because it is quite difficult to regenerate or separate the free enzyme for the next cycles of catalytic activity. Thus, more operational costs are necessary for a continuous process (Naghdi et al., 2017; Shakerian et al., 2020). In addition, larger cost is also needed when applying in large scale especially in the industry due to its poor stability (Wen et al., 2019). Due to that, enzyme is immobilised to preserve the catalytic activity of the enzyme by time and increase its resilience towards extreme operating parameters such as highly acidic or alkaline pH, high range of temperatures and disruption by chemical reagents that might cause inactivation (Jolivalt et al., 2000).

TABLE 2.2
Example of Various Immobilised Oxidoreductase Performance for the Removal of Pharmaceuticals Residues

Targeted Compound	Enzyme	Immobilisation Strategy	Process Description	Removal Efficiency & Stability	Reference
Chlortetracycline, carbamazepine and diclofenac	Laccase from *Trametes versicolor*	Covalent binding onto membrane (biochar-polyacrylonitrile)	Optimum temperature = 35°C Enzyme loading = 12.7 U/g pH = 3.6–4.0	Chlortetracycline 63%, Diclofenac 72%, Carbamazepine 48% After 10 cycles, 20% 94% after 30 days	Taheran et al. (2017)
Ibuprofen	Laccase from *Trametes versicolor*	Covalent binding onto graphene oxide	Specific enzyme activity = 72,626 U/mg pH = 11	100%	Yusuf (2020)
Carbamazepine	Laccase from *Trametes versicolor*	Adsorption onto acid-treated (by H_2SO_4/HNO_3) nanobiochar	H_2SO_4:HNO_3 (50:50, v/v)	86% After seven cycles, 6%	Naghdi et al. (2017)
Carbamazepine	Laccase from *Trametes versicolor*	Covalent binding onto polyimide aerogels	Specific enzyme activity = 8 U/g pH = 3.0	74% to 76% after seven cycles, 50%–65% after 20 days	Simón Herrero et al. (2019)
Tetracycline	Laccase from *Trametes versicolor*	Adsorption onto bentonite-derived mesoporous materials	pH = 5.0 Laccase concentration = 2 mg/mL	60% After five cycles, 30%	Wen et al. (2019)
Tetracycline and sulfonamides	Laccase from *Trametes versicolor*	Covalent binding onto biochar and stevensite	pH = 5.5–6.5 Catalytic capabilities: 1426 IU/g stevensite Catalytic capabilities: 405 IU/g biochar	69%–100% 73% after 3 months at 4°C	García-Delgado et al. (2018)

(Continued)

TABLE 2.2 (*Continued*)
Example of Various Immobilised Oxidoreductase Performance for the Removal of Pharmaceuticals Residues

Targeted Compound	Enzyme	Immobilisation Strategy	Process Description	Removal Efficiency & Stability	Reference
Paracetamol	Peroxidase from horseradish	Covalent binding onto electrospinning nanofibrous membrane (Poly (vinyl alcohol)/poly (acrylic acid)/SiO_2)	60 min at 25°C with pH 6.0 and initial 0.8 mM H_2O_2	80% After seven cycles, 40%. 60% after 30 days	Xu et al. (2015)
Hormone: Oestrogen	*Myceliophthora thermophila* and Laccase from *Trametes versicolor*	Adsorption onto treated porous polymeric IB-EC1 beads and ceramic membranes	Feasible even at very low enzyme concentrations (2.8 ABTS U/L) Immobilised laccase was best in removing EDCs within the first 6 h	91%	Becker et al. (2017)
Hormone: 17α-ethinylestradiol (EE2)	Laccase from *Pycnoporus sanguineus*	Entrapment in calcium and copper alginate–chitosan composite	Optimal conditions for LE immobilisation on Ca-beads: 1.5% (w/v) SA, 1:5 (v/v) LE/SA and 3:7 (v/v) chitosan/ion (Ca^{+2}). Optimal conditions for immobilisation on Cu-beads were 2.0% (w/v) SA, 0.5:5 (v/v) LE/SA and 3:7 (v/v) chitosan/ion (Cu^{+2})	80% After three cycles, 70%.	Garcia et al. (2019)
Hormone: 17α-ethinylestradiol (EE2)	Laccase from *Pleurotus ostreatus*	Adsorption onto *Luffa Cylindrica* fibre	Optimum pH: 3.6–4.6, Optimum temperature: 30°C and 50°C (free and immobilised enzyme)	75% After seven cycles, 25%	Lacerda et al. (2019)

2.5.1 Support Materials

Several factors that can influence the performance or catalytic activity of an immobilised enzyme include choice of carrier or support material, immobilisation method and operating parameters or conditions. Therefore, it is necessary to immobilise them on suitable support materials using proper immobilisation techniques, to maximise utilisation of enzymes for wastewater treatment. Several studies on enzymatic activity, reusability, selectivity, operational, storage and thermal stability were compared with free enzymes to evaluate the catalytic performance of immobilised enzymes (Jun et al., 2019). The support material in immobilised enzyme technology is critical to catalytic activity. It is necessary if the materials utilised for support is easily accessible, affordable and environmentally friendly (Rodrigues et al., 2013). Having a better catalytic efficiency, improved operational stability, non-toxic and resilience to severe reaction conditions and microbial assaults are all desirable support material features. The types of support materials can be chosen from organic or inorganic support, depending on the chemical composition.

The physical properties of the support materials such as their particle diameter, mechanical strength and their welling properties act as important aspects in the catalytic activity of the immobilised enzyme. For instance, materials with pores and smaller particle size will tend to have larger total surface area which in return will affect the enzyme-binding capacity. Although non-porous supports have few diffusional constraints, the enzyme-binding capacity is lower compared to porous supports which possesses higher surface area that allow more enzyme loading and protects the immobilised enzyme from the environment. Porous supports that have tunable pore distribution are advantageous for optimisation of the binding capacity. Despite inorganic carriers having many benefits (e.g., great durability against physical, chemical and microbial degradation), organic matrices are used in most industrial applications. One of the most significant variables affecting the degree of activity of an immobilised enzyme is its hydrophilic nature (Masjoudi et al., 2021).

Enzyme can be immobilised on solid supports through either physical or chemical methods. Each method that has been established has its advantages and defects. Example of physical immobilisation methods are adsorption, encapsulation or entrapment. While covalent binding or cross-linking is the most preferable technique in chemical immobilisation (Fernandez-Fernandez et al., 2013), physical immobilisation mainly by adsorption is a simple approach for immobilisation of enzymes. There is no need for chemicals addition that will change the original shape of the enzyme, which leads to higher enzyme catalytic activity (Masjoudi et al., 2021). In physical adsorption, enzymes were physically attached or adsorbed onto the support's surface by weak forces such as Van der Waals interaction, ionic interaction and hydrogen bonds. Due to the relatively weak bonding, even after a few cycles, the immobilised enzyme might desorb or leak to the environment. According to Pang et al. (2015), when laccase was immobilised on carbon nanomaterials by adsorption method, the active site on the enzyme was less likely altered or destructed. However, this method has some drawbacks especially when utilised under extreme operating conditions because most of the adsorbed enzymes had low operational stability.

Under these conditions, the enzymes might denature due to the formation of weaker bond between the enzyme and support materials.

However, even though chemical immobilisation will cause partial changes in the enzyme molecular structure, a stronger attachment to the support will allow it to be used in numerous cycles of treatment with minimal risk of leakage (Wen et al., 2019). Chemical immobilisation, especially covalent binding, is one of the most widely utilised techniques of enzyme immobilisation for wastewater treatment. Covalent bonds are formed between the support material and enzyme functional groups. Available functional groups that are usually involved in the binding of enzymes are hydroxyl, amino, tyrosine and carboxylic groups. Previous research on the immobilisation of HRP onto calcium alginate (CA) by covalent bonding has been reported by Bilal et al. (2016). An increase in the efficiency and stabilities of the enzyme catalytic were observed compared to free enzyme. A strong bond between the enzyme and support increased its resistance when undergoes harsh operating conditions. Another advantage from this method is its ability to avoid leakage of enzymes and makes it suitable for usage under batch and continuous process (Singh et al., 2011). As mentioned earlier, one of the disadvantages of this method is the possibility for a lower enzymatic activity due to deformations or destruction in the enzyme molecular structure during the immobilisation reaction (Secundo, 2013). Therefore, cross-linking reaction with glutaraldehyde which acts as a cross-linking agent is usually employed to preserve the functional and structural characteristics of enzymes in the immobilisation process, to overcome these limitations (Drioli & Giorno, 2016).

2.5.2 Operating Parameters

Apart from that, effect of several operating parameters such as pH of solution, temperature, concentrations of both the enzymes and substrate are also key parameters that will have influence on the catalytic performance of the immobilised enzyme. Several studies had shown that immobilised enzymes can demonstrate a better catalytic activity over a wider range of pH as compared to the freely form enzymes (Mohamed et al., 2013; Ali et al., 2016). Based on Matto and Husain's finding (Matto & Husain, 2009), they have proven that their immobilised turnip peroxidase on Con A wood achieved better dye decolourisation at an extensive range of pH with 85% of dye removal while the free enzyme only decolourised 55% of the dye. The pH ranges from 5 to 7 is considered as neutral pH and can be regarded as the optimum pH for both enzymes (free and immobilised enzymes). However, the enzymatic activity for free enzyme will usually decrease significantly at extreme acidic and alkaline pH, which is due to the destruction of the enzyme structures and intramolecular or intermolecular linkage breakdown. Previous studies have demonstrated that immobilised enzyme can protect and stabilise the enzymes from high pH denaturation due to the presence of greater intramolecular interactions between the support and enzyme (Kim et al., 2012; Reshmi et al., 2007). In fact, the pH of real wastewater is sometimes slightly acidic or slightly basic. Therefore, to be applied to real industrial wastewater, immobilised enzymes are more preferable as compared to free enzymes (Zhang et al., 2013).

Another operating condition is temperature. Temperature can have a major impact on the efficiency of free and immobilised enzymes. Increment in temperature will proportionally increase the enzymatic activity, resulting from the increment in the kinetic energy between the molecules. Unlike immobilised enzymes, free enzyme could not maintain the enzymatic activity in an extreme and wide range of temperature and have low thermal stability (Bayramoğlu & Arıca, 2008). A study by Gholami-Borujeni et al. (2011) have immobilised HRP on CA beads, where the immobilised HRP was preserved under a wider temperature range as compared to free enzymes. This might be attributed by the stronger intramolecular or intermolecular bond between enzymes and the support which enable it to resist the denaturation or destruction of enzymatic structures under extreme temperature ranges (Kim et al., 2016). Based on several research, 25°C–40°C is the optimum temperature for immobilised enzymes (Besharati et al., 2018; Wang et al., 2016; Lu et al., 2017). A study by Matto and Husain (2008) indicated that 40°C was found to be the optimum temperature for the enzymatic activity for both free enzymes and immobilised tomato peroxidases. However, above that temperature, it started losing its catalytic activity. This might be because of the high impact of the extreme condition that denatured the active sites of the enzyme (Arslan, 2011). Nevertheless, the catalytic effectiveness of immobilised tomato peroxidases at all temperatures was still greater than that of free enzymes.

2.6 THREE CORE VALUES IN ADVANCING BIOTECHNOLOGICAL APPROACHES IN WASTE MANAGEMENT

Economic sustainability is critical to ensure a nation's survival in the long run, especially for countries that rely much on the petroleum-based economy, such as Malaysia and many Arab nations. For many countries, discovering new economic resources is pivotal because reliance on petroleum for the nations' economy is not sustainable. Bio-based economy is one of the promising economies for the world (Schürrle, 2018). Concerning the bio-based economy, the use of biotechnological approaches is gaining momentum for the past years, thanks to universities and research institutions that have made efforts to further advance the approaches (Festel, 2018).

However, advancing biotechnological approaches in waste management need core values that can drive the progress towards balance, holistic approaches. Many industries which develop and use biotechnological approaches in waste management should be required to have clear guides on how they should move forward the approaches with considerations on multiple factors, economic, social, ethical and environmental, and not solely on the profit-making agenda. For that reason, the authors would like to propose three core values where the parties, especially industries, that develop and utilise biotechnological approaches to follow the values accordingly. The core values consist of three key aspects that are generic in nature yet have specific impacts on the waste management agenda.

The three core values are (1) inclusivity, (2) sustainability and (3) integrity. For the first core value, inclusivity means industries should be able to consult with multiple parties for them to advance the development and utilisation of biotechnological approaches by engaging with the public, governments and academia or universities. The consultations with these parties will ensure that industries will be capable of making the technologies developed relevant for various parties, especially the public. The public will need to know how the technologies produced can solve real-world problems concerning them.

Industries will also need to consult the governments if they are to ensure technologies they develop and utilise align with the needs of the country and can comply with the governments' rules and regulations regarding the technologies produced. For instance, consultation with the government agencies such as the Department of Environment will ensure treated wastewater released to the environment will protect the interest of the nation. Meanwhile, consulting with universities may make industries having partners that may be able to provide facilities and human resources, especially talents. The academia-industry relations are desirable and will make both parties benefit from strategic partnerships (Ismail & Bunyamin, 2021; Jefferies & Barnard, 2018; Sciacca & Curioni, 2018).

The second core value is sustainability (Asveld et al., 2019). It means industries will need to ensure biotechnologies they produce will be able to create positive impacts to the economy, environment and the people, on a more long-term basis than short-term. The advancement of the biotechnological approaches in waste management must not create harm to the environment and must protect the health and safety of the people, including employees of industries (Chen & Reniers, 2018).

The third value is integrity (Preston & Antonsen, 2021). This is one particular aspect of human beings that is quite challenging because integrity includes personal and group interests, specifically, industries. Integrity may mean "doing the right thing even when nobody is seeing." Integrity covers ethical dimensions (Harfouche et al., 2021). Industries will need to ensure they develop and utilise biotechnological approaches in responsible ways and will need to comply with the rules and regulations set by the government. All three core values are proposed because they are deemed essential for the industries to advance the biotechnological approaches in waste management by considering multiple factors and the interests of various parties. As industries, they are bounded by the rules and regulations and need to obey them. They need to consult the government for further clarification if they face problems regarding the uses of biotechnological approaches in waste management.

As the world has been adopting the Sustainable Development Goals (SDGs) (United Nations, 2015), all parties especially industries will need to go together with the world's agenda. Two goals in SDGs that are closely related to the use of biotechnological approaches in waste management are Industry, Innovation, and Infrastructure (SDG#9) and Responsible Consumption and Production (SDG#12). These two goals in SDGs reflect the three core values proposed. SDG#9 promotes inclusive and sustainable industrialisation, while SDG#12 promotes sustainable consumption and production patterns. Nonetheless, integrity is implicit in these two SDGs. However, it does not mean that integrity is neglected. Industries will need to comply with all rules and regulations regarding the uses of biotechnological approaches in waste management, as a manifestation of the value of integrity.

In sum, these three core values are the critical factors that can drive industries for responsible use and development of biotechnological approaches in waste management. All other parties, besides the industries, are urged to internalise and practice these three core values. Inclusivity, sustainability and integrity are the way forward for the advancement of the biotechnological approaches in waste management. The authors name these three core values "the three TYs."

2.7 ADVANCEMENT OF IMMOBILISED ENZYMES AND FUTURE PROSPECT IN WASTEWATER MANAGEMENT

The utilisation of immobilised enzymes in the wastewater management is promising due to their efficacy and effectiveness in removing various types of contaminants like dyes, phenolic compounds, heavy metals and by-products. Even though some biotechnological approaches have few limitations and challenges, their advantages and benefits remain undeniable and outstanding. Microbial cellulases are one of the techniques that have been largely used in the wastewater management since the fundamental investigation on cellulases have been commenced for decades besides its wide applications that have been technologically advanced (Wakai et al., 2019). According to Sarsaiya et al. (2019), the enzyme business world market is rapidly enlarging with approximately 7.6% of growth rate in 2012 due to the steadiness and highly dynamical behaviour of enzymes.

Recent advanced investigation on microalgae-based treatment is highlighted in many applications involving wastewater management for example by using biological approach like phycoremediation. Enzymatic algae presence in the wastewater treatment can help transforming complex dye molecules into smaller ones (Lellis et al., 2019). Such enzymes can play an important role in the reduction of dyes pollutants in wastewater to make the ecosystem less harmful (Bhardwaj & Bharadvaja, 2021). The advantages of using algae are considered vital for wastewater management due to its natural and green process as well as cost-effective. Despite of this, the performance of algae-based treatment can still be enhanced if incorporated with other advanced methods like enzyme-immobilisation technique. This is due to the extra advantages that can be obtained through this method like enzyme stabilisation, enzyme inactivation inhibition and possible microbial contamination reduction (Jun et al., 2019). Besides that, immobilisation technique that involves immobilising algae on an alginate as carrier is predicted to help decreasing the shock load and toxic that are present in the raw distillery wastewater (Solovchenko et al., 2014).

The classifications of immobilisation carriers for the enzymes can be divided into three classes which are organic carriers, inorganic carriers and composite carriers. The latest one is becoming a new trend in the new development of immobilised enzyme advancement since it is the combination of both organic and inorganic materials. According to Zhang et al. (2015), this type of carrier will lead to the integration of two types of performances that come from different materials used. For example, polyvinyl alcohol-sodium (PVA) and alginate or guar gum have been used by a group of researchers for the removal of phenol and the study has shown the complete removal of phenol as a result (Ismail & Khudhair, 2015). The utilisation of alginate as one of the materials in the carrier has more advantages since it provides more environmentally friendly impacts due to its permeability, matrix transparency and null toxicity which can give protection to the immobilised cells from any extreme conditions that can occur physically or chemically during the immobilisation process (Kadimpati et al., 2013).

The time consumption for the growth of microorganisms using conventional biological wastewater treatment can be enhanced by using the immobilisation of microbial cells method. This technique is also reported to have increased the microorganism's concentration by fixations to the carriers (Cesaro et al., 2013). An excellent result was obtained by Banerjee and Ghoshal (2016) on the efficacy of immobilisation of biomass containing phenol strains from *Bacillus cereus* using Ca-alginate carrier in petroleum wastewater. This study has shown the elimination of phenolic compounds concentration and COD level by 95%. Furthermore, the use of immobilised enzyme in the wastewater containing heavy metal ions is also showing a good trend for the future since it can enhance the stability of microorganisms used and their resistance towards the exterior extreme conditions. In one of the studies that has been reviewed, the immobilised fungus, *Penicillium citrinum* in the matrix of sodium alginate beads showed a great affinity towards copper ions removal compared to the free biomass used since the immobilised fungus showed higher copper ions removal percentage compared to the free fungus (Verma et al., 2013).

Eutrophication is one of the serious phenomena that occur in the lakes due to the excessive amounts of nutrients like phosphate, ammonium and nitrates that run into rivers and lakes. Biological treatment on these polluted lakes needs to be focused more compared to other proposed treatment methods. This is because the microalgae have a great capacity in converting nutrients in the wastewater to biomass or other bio-products (Delgadillo-Mirquez et al., 2016). A study was conducted by Kumar et al. (2018) which showed the promising results of removing phosphate and nitrates from wastewater using immobilised nitrogen fixing cyanobacterium *Gloeocapsa gelatinosa*. The removal percentages of nitrates and phosphates using immobilised bacteria were more than 80%. Besides that, incorporation of nanomaterials as carrier/support to immobilise enzymes will give a great impact on the wastewater treatment outcome. Nanotechnology has received a great attention from many industries worldwide due to their great potential in enhancing the performance and capacities of treatments. Not only the size is small, but nanomaterials also possess a lot of features like special functional groups and excellent adsorption capacities. For example, a group of researchers has incorporated magnetic mesoporous SiO_2/Fe_3O_4 hollow microspheres with immobilised laccase for the removal and biodegradation of dichlorophenol from aqueous solutions. The results recorded have shown a great potential of nanomaterials used in the study, where the removal and degradation rates of dichlorophenol were 81.64% and 52.31%, respectively (Li et al., 2016).

Moreover, the utilisation of carbon nanotubes (CNT) as support materials was also recorded as an enhancement of the immobilisation technique. Lignin peroxidase and laccase are the examples of enzymes that have been tested and immobilised onto CNT. Lignin peroxidase that has been immobilised on CNT has been tested for the application of dye degradation treatment. This study has showed a great potential of materials developed, where the catalytic efficiency and stability of the immobilised lignin peroxidase were higher than the free enzymes (Oliveira et al., 2018). Other examples are peroxidase enzyme from horseradish has also been immobilised on the nanocomposite (Sun et al., 2017) and activated carbon nanosphere (Lu et al., 2017) supports and the removal percentage of dyes and phenolic compounds recorded by these groups of researchers were 95.5% and 95.1%, respectively.

Besides functionalised CNT, the macroscopic size of CNT sheets assembly, called as Buckypaper, is also gaining serious attention from research community recently. It is due to the special properties of Buckypaper that is known to be good in thermal conductivity, chemical stability, possessing high specific surface area and good tensile strength (Liu et al., 2013). Enzyme-immobilised BP is envisaged to have a great potential and capacity as biocatalyst since these materials have eco-friendly properties, high adsorption capacity as well as good reusability and recovery performance of both enzymes and supports (Jun et al., 2019).

2.8 CONCLUSION

The enzyme immobilisation techniques in treating wastewater have a great future and showed promising outcomes in bioremediations such as dyes and phenolic compounds removal, and removal of excessive bio nutrients from pharmaceutical by-products. The key points of selecting the best strategy of developing this enzyme-immobilisation method are the choice of carriers and microorganisms itself for a particular application. Generally, the gaps between studies that have been performed by various groups of researchers always exist and open for further discussions and improvements. There is no single material that can perfectly be used for enzyme immobilisation to fit all types of pollutants treatment from wastewater. Every enzyme and carrier used in developing this wastewater treatment materials differ from each other based on their performance and particular properties, especially their cell immobilisation methods on the carriers which are adsorption, covalent bond, entrapment and encapsulation. Besides, the performances of immobilised enzymes also vary from each application depending on the different parameters that have been set up. Lastly but not least, the huge gap and challenge that need to be closed in this study is to bring the lab scales study to the real industrial scales and able to be commercialised.

ACKNOWLEDGEMENT

We highly acknowledge the Malaysian Research University Network Young Researchers Grant Scheme (R.J130000.7851.4L905) from the Ministry of Higher Education, Malaysia, and the Universiti Teknologi Malaysia for the facility support.

REFERENCES

Abdel-Shafy, H. I., & Mansour, M. S. (2016). A review on polycyclic aromatic hydrocarbons: Source, environmental impact, effect on human health and remediation. *Egyptian Journal of Petroleum*, 25(1), 107–123.

Akhtar, S., Khan, A. A., & Husain, Q. (2005). Potential of immobilized bitter gourd (*Momordica charantia*) peroxidases in the decolorization and removal of textile dyes from polluted wastewater and dyeing effluent. *Chemosphere*, 60(3), 291–301. https://doi.org/10.1016/j.chemosphere.2004.12.017.

Alibeigi-Beni, S., Zare, M. H., Chenar, M. P., Sadeghi, M., & Shirazian, S. (2021). Design and optimization of a hybrid process based on hollow-fiber membrane/coagulation for wastewater treatment. *Environmental Science and Pollution Research*, 28(7), 8235–8245.

Ali Khan, A., & Alzohairy, M. A. (2010). Recent advances and applications of immobilized enzyme technologies: A review. *Research Journal of Biological Sciences*, 5(8), 565–575. https://doi.org/10.3923/rjbsci.2010.565.575.

Ali, M., Husain, Q., Alam, N., & Ahmad, M. (2016). Enhanced catalytic activity and stability of ginger peroxidase immobilized on amino-functionalized silica-coated titanium dioxide nanocomposite: A cost-effective tool for bioremediation. *Water, Air, & Soil Pollution*, 228, 22.

Arslan, M. (2011). Immobilization horseradish peroxidase on amine-functionalized glycidyl methacrylate-g-poly(ethylene terephthalate) fibers for use in azo dye decolorization. *Polymer Bulletin*, 66, 865–879.

Asveld, L., Osseweijer, P., Posada, J.A. (2019). Societal and Ethical Issues in Industrial Biotechnology. In: Fröhling, M., Hiete, M. (eds) *Sustainability and Life Cycle Assessment in Industrial Biotechnology*. Advances in Biochemical Engineering/Biotechnology, vol 173. Springer, Cham. https://doi.org/10.1007/10_2019_100.

Bayramoğlu, G., & Arıca, M. Y. (2008). Enzymatic removal of phenol and p-chlorophenol in enzyme reactor: Horseradish peroxidase immobilized on magnetic beads. *Journal of Hazardous Materials*, 156, 148–155.

Banerjee, A., & Ghoshal, A. K. (2016). Biodegradation of real petroleum wastewater by immobilized hyper phenol-tolerant strains of *Bacillus cereus* in a fluidized bed bioreactor. *3 Biotech*, 6(2), 1–4.

Becker, D., Rodriguez-Mozaz, S., Insa, S., Schoevaart, R., Barceló, D., de Cazes, M., Belleville, M.-P., Sanchez-Marcano, J., Misovic, A., Oehlmann, J., & Wagner, M. (2017). Removal of endocrine disrupting chemicals in wastewater by enzymatic treatment with fungal laccases. *Organic Process Research & Development*, 21(4), 480–491.

Beriro, D. J., Cave, M. R., Wragg, J., Thomas, R., Wills, G., & Evans, F. (2016). A review of the current state of the art of physiologically-based tests for measuring human dermal in vitro bioavailability of polycyclic aromatic hydrocarbons (PAH) in soil. *Journal of Hazardous Materials*, 305, 240–259.

Besharati Vineh, M., Saboury, A.A., Poostchi, A.A., & Mamani, L., (2018). Physical adsorption of horseradish peroxidase on reduced graphene oxide nanosheets functionalized by amine: A good system for biodegradation of high phenol concentration in wastewater. *International Journal of Environmental Research*, 12, 45–57.

Bhardwaj, D., & Bharadvaja, N. (2021). Phycoremediation of effluents containing dyes and its prospects for value-added products: A review of opportunities. Journal of Water Process Engineering, 41, 102080.

Bilal, M., Asgher, M., Parra-Saldivar, R., Hu, H., Wang, W., Zhang, X., & Iqbal, H. M. (2017a). Immobilized ligninolytic enzymes: An innovative and environmental responsive technology to tackle dye-based industrial pollutants–a review. *Science of the Total Environment*, 576, 646–659.

Bilal, M., Iqbal, H. M., Shah, S. Z. H., Hu, H., Wang, W., & Zhang, X. (2016). Horseradish peroxidase-assisted approach to decolorize and detoxify dye pollutants in a packed bed bioreactor. *Journal of Environmental Management*, 183, 836–842.

Bilal, M., Rasheed, T., Iqbal, H. M., Hu, H., Wang, W., & Zhang, X. (2017b). Novel characteristics of horseradish peroxidase immobilized onto the polyvinyl alcohol-alginate beads and its methyl orange degradation potential. *International Journal of Biological Macromolecules*, 105, 328–335.

Bilal, M., Rasheed, T., Iqbal, H. M., & Yan, Y. (2018). Peroxidases-assisted removal of environmentally-related hazardous pollutants with reference to the reaction mechanisms of industrial dyes. *Science of the Total Environment*, 644, 1–13.

Cesaro, A., Naddeo, V., & Belgiorno, V. (2013). Wastewater treatment by combination of advanced oxidation processes and conventional biological systems. *Journal of Bioremediation & Biodegradation*, 4(8), 1–8.

Chagas, P. M. B., Torres, J. A., Silva, M. C., & Corrêa, A. D. (2015). Immobilized soybean hull peroxidase for the oxidation of phenolic compounds in coffee processing wastewater. *International Journal of Biological Macromolecules*, 81, 568–575. https://doi.org/10.1016/j.ijbiomac.2015.08.061.

Chatha, S. A. S., Asgher, M., & Iqbal, H. M. (2017). Enzyme-based solutions for textile processing and dye contaminant biodegradation—A review. *Environmental Science and Pollution Research*, 24(16), 14005–14018.

Chen, C., Reniers, G. (2018). Risk Assessment of Processes and Products in Industrial Biotechnology. In: Fröhling, M., Hiete, M. (eds) *Sustainability and Life Cycle Assessment in Industrial Biotechnology*. Advances in Biochemical Engineering/Biotechnology, vol 173. Springer, Cham. https://doi.org/10.1007/10_2018_74.

Chowdhary, P., Bharagava, R.N., Mishra, S., Khan, N. (2020). Role of Industries in Water Scarcity and Its Adverse Effects on Environment and Human Health. In: Shukla, V., Kumar, N. (eds) *Environmental Concerns and Sustainable Development*. Springer, Singapore. https://doi.org/10.1007/978-981-13-5889-0_12.

Delgadillo-Mirquez, L., Lopes, F., Taidi, B., & Pareau, D. (2016). Nitrogen and phosphate removal from wastewater with a mixed microalgae and bacteria culture. *Biotechnology Reports*, 11, 18–26.

Drioli, E., & Giorno, L. (2016). Enzyme Membrane Reactors. In: Drioli, E., Giorno, L. (eds) *Encyclopedia of Membranes*. Springer, Berlin, Heidelberg. https://doi.org/10.1007/978-3-662-44324-8_100107 EIA (2019).

Energy Information Administration, EIA projects nearly 50% increase in world energy usage by 2050, led by growth in Asia. https://www.eia.gov/todayinenergy/detail.php?id=41433.

El-Naggar, M. E., Abdel-Aty, A. M., Wassel, A. R., Elaraby, N. M., & Mohamed, S. A. (2021). Immobilization of horseradish peroxidase on cationic microporous starch: Physico-biochemical characterization and removal of phenolic compounds. *International Journal of Biological Macromolecules*, 181, 734–742. https://doi.org/10.1016/j.ijbiomac.2021.03.171.

Eurostat (2016). Accessed 4 October 2021, https://ec.europa.eu/eurostat/web/main/help/first-visit/tgm.

Farzaneh, H., Loganathan, K., Saththasivam, J., & McKay, G. (2021). Selectivity and competition in the chemical oxidation processes for a binary pharmaceutical system in treated sewage effluent. *Science of the Total Environment*, 765, 142704.

Fernandez-Fernandez, M., Sanroman, M.A., & Moldes, D. (2013). Recent developments and applications of immobilized laccase. *Biotechnology Advances*, 31, 1808–1825.

Festel, G. (2018). Economic aspects of industrial biotechnology. In *Sustainability and Life Cycle Assessment in Industrial Biotechnology* (pp. 53–74). Springer, Cham.

Fiorucci, P., Minciardi, R., Robba, M., & Sacile, R. (2003). Solid waste management in urban areas: Development and application of a decision support system. *Resources, Conservation and Recycling*, 37(4), 301–328.

García-Delgado, C., Eymar, E., Camacho-Arévalo, R., Petruccioli, M., Crognale, S., & D'Annibale, A. (2018). Degradation of tetracyclines and sulfonamides by stevensite- and biochar-immobilized laccase systems and impact on residual antibiotic activity. *Journal of Chemical Technology & Biotechnology*, 93(12), 3394–3409.

Garcia, L. F., Lacerda, M. F. A. R., Thomaz, D. V., de Souza Golveia, J. C., Pereira, M. D. G. C., de Souza Gil, E., Schimidt, F., & Santiago, M. F. (2019). Optimization of laccase–alginate–chitosan-based matrix toward 17 α-ethinylestradiol removal. *Preparative Biochemistry & Biotechnology*, 49(4), 375–383.

Gholami-Borujeni, F., Mahvi, A.H., Naseri, S., Faramarzi, M.A., Nabizadeh, R., & Alimohammadi, M. (2011). Application of immobilized horseradish peroxidase for removal and detoxification of azo dye from aqueous solution. *Research Journal of Chemistry and Environment*, 15, 217–222.

Han, Z., Liu, Y., Zhong, M., Shi, G., Li, Q., Zeng, D., Zhang, U., Fei, Y., & Xie, Y. (2018). Influencing factors of domestic waste characteristics in rural areas of developing countries. *Waste Management*, 72, 45–54.

Harfouche, A. L., Petousi, V., Meilan, R., Sweet, J., Twardowski, T., & Altman, A. (2021). Promoting ethically responsible use of agricultural biotechnology. *Trends in Plant Science*, 26(6), 546–559.

He, W., Wang, Q., Zhu, Y., Wang, K., Mao, J., Xue, X., & Shi, Y. (2021). Innovative technology of municipal wastewater treatment for rapid sludge sedimentation and enhancing pollutants removal with nano-material. *Bioresource Technology*, 324, 124675.

Ismail, A. F., & Bunyamin, M. A. H. (2021). Kerajaan, Industri Perlu Manfaatkan Kepakaran Ahli Akademik. Retrieved from https://www.bharian.com.my/rencana/komentar/2021/02/783368/kerajaan-industri-perlu-manfaatkan-kepakaran-ahli-akademik.

Ismail, Z. Z., & Khudhair, H. A. (2015). Recycling of immobilized cells for aerobic biodegradation of phenol in a fluidized bed bioreactor. *Systemics, Cybernetics and Informatics*, 13(5), 81–86.

Ivanov, V., Stabnikov, V., Stabnikova, O., & Kawasaki, S. (2019). Environmental safety and biosafety in construction biotechnology. *World Journal of Microbiology and Biotechnology*, 35(2), 26.

Jefferies, M., & Barnard, K. (2018). Rolls-Royce University Technology Centres: Relationships matter. In L. Frolund & M. Riedel, *Strategic Industry-University Partnerships: Success-Factors from Innovative Companies* (pp. 81–103). Elsevier, Britain. https://doi.org/10.1016/B978-0-12-810989-2.00005-9.

Jiang, Y., Tang, W., Gao, J., Zhou, L., & He, Y. (2014). Immobilization of horseradish peroxidase in phospholipid-templated titania and its applications in phenolic compounds and dye removal. *Enzyme and Microbial Technology*, 55, 1–6. https://doi.org/10.1016/j.enzmictec.2013.11.005.

Jolivalt, C., Brenon, S., Caminade, E., Mougin, C., & Pontié, M. (2000). Immobilization of laccase from Trametes versicolor on a modified PVDF microfiltration membrane: Characterization of the grafted support and application in removing a phenylurea pesticide in wastewater. *Journal of Membrane Science*, 180, 103–113.

Jun, L. Y., Yon, L. S., Mubarak, N. M., Bing, C. H., Pan, S., Danquah, M. K., Abduallah, E.C., & Khalid, M., 2019. An overview of immobilized enzyme technologies for dye and phenolic removal from wastewater. *Journal of Environmental Chemical Engineering*, 7, 102961–102975.

Kadimpati, K. K., Mondithoka, K. P., Bheemaraju, S., & Challa, V. R. M. (2013). Entrapment of marine microalga, *Isochrysis galbana*, for biosorption of Cr (III) from aqueous solution: Isotherms and spectroscopic characterization. *Applied Water Science*, 3(1), 85–92.

Kashefi, S., Borghei, S.M., & Mahmoodi, N.M. (2019). Covalently immobilized laccase onto graphene oxide nanosheets: Preparation, characterization, and biodegradation of azo dyes in colored wastewater. *Journal of Molecular Liquids*, 276, 153–162.

Kim, H.J., Suma, Y., Lee, S.H., Kim, J.-A., & Kim, H.S. (2012). Immobilization of horseradish peroxidase onto clay minerals using soil organic matter for phenol removal. *Journal of Molecular Catalysis B: Enzymatic*, 83, 8–15.

Kim, S., Lee, J., Jang, S., Lee, H., Sung, D., & Chang, J. (2016). High efficient chromogenic catalysis of tetramethylbenzidine with horseradish peroxidase immobilized magnetic nanoparticles. *Biochemical Engineering Journal*, 105, 406–411.

Kumar, T. P., Mandlimath, T. R., Sangeetha, P., Revathi, S., & Kumar, S. A. (2018). Nanoscale materials as sorbents for nitrate and phosphate removal from water. *Environmental Chemistry Letters*, 16(2), 389–400.

Lacerda, M. F. A. R., Lopes, F. M., Sartoratto, A., Ponezi, A. N., Thomaz, D. V., Schimidt, F., & Santiago, M. F. (2019). Stability of immobilized laccase on *Luffa Cylindrica* fibers and assessment of synthetic hormone degradation. *Preparative Biochemistry & Biotechnology*, 49(1): 58–63.

Lambert, M. R., & Skelly, D. K. (2016). Diverse sources for endocrine disruption in the wild. *Endocrine Disruptors*, 4(1), e1148803.

Lellis, B., Fávaro-Polonio, C. Z., Pamphile, J. A., & Polonio, J. C. (2019). Effects of textile dyes on health and the environment and bioremediation potential of living organisms. *Biotechnology Research and Innovation*, 3(2), 275–290.

Li, P., Miao, R., Wang, P., Sun, F., & Li, X. Y. (2021). Bi-metal oxide-modified flat-sheet ceramic membranes for catalytic ozonation of organic pollutants in wastewater treatment. *Chemical Engineering Journal*, 426, 131263.

Li, Q.-Y., Wang, P.-Y., Zhou, Y.-L., Nie, Z.-R., & Wei, Q. (2016). A magnetic mesoporous SiO_2/Fe_3O_4 hollow microsphere with a novel network-like composite shell: Synthesis and application on laccase immobilization. *Journal of Sol-Gel Science and Technology*, 78(3), 523–530.

Liu, Q., Li, M., Wang, Z., Gu, Y., Li, Y., & Zhang, Z. (2013). Improvement on the tensile performance of buckypaper using a novel dispersant and functionalized carbon nanotubes. *Composites Part A: Applied Science and Manufacturing*, 55, 102–109.

Liu, Y., Zeng, Z., Zeng, G., Tang, L., Pang, Y., Li, Z., Liu, C., Lei, X., Wu, M., Ren, P., Liu, Z., Chen, M., & Xie, G. (2012). Immobilization of laccase on magnetic bimodal mesoporous carbon and the application in the removal of phenolic compounds. *Bioresource Technology*, 115, 21–26. https://doi.org/10.1016/j.biortech.2011.11.015.

Lu, Y.M., Yang, Q.Y., Wang, L.M., Zhang, M.Z., Guo, W.Q., & Cai, Z.N. (2017). Enhanced activity of immobilized horseradish peroxidase by carbon nanospheres for phenols removal. *CLEAN–Soil, Air, Water*, 45(2), 1600077.

Lu, Y., Yan, L., Wang, Y., Zhou, S., Fu, J., & Zhang, J. (2009). Biodegradation of phenolic compounds from coking wastewater by immobilized white rot fungus *Phanerochaete chrysosporium*. *Journal of Hazardous Materials*, 165(1–3), 1091–1097. https://doi.org/10.1016/j.jhazmat.2008.10.091.

Ma, Y., & Harrad, S. (2015). Spatiotemporal analysis and human exposure assessment on polycyclic aromatic hydrocarbons in indoor air, settled house dust, and diet: A review. *Environment International*, 84, 7–16.

Margot, J., Rossi, L., Barry, D. A., & Holliger, C. (2015). A review of the fate of micropollutants in wastewater treatment plants. *Wiley Interdisciplinary Reviews: Water*, 2(5), 457–487.

Masjoudi, M., Golgoli, M., Nejad, Z. G., Sadeghzadeh, S., & Borghei, S. M. (2021). Pharmaceuticals removal by immobilized laccase on polyvinylidene fluoride nanocomposite with multi-walled carbon nanotubes. *Chemosphere*, 263, 128043.

Matto, M., & Husain, Q. (2008). Redox-mediated decolorization of Direct Red 23 and Direct Blue 80 catalyzed by bioaffinity-based immobilized tomato (*Lycopersicon esculentum*) peroxidase. *Biotechnology Journal: Healthcare Nutrition Technology*, 3, 1224–1231.

Matto, M., & Husain, Q. (2009). Decolorization of direct dyes by immobilized turnip peroxidase in batch and continuous processes. *Ecotoxicology and Environmental Safety*, 72, 965–971.

McGrane, S. J. (2016). Impacts of urbanisation on hydrological and water quality dynamics, and urban water management: A review. *Hydrological Sciences Journal*, 61(13), 2295–2311.

Mohamed, S.A., Darwish, A.A., & El-Shishtawy, R.M. (2013). Immobilization of horseradish peroxidase on activated wool. *Process Biochemistry*, 48, 649–655.

Mohammadi, M., As'habi, M. A., Salehi, P., Yousefi, M., Nazari, M., & Brask, J. (2018). Immobilization of laccase on epoxy-functionalized silica and its application in biodegradation of phenolic compounds. *International Journal of Biological Macromolecules*, 109, 443–447. https://doi.org/10.1016/j.ijbiomac.2017.12.102.

Naghdi, M., Taheran, M., Brar, S. K., Kermanshahi-Pour, A., Verma, M., & Surampalli, R. Y. (2017). Immobilized laccase on oxygen functionalized nanobiochars through mineral acids treatment for removal of carbamazepine. *Science of the Total Environment*, 584–585, 393–401.

Nematollahi, M. J., Keshavarzi, B., Mohit, F., Moore, F., & Busquets, R. (2022). Microplastic occurrence in urban and industrial soils of Ahvaz metropolis: A city with a sustained record of air pollution. *Science of the Total Environment*, 819, 152051.

Nielsen, K., Kalmykova, Y., Strömvall, A. M., Baun, A., & Eriksson, E. (2015). Particle phase distribution of polycyclic aromatic hydrocarbons in stormwater—using humic acid and iron nano-sized colloids as test particles. *Science of the Total Environment*, 532, 103–111.

Oliveira, S. F., da Luz, J. M. R., Kasuya, M. C. M., Ladeira, L. O., & Junior, A. C. (2018). Enzymatic extract containing lignin peroxidase immobilized on carbon nanotubes: Potential biocatalyst in dye decolourization. *Saudi Journal of Biological Sciences*, 25(4), 651–659.

Pal, A., He, Y., Jekel, M., Reinhard, M., & Gin, K. Y. H. (2014). Emerging contaminants of public health significance as water quality indicator compounds in the urban water cycle. *Environment International*, 71, 46–62.

Pang, R., Li, M., & Zhang, C. (2015). Degradation of phenolic compounds by laccase immobilized on carbon nanomaterials: Diffusional limitation investigation. *Talanta*, 131, 38–45.

Preston, C., & Antonsen, T. (2021). Integrity and agency: Negotiating new forms of human-nature relations in biotechnology. *Environmental Ethics*. 43(1), 21-41. https://doi.org/10.5840/enviroethics202143020.

Qiu, X., Wang, Y., Xue, Y., Li, W., & Hu, Y. (2020). Laccase immobilized on magnetic nanoparticles modified by amino-functionalized ionic liquid via dialdehyde starch for phenolic compounds biodegradation. *Chemical Engineering Journal*, 391. https://doi.org/10.1016/j.cej.2019.123564.

Ranjan, B., Pillai, S., Permaul, K., & Singh, S. (2019). Simultaneous removal of heavy metals and cyanate in a wastewater sample using immobilized cyanate hydratase on magnetic-multiwall carbon nanotubes. *Journal of Hazardous Materials*, 363, 73–80.

Reshmi, R., Sanjay, G., & Sugunan, S. (2007). Immobilization of α-amylase on zirconia: A heterogeneous biocatalyst for starch hydrolysis, *Catalysis Communications*, 8, 393–399.

Rodrigo-Comino, J., López-Vicente, M., Kumar, V., Rodríguez-Seijo, A., Valkó, O., Rojas, C., … & Panagos, P. (2020). Soil science challenges in a new era: A transdisciplinary overview of relevant topics. *Air, Soil and Water Research*, 13, 1178622120977491.

Rodrigues, R.C., Ortiz, C., Berenguer-Murcia, Á., Torres, R., & Fernández-Lafuente, R. (2013). Modifying enzyme activity and selectivity by immobilization. *Chemical Society Reviews*, 42, 6290–6307.

Sany, S. B. T., Hashim, R., Salleh, A., Rezayi, M., Karlen, D. J., Razavizadeh, B. B. M., & Abouzari-Lotf, E. (2015). Dioxin risk assessment: Mechanisms of action and possible toxicity in human health. *Environmental Science and Pollution Research*, 22(24), 19434–19450.

Sarsaiya, S., Jain, A., Awasthi, S. K., Duan, Y., Awasthi, M. K., & Shi, J. (2019). Microbial dynamics for lignocellulosic waste bioconversion and its importance with modern circular economy, challenges and future perspectives. *Bioresource Technology*, 291, 121905.

Schürrle, K. (2018). History, current state, and emerging applications of industrial biotechnology. In *Sustainability and Life Cycle Assessment in Industrial Biotechnology* (pp. 13–51). Springer, Cham.

Sciacca, C., & Curioni, A. (2018). Building global innovation ecosystem through public private partnerships: How IBM has leveraged academic collaboration for 70+ Years. In L. Frolund & M. Riedel, *Strategic Industry-University Partnerships: Success-Factors from Innovative Companies* (pp. 59–79). Elsevier, Britain. https://doi.org/10.1016/B978-0-12-810989-2.00004-7.

Secundo F. (2013). Conformational changes of enzymes upon immobilization, *Chemical Society Reviews*, 42, 6250–6261.

Shakerian, F., Zhao, J., & Li, S.P. (2020). Recent development in the application of immobilized oxidative enzymes for bioremediation of hazardous micropollutants: A review. *Chemosphere*, 239, 124716.

Silva, E. N., Cantillo-Castrillon, M., Dantas, T. M., Mesquita, Y. M., Maia, D. A., Bastos-Neto, M., … & Azevedo, D. C. (2021). Siloxane adsorption by porous silica synthesized from residual sand of wastewater treatment. *Journal of Environmental Chemical Engineering*, 9(2), 104805.

Simón Herrero, C., Naghdi, M., Taheran, M., Brar, S., Romero, A., Valverde, J., Ramirez, A.A., … & Sánchez-Silva, L. (2019). Immobilized laccase on Polyimide Aerogels for removal of carbamazepine. *Journal of Hazardous Materials*, 376, 83–90.

Singh, R. K., Zhang, Y. W., Jeya, M., & Lee, J. K. (2011). Covalent immobilization of β-1, 4-glucosidase from Agaricus arvensis onto functionalized silicon oxide nanoparticles. *Applied Microbiology and Biotechnology*, 89, 337–344.

Solovchenko, A., Pogosyan, S., Chivkunova, O., Selyakh, I., Semenova, L., Voronova, E., … & Kirpichnikov, M. (2014). Phycoremediation of alcohol distillery wastewater with a novel *Chlorella sorokiniana* strain cultivated in a photobioreactor monitored on-line via chlorophyll fluorescence. *Algal Research*, 6, 234–241.

Sun, H., Jin, X., Long, N., & Zhang, R. (2017). Improved biodegradation of synthetic azo dye by horseradish peroxidase cross-linked on nano-composite support. *International Journal of Biological Macromolecules*, 95, 1049–1055.

Taheran, M., Naghdi, M., Brar, S. K., Knystautas, E. J., Verma, M., & Surampalli, R. Y. (2017). Covalent immobilization of laccase onto nanofibrous membrane for degradation of pharmaceutical residues in water. *ACS Sustainable Chemistry & Engineering*, 5(11): 10430–10438.

Temesgen, A., Storsletten, V., & Jakobsen, O. (2021). Circular economy–reducing symptoms or radical change? *Philosophy of Management*, 20(1), 37–56.

United Nations (2015). The 17 Goals. Retrieved from https://sdgs.un.org/.

Verma, A., Singh, A., Bishnoi, N. R., & Gupta, A. (2013). Biosorption of Cu (II) using free and immobilized biomass of *Penicillium citrinum*. *Ecological Engineering*, 61, 486–490.

Vineh, M. B., Saboury, A. A., Poostchi, A. A., & Ghasemi, A. (2020). Biodegradation of phenol and dyes with horseradish peroxidase covalently immobilized on functionalized RGO-SiO_2 nanocomposite. *International Journal of Biological Macromolecules*, 164, 4403–4414. https://doi.org/10.1016/j.ijbiomac.2020.09.045.

Wakai, S., Nakashima, N., Ogino, C., Tsutsumi, H., Hata, Y., & Kondo, A. (2019). Modified expression of multi-cellulases in a filamentous fungus *Aspergillus oryzae*. *Bioresource Technology*, 276, 146–153.

Wang, H., Li, S., Li, J., Zhong, L., Cheng, H., & Ma, Q. (2020). Immobilized polyphenol oxidase: Preparation, optimization and oxidation of phenolic compounds. *International Journal of Biological Macromolecules*, 160, 233–244. https://doi.org/10.1016/j.ijbiomac.2020.05.079.

Wang, S., Fang, H., Yi, X., Xu, Z., Xie, X., & Tang Q. (2016). Oxidative removal of phenol by HRP-immobilized beads and its environmental toxicology assessment. *Ecotoxicology and Environmental Safety*, 130, 234–239.

Wen, X., Zeng, Z., Du, C., Huang, D., Zeng, G., Xiao, R., Lai, C., Xu, P., Zhang, C., Wan, J., Hu, L., Yin, L., Zhou, C., & Deng, R. (2019). Immobilized laccase on bentonite-derived mesoporous materials for removal of tetracycline. *Chemosphere*, 222, 865–871.

Xu, R., Si, Y., Li, F., & Zhang, B. (2015). Enzymatic removal of paracetamol from aqueous phase: Horseradish peroxidase immobilized on nanofibrous membranes. *Environmental Science and Pollution Research*, 22(5), 3838–3846.

Yusuf, Y. (2020). The utilization of laccase-functionalized graphene oxide as an effective biodegradation of pharmaceutical industry waste: Diclofenac and ibuprofen. *Systematic Review Pharmacy*, 11(1), 536–544.

Zhang, D.-H., Yuwen, L.-X., & Peng, L.-J. (2013). Parameters affecting the performance of immobilized enzyme. *Journal of Chemistry*.

Zhang, X., You, S., Ma, L., Chen, C., & Li, C. (2015, 28-29 December). The application of immobilized microorganism technology in wastewater treatment. In 2015 *2nd International Conference on Machinery, Materials Engineering, Chemical Engineering and Biotechnology* Chongqing, China, (pp. 103–106). Atlantis Press.

Zdarta, J., Jankowska, K., Bachosz, K., Degórska, O., Kaźmierczak, K., Nguyen, L. N., Nghiem, L. D., & Jesionowski, T. (2021). Enhanced wastewater treatment by immobilized enzymes. *Current Pollution Reports*, 7(2), 167–179. https://doi.org/10.1007/s40726-021-00183-7.

3 Value-Added Products from Microalgae

A. Ayush Kumar, Vinodini Elango, Aayush Kumar Choudhary, Ojshwi Prakash, M. Premalatha, V. Mariappan, Godwin Glivin, and N. Kalaiselvan
National Institute of Technology

Joseph Sekhar Santhappan
University of Technology and Applied Sciences

CONTENTS

3.1 INTRODUCTION

Microalgae are unicellular photosynthetic microorganisms that convert sunlight, water, and carbon dioxide into algal biomass in saline or freshwater environments. They are a source of biofuels, bioactive pharmaceutical compounds, and food ingredients that are renewable, sustainable, and cost-effective. A number of species of microalgae have an excellent diverse pharmacological quality. Biofuels are a substitute for liquid fossil fuels in terms of price, renewability, and pollution. Microalgae have a high capacity for converting CO_2 from the atmosphere into beneficial products

DOI: 10.1201/9781003188292-3

including carbohydrates, lipids, and other bioactive compounds (Khan et al., 2018). Despite the fact that microalgae are feasible producers of biofuels and biopharmaceuticals in particular, there are substantial constraints and obstacles to address before the technology can go from the pilot to the industrial stage (Stengel and Connan, 2015). Microalgae represent a large group of diverse microorganisms primarily including the likes of blue-green algae which is a cyanobacterium with no defined nuclei (prokaryotic), and photosynthetic protists which are eukaryotic by cell configuration and component segmentation and utilize light energy for the synthetization of organic molecules (Singh and Saxena, 2015). Microalgae have been pictured as a vital resource in the manufacture of the value-added components focused but not limited to the biochemical, nutraceuticals which represent food sources with added health benefits alongside with the promised nutritional value, and Active Pharmaceutical Ingredients (APIs) in pharmaceutical sector (Ravi et al., 2012). Hence, the cultivation is targeted for the implementation at a large scale in food supplements, feed ingredients, cosmetic, and pharmaceutical applications. Some of the species of algae are invested in the wastewater treatment operations known to have favorable cultivation environments in wastewater (Mohsenpour et al., 2021).

In the present universal challenges of global warming and energy crisis, the paradigm shift in the domain of energy generation has opened new avenues for microalgal involvement catalyzing the exploration for hydrocarbon and oil production (Ahmad et al., 2011), sequestration of carbon dioxide and energy resource (Singh and Ahluwalia, 2013). Microalgae are photosynthetic organisms tipped to have high adaptability to changing environments. The lower land use in the cultivation boosts its stocks as compared to the energy crops alternative (Gerbens-Leenes et al., 2014), exponential growth rate coupled with high lipid production, and high fixation rates of carbon dioxide characterize microalgae. The ability to thrive in poor water quality allows the cultivation and treatment of agricultural, industrial, and municipal wastewater. The microalgae have high recovery potential so they can be utilized for recovering phosphorus and N_2 from wastewater streams, thus improving the wastewater quality (Gardner-Dale et al., 2017). Microalgal biomass allows the production of diverse fuels including biogas, biodiesel, and bioethanol. Algae are also being pushed as effective resources for polyunsaturated fatty acids (PUFA). Humans and animals have been diagnosed as lacking in enzymes that have the ability to synthesize PUFA's with carbon atoms in excess of 18, and must obtain that from food also referred to as essential fatty acids (Glivin and Sekhar, 2020; Glivin et al., 2021a; Khozin-Goldberg et al., 2016). Omega 3, a group of essential fatty acids, is on its upsurge catching the eyeballs of nutritionists, as it holds a carbon double bond in the third position from the methyl end. Fish oils are rich source of UFA's, and fish ultimately obtain this PUFA from algae (Ryckebosch et al., 2012). There are various technologies being developed and in practice which are under implementation for the biofuel production from the microalgae resources. The full-scale cultivation faces challenges regarding the feasibility on technical grounds and economic complexities. The difficulty in controlling the optimum conditions for the algal growth presents major roadblocks in the scale up of the cultivation system. In the existing models, the energy required for the cultivation exceeds the energy generated from the produced algae (Lee et al., 2015).

3.2 ALGAL FEEDSTOCK

Depending on the cellular structure, algal biomass can be broadly classified into microalgae and macroalgae. As evident from the name, macroalgae are multicellular organisms comprising red, green, and brown algae. Macroalgae have a greater potential to detoxify pollutants due to their size, as their bigger surface area may give a wider biosorption area for hazardous chemicals. Furthermore, microalgae are important feedstocks for sustainable energy sources like bioethanol, biodiesel, and biogas. They possess plant-like characteristics comprising a lamina, the stipe, and holdfast. Green, Red, and Brown seaweed types store Starch, Glucan, and Laminarin as primary polysaccharides with minor amounts of Xylan and Mannan for red seaweed and Mannitol for brown algae (Tang et al., 2015). There are preliminary stage analyses to evaluate the microalgal strains of *Dunaliella, Haematococcus,* and *Botryococcus* for the production of value addition products, lipids, and hydrocarbons. Figure 3.1 shows the different energy-related applications of algae.

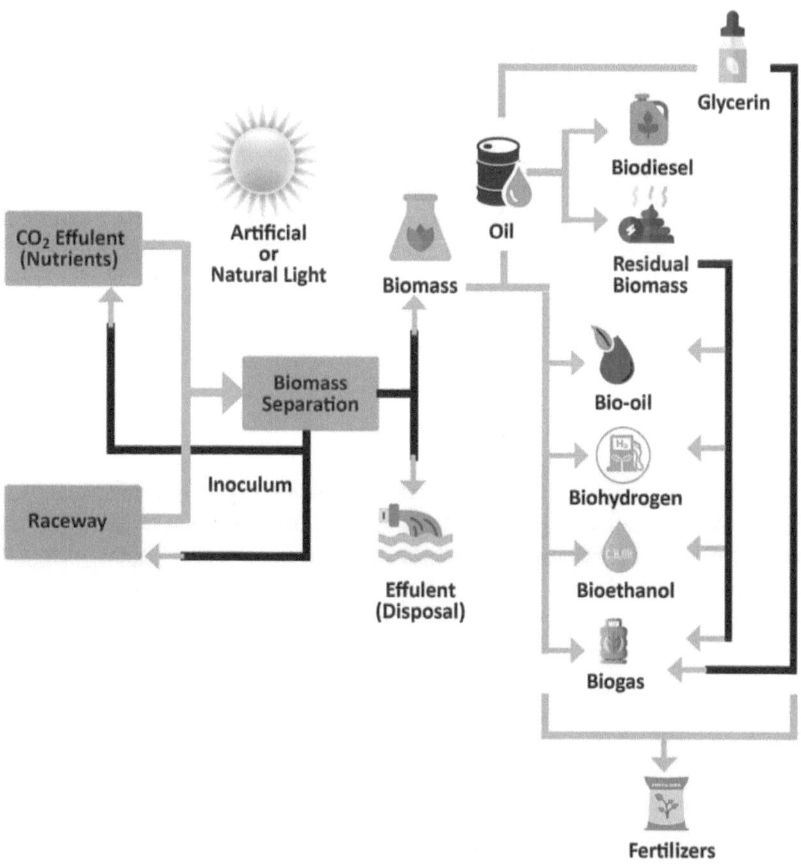

FIGURE 3.1 Algae – bioenergy applications.

It has the ability to develop quickly and produce oil throughout the year. Microalgae biomass was first suggested as a feedstock for biofuel production, and it gained early commercial interest. Microalgae are less in number and not much research has been carried out in cultivation of these unicellular forms. For biodiesel production, PUFAs must be cultivated from these microalgae. But they present as a sustainable feedstock and act as base substrates in several utilities like biodiesel and bioalcohol production. They are energy rich but the exact mechanism of growth is not widely researched and achieving a viable production process is still a challenge (Amaro et al., 2017; Kalaiselvan et al., 2022).

3.3 BIODIESEL

Algae contain 20%–80% oil, which can be turned into a variety of fuels including kerosene oil and biodiesel. The generation of diesel from algae is both cost-effective and simple (Ianda et al., 2022). Several species, including tribonema, ulothrix, and euglena, have high biodiesel potential. Biofuels are liquid fuels made from biomass from various agricultural and forest products, as well as a biodegradable component of industrial waste. Algae are increasingly being studied with a potential of becoming the world's primary source of biofuel generation. They are thought to be the safest, non-competitive, and fastest growing organisms among those that could be utilized to make biodiesel. They have the ability to develop without much care for waste nutrients, and are regarded as the superior source of biodiesel production because other sources can cause food issues because they mostly include plants that are utilized for food (Ferreira Mota et al., 2022). Moreover, biodiesel contents of crops are less sustainable and less in quantity as compared with algae. Algae can efficiently remove hazardous components from water, making it useful in the treatment of wastewater. Their ability to cleanse wastewater and provide abundant biodiesel makes them suited for large-scale production.

3.4 BIO-OIL

Bio-oil has been proposed as a potential alternative energy source for use in fuel applications (Lim and Yusup, 2022). Pyrolysis and hydrothermal liquefaction are the two main techniques for producing bio-oil from biomass at the moment. Bio-oil has unfavorable qualities such as high oxygen concentration and acidity, necessitating its upgrading for use as a fuel. All bio macromolecules (carbohydrate, protein, and lipid) are broken down into an organic liquid phase called bio-oil during bio-oil manufacturing. Bio-oil is a possible substitute for crude oil in the production of transportation fuels and the extraction of important compounds. As plant biomass contains tiny levels of sulfur, bio-oils are CO_2/GHG neutral with little or zero SOx emissions. As a result, bio-oils are less polluting and cleaner than fossil fuels. Bio-oil, on the other hand, has a number of undesirable qualities (such as high viscosity, corrosiveness, and poor heating value) that limit its use as a liquid fuel. As a result, upgrading bio-oil is required before it can be utilized as a liquid fuel or a chemical feedstock for biorefineries to extract valuable chemicals.

3.5 BIOGAS

Biogas production from algae by anaerobic digestion has aroused interest due to the case of excessive polysaccharides (agar, alginate, carrageenan, laminaran, and mannitol) with zero lignin and low cellulose content. Generally, seaweeds are thought to be a suitable fuel for biogas production. Several researchers have proved the fermentation of various algae species for biogas production, including *Scenedesmus*, *Spirulina*, *Euglena*, and Ulva (Behera et al., 2015). The ability to adapt to varying bicarbonate concentrations in the growth media, salinity conditions, and varying nitrogen sources of organic and inorganic nature are the key factors for the evaluation of the aforementioned strains (Glivin et al., 2021b; Ravi et al., 2012). Microalgae are one of the most efficient ways to generate renewable energy.

3.6 PRETREATMENTS

Some green algae species, such as *Spirogyra* and *Chlorococcum*, have a lot of polysaccharides in their cell walls. Microalgae like *C. vulgaris* contain about 37% starch by dry weight, making it the ideal resource of bioethanol with a conversion efficiency of 65%. Polysaccharide-based biomass requires extra processing before fermentation, such as pretreatment and saccharification. Algal biomass pretreatment involves degrading or disrupting the biomass in order to change, accumulate, and process the carbohydrates and lipids it contains. Biomass pretreatment is a bottleneck and possibly costly step in the manufacture of biofuels on a big scale. Although various methods for pretreatment of algal biomass have been documented, there is currently no ideal, highly productive method (Martin Juárez et al. 2021). Researchers must devise practical and cost-effective biomass pretreatment technologies for bioethanol production that are optimized for various feedstocks. Saccharification and fermentation can be done simultaneously using an amylase enzyme-producing strain to produce ethanol in a single process. The technology can produce bioethanol from microalgae and is comparable to first-generation technologies that use corn-based feedstocks. Pretreatment is an important step that makes biomass more available to monosaccharide-releasing enzymes. To convert polymers contained in cell walls to simpler ones, acid pretreatment is widely utilized. The pretreatment requires very little energy and is also a very efficient process. Algal biomass can be converted into a viable energy source via several processes (Fu et al. 2021). Chemical pretreatment processes include the treatment with acids, alkalis, and reactions like hydrolysis, etc. Milling, ultrasonication, and other mechanical operations can also be used for treating biomass. Lately, biological methods like enzymes and biodegradation are also being used along with several hybrid approaches combining different permutations of the aforementioned processes. Process parameters like temperature, pressure, catalyst concentration, and mechanical characteristics deeply impact the efficiency of the process, and these can be altered to yield value-added products. Ultrasonication, microwaves, and beating have all been utilized by certain researchers to break down algal biomass. To minimize chemical waste and optimize the pretreatment process, chemical and mechanical technologies can be combined. They do not pollute the environment; nevertheless, because of energy use, they raise prices (Siddiki et al., 2022).

The genetic modification of the microalgae is regarded as the best way to improve the yield of the products at a reduced cost (Schiano di Visconte et al., 2019). Higher lipid and carbohydrate synthesis, higher H_2 outputs, and the conversion of important metabolic intermediates to fungible biofuels have all been achieved. Photosynthetic microorganisms are gaining a lot of interest in these efforts due to their relatively high photosynthetic conversion efficiencies, varied metabolic capabilities, faster rate of growth, and ability to store or secrete energy-rich hydrocarbons. In contrast to cyanobacteria, eukaryotic microalgae have several metabolic characteristics that are important for biofuel production, such as the accumulation of large amounts of triacylglycerol, storage starch synthesis similar to that found in higher plants (amylopectin and amylose), and the ability to efficiently couple photosynthetic electron transport to H_2 production (Radakovits et al., 2010). Although genetic engineering to improve energy production phenotypes in eukaryotic microalgae is still in its early stages, microalgal model systems have recently made significant progress in the development of genetic manipulation tools, and these organisms are now being used to manipulate central carbon metabolism (Radakovits et al., 2010).

The lack of cell differentiation unwinds the complexity of genetic manipulation as compared to that in the higher plants. The growth observes six different phases in any batch culture for microalgae growth. The six phases are as follows: lag phase where the growth is delayed in the presence of the non-viable cells or while adjusting to the new environments, exponential phase where cells have the ability to grow and divide as an exponential function of time. The cell division slows down in the linear phase growth regime, the declining growth phase observes the reduction in the cell division rate, the stationary phase as evident reaches a zero-growth rate, and the death phase observes the rapid decline in the cell concentration (Lee et al., 2015).

3.7 FACTORS AFFECTING THE BIOMASS CONVERSION

There are several factors that affect the conversion of algae into biofuel and value-added products. The most important of these are light energy, nutrient concentration, pH, salinity, temperature, flora and fauna around, etc. These affect the metabolism of algae and hence determine the efficiency of the process involved. If the metabolism process is photoautotrophic, light is the single energy source, and the concentration and growth of algae depend singularly on the intensity of light. High intensity is desired, and for *C. vulgaris*, the minimum light intensity was determined to be 265 $mmol/m^2/s^1$ (Tang et al., 2015).

Algae biofuels have been praised for their fast productivity growth, increased oil content, and low growth density. However, there are a number of obstacles to overcome before algae can mature as a commercially viable platform to offset petroleum and, as a result, limit CO_2 emissions. These concerns range from determining how and where algae can be grown to enhancing oil extraction and fuel processing.

3.8 VALUE-ADDED PRODUCTS

Due to the self-synthesis of pigments, microalgae are capable of producing several compounds like amino acids, enzymes, metabolites, etc. which can be widely used in several

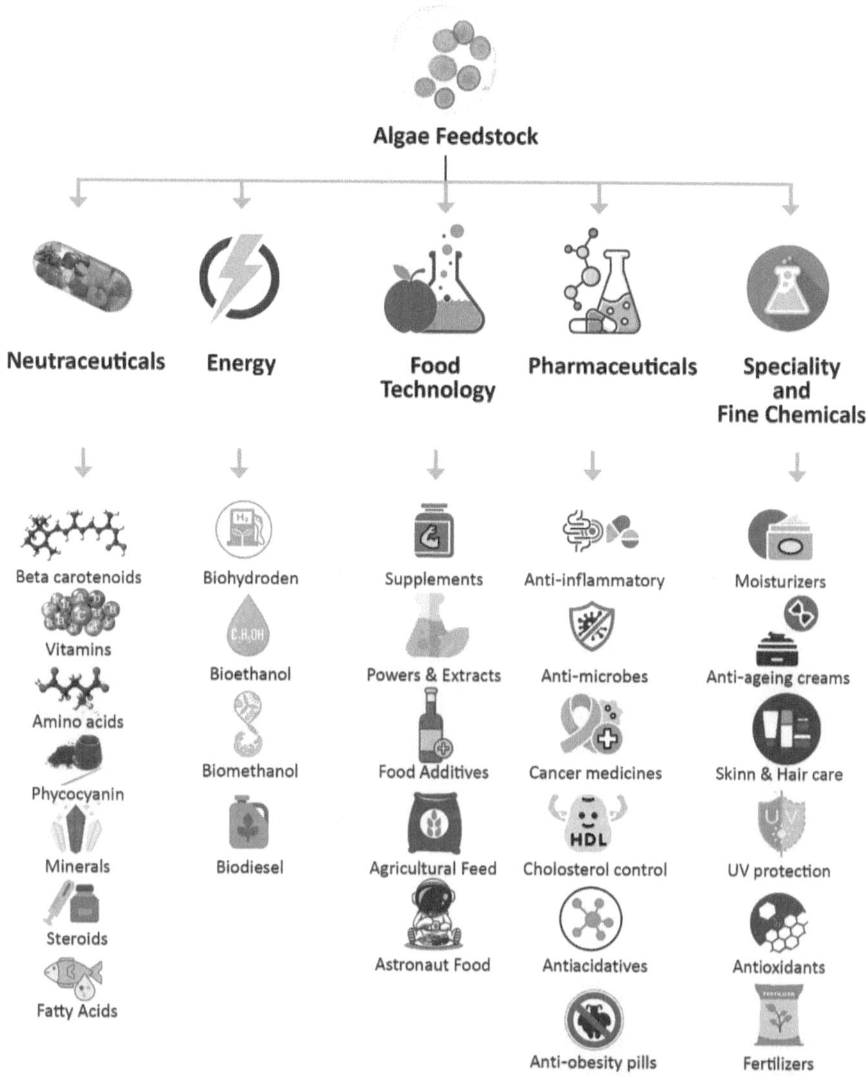

FIGURE 3.2 Value-added products from algae.

industries ranging from cosmetics to pharmaceutical and food industry. They are also economically viable because they do not compete with land and other biological entities for growth and can wholly replace synthetic chemical-based raw materials in product industry. Figure 3.2 shows the different value-added products from Algal feedstock.

Microalgal species have the ability to produce a variety of health-related products, including anti-cancer drugs, cholesterol-lowering agents, skin-health-improving agents, and anti-microbial agents, among others. It's used in cosmetics and other skin care products, and in medical applications, to shield skin from sunburn. Microalgae contain a high amount of physiologically active metabolites, which are used in pharmaceutics and also are nutritionally important. In the cosmetic industry, microalgal biomass such as Arthrospira and Chlorella are commonly employed as thickening agents, water-binding agents, and antioxidants. Microalgal helps in extracting from *Chondrus crispus*, *Mastocarpusstellatus*, *Ascophyllum nodosum*, *Alaria esculenta*, *Spirulina platensis*, *Nannochloropsis oculata*, *Chlorella vulgaris*, and *Dunaliella salina* are frequently used in value-added products including such face and skin care products, anti-aging creams, refreshing care products, emollients, and anti-irritants. Microalgae produce a variety of organic metabolites to defend themselves from UV radiation, including sporopollenin, scytonemin, and mycosporine-like amino acids. Value-added products are used in therapeutics, treatments, human nutrition, functional foods, antibiotics, and green plastics, to name a few. Because microalgae do not compete for land to create diverse value compounds, they are an ideal feedstock. Pigments, antioxidants, and other high-value chemical compounds are used as commodities in a range of commercial industries (Morales-Sánchez et al., 2017). These products are being tested as a potential substitute for chemical-based commercial products that are used as a raw material in a variety of industries (Kothari et al., 2017).

3.8.1 Pharmaceutical

The search for antibiotics and pharmacologically active chemicals in microalgae, particularly cyanobacteria (blue-green algae), has gotten a lot of attention in the previous decade. Several pharmaceutical products can be obtained with microalgae cultivation in the process of producing biomass. Cosmetic products like skin care creams, sunscreen, dermatological treatment products, and emollients can be obtained from *Chlorella* and *Arthrospira*. Several species of microalgae produce organic chemicals which are useful in resistance to UV radiation (Kothari et al., 2017). Algae-derived pharmaceuticals come in a variety of forms. Antimicrobials, antivirals, and antifungals, as well as neuroprotective compounds, therapeutic proteins, and medicines, are just a few examples.

3.8.2 Antimicrobials, Antivirals, and Antifungals

Anti-microbial activity is found in both microalgae and macroalgae, which are used in the pharmaceutical industry. Various strains of cyanobacteria have been found to produce intracellular and extracellular compounds having antibacterial, antifungal, and antiviral properties. The presence of volatile molecules, certain phenols, free fatty acids, and their oxidized derivatives may be responsible for the algae's biological activities. There have been numerous reports of macroalgae-derived chemicals that exhibit antibacterial, antiviral, anti-neoplastic, antifouling, anti-inflammatory, cytotoxic, and antimitotic properties (Ramkumar et al. 2017). Anti-pathogenic properties of red and brown macroalgae extracts show promise for use in fish farming.

3.8.3 Neuroprotective Products

Microalgae and macroalgae are both neuroprotective substances that help nerve cells live longer. *Spirulina platensis* could help researchers discover new treatments for neurological diseases including Alzheimer's and Parkinson's. Several macroalgae have been discovered to have therapeutic potential in the treatment of neurodegenerative illnesses caused by neuroinflammation. Microalgae are known to produce a variety of therapeutically useful bio compounds that can be extracted from the biomass or released into the media extracellularly. Proteins, polysaccharides, lipids, vitamins, enzymes, sterols, and other pharmacological and nutritionally significant chemicals can all be found in these bacteria, and they can all be exploited economically. Anti-microbial, antiviral, anticoagulant, antioxidant, antifungal, anti-inflammatory, and anti-cancer activity have been discovered in bioactive compounds from well-studied algal forms such as *Arthrospira* (Spirulina), *Botryococcus braunii, Chlorella vulgaris, Dunaliella salina, Haematococcus pluvialis*, and Nostoc. Antibacterial, antifungal, antiviral, anti-cancer, antihuman immunodeficiency virus (HIV), anti-inflammatory, antioxidant, antimalarial, herbicidal, and immunosuppressive properties have been reported in prokaryotic blue-green algae (cyanobacteria) (Bhattacharjee, 2016).

3.8.4 Food Technology

Microalgae can be used to produce several products beneficial in food industry like coloring pigments, fats, amino acids, antioxidants, etc. Several chemical dyes can be replaced with pigments like astaxanthin, lutein, phycocyanin, etc. which are produced naturally from algae. Microalgae have a number of advantages over land plants when compared to other feedstocks, including: (1) cost-effective CO_2 conversion through photosynthesis; (2) fast growth rate efficiency in a few days (3–5 days) blended with a very short harvesting cycle (8–10 days); and (3) the ability to develop in non-agricultural land (e.g., seashore lands, desert, or semiarid regions) using salt water (saline). Owing to its excellent, microalgae are good possibilities for commodity supply, including both food and non-food commodities. Microalgae are also great candidates for modern "nutraceutical" or "functional food" due to their ability to synthesize key products such as carotenoids, long-chain fatty acids, sugar, essential and non-essential amino acids, enzymes, vitamins, and minerals. Algae also contain yellow, red, or orange pigment, carotenoids which possess beta carotene which is converted to vitamin A by the human body (Milledge, 2011). Carotenoids are further used as colorants in food and as supplements for animal and human feed. Although the carotenoid percentage is around 0.1%–0.2%, when *Dunaliella* is allowed proper conditions to grow under increased light intensity and high salinity it has the ability to get around 14% of beta carotene. The generation of bioactive chemicals with potential health benefits is one of microalgae's primary properties.

3.8.5 Specialty Chemicals

As a way to advance sustainable manufacturing, algal bioproducts can be used as raw materials for several specialty chemicals. Several valuable products of different families like alcohols, ether, and polymers can be obtained economically from microalgae. By suitable optimization and implementation of feedstock selection, cultivation, harvesting, and liquid extraction, several desirable products can be obtained (Gong and You, 2015). As microalgae are large producers of carotenoids, lipids, and other alcohols, the carbon from these organisms can be used in processes requiring carbon for producing secondary products like fructose, etc. Astaxanthin, another carotenoid derived from algae, finds its application in fish farming, antioxidants, or dietary supplements (Ambati et al., 2014). It intends to transform it into speciality compounds by breaking open—but not digesting—the microalgae using a proprietary blend of enzymes. "The intracellular lipids, proteins, and carbohydrates are released, resulting in a filtrate containing monosaccharides and soluble proteins, as well as a precipitate containing lipids, insoluble proteins, and algal cell walls," says CEO Kelvin T. Okamoto (Sharma and Sharma, 1994).

3.8.6 Biopolymers

Algae can also be used as a precursor for biopolymer production. This is because of the presence of a variety of products like polysaccharides, amino acids, fats, polymers, carbohydrates, etc. Biopolymers have recently been recognized as a viable alternative to fossil-based polymeric materials, which raises a number of environmental issues. Biopolymers can be made from a variety of biological sources, including plants, animals, agricultural waste, and bacteria. Microalgae (and certain cyanobacteria) appear to be two of the most promising sources of polyhydroxyalkanoates (PHAs), cellulose, carbohydrates (especially starch), and proteins for the production of bioplastics, according to studies. They also include a considerable quantity of structural biopolymers, such as proteins and carbohydrates, in addition to these nutritious components. These structural biopolymers could have intriguing technological functions in food items, such as acting as a texturizer, stabilizer, or emulsifier, for example. The lower the number of structural biopolymers, such as proteins and carbohydrates, the higher the lipid content of microalgal biomass (Bernaerts et al., 2019).

The value of a particular feedstock of algae is determined by the composition and the percentage of proteins, lipids, carbohydrates, etc. Out of these, biopolymers can also be extracted from some species of algae and they are desirable because of novel applications in packaging, food technology, medicine, etc. Also finding use in drug delivery and other biomedical applications, biopolymer industry is revolutionizing the usage of algae. Polyhydroxy alkanoates, Polyhydroxy butarate, Polyhydroxy Butyrate -CO- B-Hydroxy Valerate (PHBV) and Polylactic Acid (PLA) are some of the commercially used polymers that can be obtained using algae. The biopolymer is commonly referred to as "bioplastic." Regardless of the fact that bioplastic is biodegradable, this does not indicate that the polymer is made from biological resources. Some petroleum-based polymers, such as polycaprolactone and poly (butylene succinate), are biodegradable. The term "bio-based polymer" refers to materials made from renewable resources. Some bio-based polymers, on the other hand, are not biodegradable. Although this contradiction in terminology, the polymer derived from renewable resources will be the focus. To obtain biopolymers from renewable resources, there are three main methods: (1) polymers derived from biomass (naturally occurring polymers), (2) polymers made by microorganisms, and (3) polymers made from bio-derivative monomers (Özçimen et al., 2017).

3.9 CONCLUSION

The sustainable future of microalgae is reassured by its potential to sequester CO_2. Regardless of the fact that microalgae are essential for bioenergy generation, there are some concerns concerning the environmental implications of large-scale microalgae cultivation. From ammonia to much more sophisticated biologically active molecules like polypeptides and polysaccharides, algae produce a wide range of hazardous substances. Other natural species in the surrounding ecosystem may be harmed by these pollutants. Their impact on other native species can be abrupt or prolonged. Toxin production is highly variable depending on the species and the surrounding environment. As a result, effective algae selection for biomass cultivation is critical in the algal-based industrial sector to avoid algal toxicity. In the following years, the market price and potential are predicted to double, indicating a promising future for economic growth. In the years ahead, a promising ecosystem for algal-based value-added items is projected to explode. To meet its current and long-term food and liquid fuel production demands, microalgal strains can be genetically modified and metabolically transformed. The energy input and production cost present tough challenges for the application in the industrial sector. These issues need resolution to make the products more viable from a commercial viewpoint. The feasibility can be enhanced on the technological and economical fronts under the condition that bioproducts can be prepared from the applied algae. Long-term sustainability and environmental benefits must be kept as an aim for all the phases of exploitation of algae (Siddiki et al., 2022). The future implementation plans should be centered around the application in the developing countries ensuring stability on food and energy foregrounds, in the biofuel industries, and pharma and cosmetic sectors. The appropriate organism needs to be determined for the successful implementation of a biofuel production system. The lipid, protein, and carbohydrate composition analysis form the basis of the selection of the organism for biofuel and value-added products manufacture. The combination of genetic manipulation and strain selection is essential to the development of future technologies considering the cost effectiveness, downstream technologies, biomass productivity among the other key features.

REFERENCES

Ahmad, Abdul Latif, N. H. Mat Yasin, C. J. C. Derek, and J. K. Lim. 2011. "Microalgae as a Sustainable Energy Source for Biodiesel Production: A Review." *Renewable and Sustainable Energy Reviews* 15(1): 584–93.

Amaro, Helena M., I. Sousa-Pinto, Francisco Xavier Malcata, and A. Catarina Guedes. 2017. "Microalgal Fatty Acids—From Harvesting until Extraction." In *Microalgae-Based Biofuels and Bioproducts*, pp. 369–400. Elsevier.

Ambati, Ranga Rao, Phang Siew-Moi, Sarada Ravi, and Ravishankar Gokare Aswathanarayana. 2014. "Astaxanthin: Sources, Extraction, Stability, Biological Activities and Its Commercial Applications—A Review." *Marine Drugs* 12(1): 128–52.

Behera, Shuvashish et al. 2015. "Scope of Algae as Third Generation Biofuels." *Frontiers in Bioengineering and Biotechnology* 2: 90.

Bernaerts, Tom M. M. et al. 2019. "The Potential of Microalgae and Their Biopolymers as Structuring Ingredients in Food: A Review." *Biotechnology Advances* 37(8): 107419.

Bhattacharjee, Meenakshi. 2016. "Pharmaceutically Valuable Bioactive Compounds of Algae." *Asian Journal of Pharmaceutical and Clinical Research* 9: 43–47.

Ferreira Mota, Gabrielly et al. 2022. "Biodiesel Production from Microalgae Using Lipase-Based Catalysts: Current Challenges and Prospects." *Algal Research* 62: 102616.

Fu, Qian et al. 2021. "Kinetics of Hydrolysis of Microalgae Biomass during Hydrothermal Pretreatment." *Biomass and Bioenergy* 149: 106074.

Gardner-Dale, D. A., I. M. Bradley, and J. S. Guest. 2017. "Influence of Solids Residence Time and Carbon Storage on Nitrogen and Phosphorus Recovery by Microalgae across Diel Cycles." *Water Research* 121: 231–39.

Gerbens-Leenes, P. W., L. Xu, G. J. De Vries, and Arjen Ysbert Hoekstra. 2014. "The Blue Water Footprint and Land Use of Biofuels from Algae." *Water Resources Research* 50(11): 8549–63.

Glivin, Godwin et al. 2021a. "Conversion of Biowaste to Biogas: A Review of Current Status on Techno-Economic Challenges, Policies, Technologies and Mitigation to Environmental Impacts." *Fuel* 302: 121153.

Glivin, Godwin et al. 2021b. "Comparative Study of Biogas Production with Cow Dung and Kitchen Waste in Fiber-Reinforced Plastic (FRP) Biodigesters." *Materials Today: Proceedings* 52: 2264–67.

Glivin, Godwin, and S. Joseph Sekhar. 2020. "Waste Potential, Barriers and Economic Benefits of Implementing Different Models of Biogas Plants in a Few Indian Educational Institutions." *BioEnergy Research* 13(2): 668–82.

Gong, Jian, and Fengqi You. 2015. "Value-Added Chemicals from Microalgae: Greener, More Economical, or Both?" *ACS Sustainable Chemistry & Engineering* 3(1): 82–96.

Ianda, Tito Francisco et al. 2022. "Techno-Economic Modeling to Produce Biodiesel from Marine Microalgae in Sub-Saharan Countries: An Exploratory Study in Guinea-Bissau." *Biomass and Bioenergy* 158: 106369.

Kalaiselvan, N et al. 2022. "A Waste to Energy Technology for Enrichment of Biomethane Generation: A Review on Operating Parameters, Types of Biodigesters, Solar Assisted Heating Systems, Socio Economic Benefits and Challenges." *Chemosphere* 293: 133486.

Khan, Muhammad Imran, Jin Hyuk Shin, and Jong Deog Kim. 2018. "The Promising Future of Microalgae: Current Status, Challenges, and Optimization of a Sustainable and Renewable Industry for Biofuels, Feed, and Other Products." *Microbial Cell Factories* 17(1): 1–21.

Khozin-Goldberg, Inna, Stefan Leu, and Sammy Boussiba. 2016. "Microalgae as a Source for VLC-PUFA Production." In *Lipids in Plant and Algae Development*, pp. 471–510. Springer.

Kothari, Richa et al. 2017. "Microalgal Cultivation for Value-Added Products: A Critical Enviro-Economical Assessment." *3 Biotech* 7(4): 1–15.

Lee, Eunyoung, Mehregan Jalalizadeh, and Qiong Zhang. 2015. "Growth Kinetic Models for Microalgae Cultivation: A Review." *Algal Research* 12: 497–512.

Lim, Huei Yeong, and Suzana Yusup. 2022. "Technology to Convert Biomass to Biooil: Challenges and Opportunity." In *Biofuels and Bioenergy*, pp. 25–40.

Martin Juárez, Judit et al. 2021. "Evaluation of Pretreatments for Solubilisation of Components and Recovery of Fermentable Monosaccharides from Microalgae Biomass Grown in Piggery Wastewater." *Chemosphere* 268: 129330.

Milledge, John J. 2011. "Commercial Application of Microalgae Other than as Biofuels: A Brief Review." *Reviews in Environmental Science and Bio/Technology* 10(1): 31–41.

Mohsenpour, Seyedeh Fatemeh et al. 2021. "Integrating Micro-Algae into Wastewater Treatment: A Review." *Science of the Total Environment* 752: 142168.

Morales-Sánchez, Daniela, Oscar A. Martinez-Rodriguez, and Alfredo Martinez. 2017. "Heterotrophic Cultivation of Microalgae: Production of Metabolites of Commercial Interest." *Journal of Chemical Technology & Biotechnology* 92(5): 925–36.

Özçimen, Didem, Benanİnan, OgünMorkoç, and Aybüke Efe. 2017. "A Review on Algal Biopolymers." *Journal of Chemical Engineering Research Updates* 4: 7–14.

Radakovits, Randor, Robert E. Jinkerson, Al Darzins, and Matthew C. Posewitz. 2010. "Genetic Engineering of Algae for Enhanced Biofuel Production." *Eukaryotic Cell* 9(4): 486–501.

Ravi, Sarada et al. 2012. "Influence of Different Culture Conditions on Yield of Biomass and Value Added Products in Microalgae." In *Dynamic Biochemistry and Process Biotechnology and Molecular Biology*, pp. 77–85.

Ryckebosch, Eline, Charlotte Bruneel, Koenraad Muylaert, and Imogen Foubert. 2012. "Microalgae as an Alternative Source of Omega-3 Long Chain Polyunsaturated Fatty Acids." *Lipid Technology* 24(6): 128–30.

Schiano di Visconte, Gino, Andrew Spicer, Christopher J. Chuck, and Michael J. Allen. 2019. "The Microalgae Biorefinery: A Perspective on the Current Status and Future Opportunities Using Genetic Modification." *Applied Sciences* 9(22): 4793.

Sharma, Ashish, and Dipak Sharma. 1994. "Souvenir." In *National Symposium on Mushroom, NCMR & T. Solan*, pp. 40–41.

Siddiki, Sk Yasir Arafat et al. 2022. "Microalgae Biomass as a Sustainable Source for Biofuel, Biochemical and Biobased Value-Added Products: An Integrated Biorefinery Concept." *Fuel* 307: 121782.

Singh, Jasvinder, and Rakesh Chandra Saxena. 2015. "An Introduction to Microalgae: Diversity and Significance." In *Handbook of Marine Microalgae*, pp. 11–24., Elsevier.

Singh, Uday Bhan, and A. S. Ahluwalia. 2013. "Microalgae: A Promising Tool for Carbon Sequestration." *Mitigation and Adaptation Strategies for Global Change* 18(1): 73–95.

Stengel, Dagmar B., and Solène Connan. 2015. "Marine Algae: A Source of Biomass for Biotechnological Applications." In *Natural Products from Marine Algae*, pp. 1–37, Springer.

Tang, Yuting et al. 2015. "Microalgae as a Feedstock for Biofuel Precursors and Value-Added Products: Green Fuels and Golden Opportunities." *BioResources* 11(1).

[illegible]

4 Cleanup of Marine Oil Spills through Bioremediation Method

Farah Shahirah Mohd Fairuz, Nur Fatien Muhamad Salleh, and Nurasmat Mohd Shukri
Universiti Sains Malaysia

Muhammad Hilman Abdul Mustapa, and Wan Nur Aini Wan Mokhtar
Universiti Kebangsaan Malaysia

Nur Afiqah Badli
Universiti Teknologi Malaysia

CONTENTS

4.1 INTRODUCTION

Control of oil spills is an important part of the contingency plan for oil spills (Jha et al., 2008). The potential of pollution is undoubtedly growing due to the rapid improvement of the oil industry. The occurrence of marine oil spills can be explained as the discharge of liquid petroleum hydrocarbons into the ocean or coastal areas caused by human activities (Li et al., 2016). The contamination of marine due to oil spills occurred from broken pipes, leaking underground storage tanks, ship collisions

DOI: 10.1201/9781003188292-4

or floods, overfilling of gas tanks, oil-contaminated road run-off, parking lots during rainstorms, and the spills of heavier fuels, refined petroleum products, and any oily white refuse or waste oil as well (Lee et al., 2015).

The organism in water, including plants and animals, will be affected by the oil spills since oil and water do not mix. When the oil spills into the sea or marine, it then forms a thin layer on top of the water, acting as a lid containing an emulsion of oil in water or a floating film, and prevents plants and animals living in water from breathing. In addition, oil spills can harm the quality of the air. For instance, crude oil entering waterways from spills or runoff contains polycyclic aromatic hydrocarbons (PAHs), the most toxic components of oil (Lim and Huang, 2007).

However, the effects of hydrocarbon released at sea are influenced by the location of the occurrence and its subsequent proximity to environmentally sensitive areas and organisms (Lee et al., 2015). Besides that, marine oil spills can cause environmental, economic, and socioeconomic impacts including mortality and degradation of marine organisms, interruption of commercial, recreational fisheries, coastal tourism, and total amount of liability and compensational funds.

In Malaysia, oil spill cases happened when water was discharged from the vessels at 43.14% and followed by from the unknown sources at 39.22% The famous oil spill incidents that happened in the world have entirely been considered to be a consequence of both direct and indirect human factor weaknesses (Fingas, 2011).

According to the Department of Environment (DOE) and the Marine Department, oil spill incidents accounted for 43.13%, or 22 out of 51, of all oil spill incidents in Malaysia between 2014 and 2016. Over 1 billion gallons of oil have been leaked globally in the previous decade, with 6 million tons entering the oceans each year. Oil spills are widespread, and many little accidents go unreported, especially in places where environmental regulations or standards are unenforceable, minimal, or non-existent (Zhang et al., 2019).

Cleaning and recovery from oil spills is challenging and depends on several aspects such as the temperature of the water affecting biodegradation and evaporation, type of oil, and shorelines as well as beaches involved. Oil spill remediation, as well as its effects on marine environments, is largely dependent on a thorough understanding of the oil weathering reactions that control spilled oil's behavior and fate, as well as the chemical composition and bulk properties of the spilled oil (Lee et al., 2015). A multitude of physical and chemical reactions may occur when oil travels through the maritime environment including oil dissolution, evaporation, photo-oxidation, biodegradation, and emulsification/dispersion. In this short review, we will discuss on the sources of oil spills in Malaysia and study the previous bioremediation method to curb of marine oil spills.

4.2 SOURCES OF OIL SPILLS OCCUR IN MALAYSIA

This chapter reviews literature based on the aspects of oil spill incidents and how they affected the human, wildlife, and environment. Besides, it also discusses the conventional method used to clean up the oil spill.

An oil spill is a phenomenon that happens from time to time. It is challenging to exclude petroleum activities because of petroleum exploitation, exploration, movement of crude oil from place to place, and oil installation failure. Its consequences on the environment are detrimental because of the environmental degradation it causes and its effect on things of value in the environment. An oil spill happened when a ship released petroleum liquids into the water, either deliberately or accidentally, causing damage to the earth's environment. The release of toxic substances such as oil into the sea can cause severe damage to crops, fisheries, and other seafood sources such as fish, crabs, and others (Abayomi et al., 2017).

4.2.1 Oil Spills in Malaysia and Global

The increase in automotive industry in Malaysia caused the oil spill incident that happened in the country. The oil spill that occurred in the nation has numerous consequences for human life, the environment, and the country itself, because it is a serious situation to which we must pay attention. One study in Peninsular Malaysia shows that the oil spill incident cases happened from 2014 until 2016. Tables 4.1–4.3 list the incident of oil spills that happened in Malaysia water which comprised of incident date, location, source, level of incident, time, and related agencies involved during cleanup activities in Peninsular Malaysia (Ishak et al., 2019).

Oil spill incidents impacted both marine habitats and fresh water. It impacts a diverse range of subsurface organisms and surface resources, all of which are linked to a complicated food chain that includes human food resources. Oil spills may pollute the environment in a variety of ways, including physical damage to animals and their habitats (such as covering mammals or birds in an oil layer) and the toxicity of the oil itself, which can kill exposed creatures. Several factors influence the

TABLE 4.1
The Oil Spill Incident from 2014

Month	Locations	Sources	Agencies Involvement
January	Fishing jetty, Tanjung Belungor, Kota Tinggi, Johor	Crude oil discharged from MTO from an unknown source	DOE, Fishermen
February	Teluk Cempedak Beach, Pahang	Tarball spill at Teluk Cempedak coastal beach	DOE
May	Teluk Batik, Perak	Spill oil at Teluk Batik beach from an unknown source	DOE
June	Sepanggar, Kota Kinabalu, Sabah	Spill oil at Perairan Sepangar, Kota Kinabalu from unknown source	DOE
September	Kampung Tanjung Buai, Kota Tinggi, Johor	Oil sheen at fish nets from unknown source	DOE
October	Sg. Buntu Pengerang	Tar Ball at Sg. Buntu, Pengerang, Johor from unknown source	DOE
November	Pengerang, Kota Tinggi, Johor	Oil spill at Pengerang Jetty from unknown source	DOE

MMEA, Malaysian Marine Enforcement Agency.

TABLE 4.2
Oil Spill Incident from 2015

Date	Locations	Sources	Agencies Involvement
March	Teluk Cempedak Beach and Tembeling Resort, Pahang	Discharge oil at the beach from an unknown source	DOE
	Kemasik Beach, Kemaman, Terengganu	Discharge oil at the beach from an unknown source	DOE
	Sepat Beach, Kuantan, Pahang	Discharge oil at the beach from an unknown source	DOE
	Tenggol Island, Dungun, Terengganu	Discharge oil at the beach from an unknown source	DOE
April	Lang Tengah Island, Setiu, Terengganu	Discharge oil at the beach from an unknown source	DOE
	Tenggol Island, Dungun, Terengganu	Discharge oil at the beach from an unknown source	DOE
July	Pengerang Terminal, Pengerang, Kota Tinggi, Johor	Discharge oil at the beach from an unknown source	DOE
August	Tanjug Piai, Pontian, Johor	Discharge oil at the beach from an unknown source	DOE
	Teluk Brunei, Sabah	Discharge oil at the beach from an unknown source	DOE
November	Asian Supply Base Jetty, Labuan	Discharge oil at the beach from an unknown source	DOE
December	Cendera Mata Village, Jalan Batu Api, Sandakan, Sabah	Fire vessel from engine problem	DOE

MMEA, Malaysian Marine Enforcement Agency.

severity of an oil spill's impact, including the oil's physical properties, whether it is petroleum-based or not, and the spilled oil's eventual fate (EPA, 2016).

Several types of freshwater and marine habitats seen in nature have variable sensitivity to the detrimental effects of oil pollution, as well as varying recovery capacities. Although certain species may be severely injured or killed as a result of coming into contact with oil in a spill, other effects are generally more subtle and last longer. Freshwater species, for example, are at risk of being suffocated by the oil carried by the current or of being progressively poisoned by long-term exposure to oil trapped in shallow water or stream beds. Furthermore, the oil spill has the potential to be disastrous for birds and mammals (EPA, 2016).

Table 4.1 showed that in 2014, most of the oil spill incidents in Peninsular Malaysia occurred due to fuel discharged from the ship, unknown sources, crude oil discharged, tarball spills, ship collisions, and oil spills from sinking vessels (Ishak et al., 2019).

Table 4.2 shows that in 2015 the oil spill incident occurred due to ship collision, fuel oil discharge from the ship, discharge oil at beach from unknown sources, fire vessel engine problem, and pipe leakage (Ishak et al., 2019).

TABLE 4.3
The Oil Spill Incident from 2016

Date	Locations	Sources	Agencies Involvement
January	Tg Leman Beach Resort, Mersing, Johor	Tarball from an unknown source	DOE
March	Desaru Beach, Kota Tinggi, Johor	Spill oil patch at the coastal area from an unknown source	DOE
April	Lang Tengah Island, Terengganu	Tarball from an unknown source	DOE
	Beserah Beach, Kuantan, Pahang	Spill oil patch at the coastal from an unknown source	DOE
July	Tioman Island, Pahang	Oil spill from an unknown source	DOE
	Tanjung Pelepas Port, Johor	Oil spill from an unknown source	DOE
August	Tanjung Batu, Coastal, Tawau, Sabah	Oil spill from an unknown source	DOE
	ATB Terminal, Sg Pulai, Johor	Oil spill from an unknown source	DOE
	Morib Beach, Selangor	Oil spill from an unknown source	DOE
September	Pangkor Jetty, Perak	Oil spill from an unknown source	DOE
November	Gaya Island, Sabah	Tarball discharge from unknown source	DOE

MMEA, Malaysian Marine Enforcement Agency.

However, Table 4.3 shows that in 2016, the oil spill incidents happened due to oil discharged from vessels, ship collisions, pipeline leakage, overboard discharged leakage, tarball discharge, and unknown source (Ishak et al, 2019).

Based on the source of oil spill incidents from the Malaysian Marine Enforcement Agency, there are still the same sources that polluted the water, which happened from 2014 to 2016. These incidents showed that an oil spill is a serious case that needs to be given full attention to eliminate oil spill incident cases.

There is also a global trend in oil spills from tankers. Then, the other analysis is looking at historical and current data to see if there are any trends or patterns in the frequency of oil spills. It is based on spills higher and lower than 700 tons because sufficient data is available for these spill volume categories. Around 80% of spills documented since 1970 have been minor (700 tons), which has dropped substantially during the previous 51 years. In the decade 2010–2019, the yearly average was 1.8 spills, which is less than a tenth of the average in the decade 1970–1979. The forecast for the next 10 years is unknown, but the fact that no major leaks occurred in the first year of the new decade is promising. According to reports, the 1970s accounted for 52% of all big spills in the previous five decades, whereas the current decade accounted for only 4%. It's important to note, although, that when data is analyzed per decade rather than yearly, the gradual decline in the number of big spills is considerable (International Tanker Owners Pollution Federation, 2021).

Sorbents must have two important characteristics: oil-attractive (oleophilic) and water repellent (hydrophobic) for use in the fight against oil spills (Natasha, 2006). Even though the sorbents may be used as a single cleaning method for small spills, they are the most used to remove final traces of oil or in areas where skimmers cannot be reached (Xiang, 2011). Sorbent materials that are being used for oil removal must be disposed of in compliance with authorized local, state, and federal regulations. Any oil that has been removed from sorbent materials must also be disposed of or recycled properly to prevent further contamination. Nowadays, there is growing interest in finding cheap, abundant, and efficient natural organic sorbent materials mainly from agriculture or biomass for oil spill removal in water. A wide variety of cellulose materials such as kapok have shown good results, making them potential candidates for oil spill treatment. As a result, biomass-based oil spill cleanup is one of the most widely utilized methods, in which synthetic sorbent materials such as polypropylene are employed to capture oil from seawater. This study was done using the same approach to identify a natural and biodegradable sorbent to replace the present one.

4.2.2 Remediation Method to Curb Oil Spills

Marine oil spills clean-up is the most critical issue, and a variety of oil clean-up techniques have been utilized to prevent oil spills in marine waters. The four basic categories of methods currently available are physical, chemical, thermal, and biological clean-up.

4.2.2.1 Physical Remediation Method

Physical techniques are typically applied to remove oil spills in aquatic ecosystem. The majority of these techniques are used as a barrier to prevent oil spills from spreading by modifying their physical or chemical properties. Oil spills are controlled using various barriers, including booms, skimmers, and adsorbent materials (Dhaka and Chattopadhyay, 2021).

Booms are an oil spill response tool that acts as a barrier to oil movement, preventing the spill from spreading. Fence booms, curtain booms, and fire-resistant booms are the three types of booms (Dave and Ghaly, 2011). Fence booms are structures constructed of stiff or semi-rigid materials that are lightweight, require minimal storage, are user-friendly, and can be used with any oil. However, they have drawbacks, including poor stability in heavy winds, limited towing flexibility, and poor performance in rough seas (Hoang et al., 2018). Meanwhile, curtain booms are impermeable, and non-absorbent with floating structures. It is reliable in clam water and has high towing flexibility but is hard to wash and store. Fire-resistant booms are made of fire-resistant metal that can focus an adequate volume of oil to burn efficiently at temperatures as high as 1,093°C. It is frequently used in combination with thermal methods (Ventikos et al., 2004). Although it has the potential to shield the beach from an oil fire, it is heavy and bulky, making it even harder to move (Dave and Ghaly, 2011).

In combination with booms, skimmers can be used to curb oil spills on the surface of the water without affecting the oil's characteristics, allowing it to be recycled (Kumari et al., 2019). Weir, oleophilic, and suction skimmers are the three types of skimmers (Nomack and Cleveland, 2010). Skimming performance is dependent on the kind of oil spill, thickness, water particles, geography, and climate. It works best in a quiet environment. Floating debris can block the pipes in the water. Weir skimmers work like a dam, collecting oil from the water's surface. They operate best with less viscous oil, have a lower density, and non-emulsion oil. However, on the other hand, they function inefficiently with oil emulsion and are frequently clogged and jammed by floating debris (Jensen et al., 1995). The example of oleophilic skimmers are ropes, drums, discs, belt skimmers, and brushes. Prior to getting collected in a tank, the oil that adheres to the material's surface can be wiped off. Because of their oleophilic nature, they can absorb 90% of the oil in water. Despite this, they are unable to curb oil that has been mixed with dispersants, and trash separation needs to be done manually. Suction skimmers operate similarly to a vacuum pump equipped with an air vent system, sucking up oil via broad floating heads and transferring it to tanks. Highly effective at managing a wide variety of oil viscosity. They are most used to recover oil from beaches, restricted locations, or remove oil from land surfaces. However, it is prone to becoming clogged with debris and requiring competent operators, and it is not recommended for use with combustible oil products, which might lead to an explosion (OSS, 2010).

The hydrophobic adsorbent is very useful in controlling oil spills because it cleans up the remaining oil after skimming. It promotes complete oil removal by converting oil from liquid to semi-solid. Natural organics, synthetics, and inorganics are all effective adsorbent materials for oil spill clean-up. Peat moss and vegetable fibers are natural adsorbents with a 3–15 times adsorption capability from its weight (Banerjee et al., 2006). Natural organic adsorbents are labor demanding, absorb water and oil, sink, and are difficult to retrieve after being placed over oil spill water and must be removed (Nomack and Cleveland, 2010). Water may absorb 4–20 times an inorganic adsorbent's weight (Alther, 2002). Some natural inorganic adsorbents, such as clay and vermiculite, are loose materials that are difficult to apply under windy conditions, and some are connected with possible health hazards if inhaled. Because they are primarily used as commercial sorbents, synthetic adsorbents have both hydrophobic and oleophilic characteristics. Besides, it has 70–100 times adsorption capacity per weight. The main disadvantages of absorbents are storage and their nonbiodegradability (Dave and Ghaly, 2011).

4.2.2.2 Chemical Remediation Method

Solidifiers and dispersants are two chemical techniques for cleaning up an oil spill. Surfactants are used in dispersants, which can break down oil spills into tiny droplets and transfer them into the water column, where they are swiftly diluted and destroyed. Dispersants are frequently employed by spraying the chemical into the water and mixing it thoroughly with the wind or the propeller of a boat (Lessard and Demarco, 2000). Dispersants such as Corexit 9500 remove up to 90% of spilled oil and are affordable than physical methods (Holakoo, 2001). It also improves natural biodegradation by increasing surface area, prevents the formation of oil-water emulsions, reduces the likelihood of oil adhering to surfaces, and speeds up treatment. The kind of oil and atmospheric and oceanic conditions influence the efficiency of dispersants (Nomack and Cleveland, 2010). The flammability of most dispersants, on the other hand, poses a risk to human health during application and may harm marine life.

Meanwhile, solidifiers are hydrophobic polymers that react with the oil to transform it from a liquid to a solid rubber-like condition easily removed through physical methods. Solidifiers include dry granular and semi-solid materials. Due to the mixing energy generated by solidifiers, they can be employed only in moderately waved oceans (Nomack and Cleveland, 2010). A solidifier's efficiency is dependent on the type and composition of oil. Solidifiers have not been widely employed in the past due to the challenge of recovery and are less efficient than dispersants (Fingas et al., 1995).

4.2.2.3 Thermal Remediation Method

Thermal remediation techniques used to recover spilled oil since the late 1960s are a quick and straightforward method requiring minimal specialist equipment and greater oil removal efficiency. In calm wind circumstances, this technique of oil spill reaction works well, and it immediately burns the spills of light refined products or fresh oils without causing negative effects to the marine organism. The residue produced from this technique would sink, then cover the bottom of the sea. The thickness of the oil and the availability of sufficient oxygen are critical factors in the effective operation of the burning process (Buist et al., 1999).

Different types of agents can be used to provide enough oxygen to the fire: combustion agents and keep the oil burning, which include light crude oils and gasoline, and wicking agents such as glass beads, wood, and straw (Fingas et al., 1990). Burning agents are used to keep the oil burning to ensure that the fire receives sufficient oxygen. Thermal remediation is an effective technique for oil spills. However, there are significant obstacles to its widespread use, including the fear of causing secondary fires, long-term alteration of aquatic life and animals near the burning site, as well as negative effects to human health and the environment from the by-products of burning, which are carbon monoxide, carbon dioxide, volatile organic compounds, polynuclear aromatic hydrocarbon, and nitrogen oxide (Buist et al., 1999).

4.2.2.4 Biological Remediation Method

Microorganisms digest and metabolize chemical compounds as part of the bioremediation process, which restores the environmental ecosystem. The purpose of this method is to speed up the natural degradation process, in which microbes convert organic compounds to cell biomass and release by-products like water, carbon dioxide, and heat (Atlas and Cerniglia, 1995). Microorganisms that can degrade hydrocarbons have naturally existed at the marine oil spill sites. In the marine ecosystem, bacteria are the most common hydrocarbon degraders. At various stages of bioremediation, different microorganisms prevail, and then when hydrocarbons are decomposed, the microbial species convert from alkanes to aromatic hydrocarbons (Sugai et al., 1997).

Oil content, the amount of prior degradation, duration, and nutrient accessibility all influence oil spill biodegradation in the marine environment (Zahed et al., 2010). Nitrogen and phosphorus, which are required to grow bacteria, are always in low concentrations in aquatic environments. Therefore, the natural degradation of oil spills does not proceed at a feasible rate due to nutrient limitation (Atlas, 1995). The biodegradation process will be hindered as the initial concentration of spilled oil is higher, resulting in a prolonged reaction time of up to 4 weeks (Zahed et al., 2010). Temperature and oxygen are important environmental factors because temperature affects crude oil content and dissolved oxygen affects microorganism activity (Yang et al., 2009). To make bioremediation effective, polluted seawater must be separated from hydrocarbon-degrading microorganisms, and fertilizers, dispersants, or both must be added to speed up the natural degradation process. According to Bragg et al. (1994) and Atlas, fertilizer usage did not result in algal blooms and had no acute toxicity on sensitive species examined. Moreover, non-biodegradable complex components of crude oil are transformed into asphaltic wastes, which enclose and destroy marine life in a specific region. Bioremediation also eliminates the toxicity of petroleum hydrocarbons in the environment's biota.

Durval et al. (2020) reported that the biosurfactant is compatible and has the potential for the bioremediation of damaged maritime environments caused by oil spills. A novel biosurfactant from *Bacillus cereus* was developed to establish its application as a marine bioremediation agent. In the form of microbial tensioactive molecules known as biosurfactants, biotechnology can play a critical role in the treatment process. These characteristics make it possible to use it in environmental applications, including oil spill treatment. The use of biosurfactants has been shown to have a lower environmental impact than conventional surfactants, be biodegradable, and are less toxic. A variety of bacteria and yeasts produce biosurfactants. Bioremediation offers significant advantages in the clean-up of marine oil spills due to its green technology and cost-effective qualities. Bioremediation is significantly less expensive than other clean-up approaches.

4.2.3 Analytical Bioremediation Method to Oil Spill

Several researchers have investigated to address the best method for bioremediation on contaminated marine sediments. Generally, there are two biological processes known as biostimulation and bioaugmentation that have been used to remediate the oil spills. This method is useful for removing two major components in oils: polar hydrocarbon and PAH. The aliphatic hydrocarbons can be easily degraded by microorganisms, whereas the long-chain, branched, or cyclic chain hydrocarbons are more resistant to bioremediation (Maletic et al., 2011). Biostimulation is one of the remediation methods by adding nutrients such as nitrogen and phosphorus to adjust environmental conditions and promote the growth of microorganisms for biodegrading oil. This nutrient can become a control agent for the growth of native microorganisms. The high nutrient content can accelerate the growth of microorganisms; thus the rate of biodegradation also increased.

Bioventing is the process of in-situ biodegradation for biostimulation, in which microorganisms (fungus, bacteria, and yeast) take in oxygen via the soil. Herbicides, pesticides, and non-halogenated volatile organic chemicals are removed from the soil via bioventing (Seyyed et al., 2020). The addition of hydrogen peroxide and pure oxygen to the soil has overcome the contaminants' inefficient air permeability, providing enough oxygen for aerobic biodegradation and the growth of indigenous microorganisms, as well as enhancing the contaminants' catabolic activity (Ossai et al., 2014). Mancera-López et al. (2008) identified and used fungi such as *Penicillium*,

Fusarium, and *Rhizopus* species in the bioremediation of petroleum hydrocarbon polluted soil and sediments. According to Agarry and Latinwo (2015), bioventing on contaminated soil for 28 days with brewery effluents as organic agents can produce a clearance efficacy of up to 91.5%. Another research revealed that for diesel-contaminated soil restoration, the removal efficiency of up to 85% may be achieved in 60 days without the use of soil amendments (Thomé et al., 2015).

The autochthonous microorganism achieved 55% total petroleum hydrocarbon (TPH) removal of bitumen biodegradation with inorganic fertilizer and hydrogen peroxide used in the soil (Agarry et al., 2014). However, the reduction of TPH content will not influence the residual toxicity in the soil. The effect of temperature in the biostimulation method is crucial for mesophilic microorganisms. Other commercial fertilizers' efficacy, as well as other common techniques like bioventing, is yet unknown and undocumented (Díaz Sanz et al., 2015). Surfactant and dispersant biological and chemical properties can promote the development of hydrocarbon degraders by enhancing the bioavailability of hydrocarbon compounds. The dioctyl, glycols, light petroleum distillates, and sulfosuccinate in the dispersants can function as a microbial growth substrate. The dispersant was employed to encourage the enrichment genera for Dilbit degradation (Schreiber et al., 2019). To improve aromatic component degradation, biosurfactant must provide a favorable environment for microorganisms to grow on heteroatomic polyaromatic compounds. Deziel et al. (1996) described the synthesis of surface-active substances by a soil *Pseudomonas* strain that required a high -C/-N ratio and a low iron content.

In contrast, bioaugmentation is the addition of microorganisms capable of directly biodegrade the oil, including the microorganism that already exists at contaminated sites or new species. The bioaugmentation technique requires a longer acclimatization period (cold climates), a small number of particular petroleum hydrocarbon degraders, and the presence of recalcitrant compounds (Seyyed et al., 2020). The inclusion of a resistant degrader strain, emulsifier for generating strains, genetically modified microorganism, and a variety of consortia and microorganisms is the most common way employed in bioaugmentation. All of the methods described are relying on microbial populations' capacity to survive, environmental stability, and enzyme activity (Hosokawa et al., 2009). However, through bioremediation, the microorganism can degrade the contaminated oil, and there is still no single species of microorganism to degrade all the carbon components in oil completely. Each species of microorganism has its own roles and ability, either good in degrading alkane or toward aromatics. The fungal community that has been reported has the ability to transform PAH (six or more aromatic rings) and the asphaltene (Hernández-López et al., 2016). The biodegradation of asphaltenes and resin can be done by using bacterial strains such as *Bacillus* sp., *Corynebacterium* sp., *Revibacillus* sp., and *Staphylococcus* sp. (Seyyed et al., 2020). However, biodegradation kinetics and removal percent of asphaltene were lower than the other crude oil components. Therefore, much research has been reported toward the clean-up of oil spills using bioremediation.

The biostimulation and bioaugmentation also have their limitation to perform well in the biodegradation of hydrocarbons. One of the factors is abiotic which includes nutrients, oxygen, salinity, pH, and temperature. The biodegradation process can be decreased when the factors do not achieve the optimal conditions for microbial growth to utilize carbon as their source of energy. The low levels of phosphates and nitrogen are the most rate-limiting factors effecting in microbial degradation of hydrocarbons (Santos et al., 2011). The degradation of hydrocarbon can occur over a wide temperature range. An increase in temperature could increase the rate of oil degradation in soil, and the faster degradation rates occur at a temperature between 30°C and 40°C. Furthermore, the properties of oils, such as viscosity and volatility, change with varying temperature (Tyagi et al., 2010). The solubility of oil components is different and the short-chain alkanes are more soluble at a lower temperature while low molecular-weight aromatics are favorable at high temperature. The microorganism was unable to change the temperature the same way as the indigenous population of microorganism is mainly caused by changing temperature. Moreover, the extreme temperature can impact the rate of degradation of oil, which become slower or inhibit the degradation due to high toxicity of certain hydrocarbon at high temperature (Mohan et al., 2006).

Besides the temperature factors on bioremediation, the sufficient oxygen content in the soil is crucial for most microorganisms in actively degrading the oil pollutant (Santos et al., 2011). The degradation of saturated hydrocarbon and aromatic compounds by the microorganism requires sufficient oxygen. The high-energy area such as the area with tidal flow and wave action usually has sufficient oxygen. In contrast, the low-energy area (salt marshes, intertidal, mudflats, etc.) face limiting oxygen. The limiting of oxygen will cause insignificant microbial degradation when limiting nutrients or amount of microorganisms (Prince, 2010). Additional high nutrients over the acceptable content cause the creation of alga blooms. The formation of alga booms will consume the oxygen within the environment and create an anaerobic environment. Thus, the activity of microbial degradation toward oil will decrease. The salinity and pH influenced the biodegradation of oils by microorganisms. The microbial population change with the change in salinity; thus, diversity will be decreased. The degradation rates of hydrocarbon decrease when the salinity was higher due to inhibition of degradation of PAHs (Lu et al., 2011). The pH in the environment is variable depending on the location, in which pH in wetlands is lower but in mineral soils slightly higher pH. The solubility of nutrients such as ammonia in the environment causes changes in pH levels (Radwan, 2008). The microorganism degradation is more favorable in slightly alkaline conditions, thus showing the unsuccessful degradation in lower pH at salt marshes, wetlands, and mangroves (Mercer and Trevors, 2011).

The microorganism that has been introduced must be capable of surviving and proliferating in the environment. The ability to compete with the indigenous microorganism is important in order to avoid predation and requires acclimating the contamination, including temperature, pH, and water content (Hosokawa et al., 2009). The new microorganism needs to be the same species as the species found in the contaminated soil. Furthermore, utilizing indigenous microorganisms could enhance the ability to survive and degrade the oil efficiently, especially in the later degradation process when the oil concentration becomes toxic to the indigenous microbial community. The efficiency of samples and techniques that have been developed via bioremediation can be determined through the rate of biodegradation, toxicity, and specific compound classes. The most physicochemical factors in the activity of microbial groups are metal, nutrition, and temperature (Seyyed et al., 2020). The aboriginal bacterial consortium used in the Penglai 19-3 oil spill accident shows that the relative degradation values of TPH are 51.29% (Chuanyuan et al., 2018). In terms of biodegradation rate, this bacterium prefers to saturate hydrocarbon (alkanes) about 67.85%–77.29% compared to aromatic about 47.13%–57.21% only. Others, such resins and asphaltenes, show no significant difference. The saturated hydrocarbon fractions show the fastest and favorable degradation compared to others.

Besides that, biosurfactants' use to degrade the crude oil spill also gets more attention due to their efficient removal of contaminants. Biosurfactants have several good properties such as foam formation, emulsifications, phase separation, humectation, crude oil viscosity reduction, and surface activity. These properties enhance the microbial cells to grow on the hydrocarbon substrates, increasing their bioavailability and ability to utilize the hydrocarbons (Bao et al., 2012). Generally, biosurfactant consists of two parts which are hydrophilic and hydrophobic part (known as amphipathic). The hydrophobic part comprises fatty acids with carbon chain from C8 to C18. In contrast, the hydrophilic part comprises esters such as hydroxyl, phosphate, carboxylic, and other complex moieties such as sugar proteins (Singh et al., 2019). Sakthipriya et al. (2015) reported the production microorganism of "*Bacillus subtilis*" by biosurfactant from the polymer dumpsite. "*Bacillus subtilis*" show great potential for oil spill treatment with good properties of high microbial adherence, emulsification activity, surface tension reduction, stability toward extreme environment conditions, production of a higher amount of biosurfactant, high rate of degradation, and viscosity reduction. Through the process of biodegradation, the important thing and the main requirement needed is the growth of bacteria. The analysis shows the growth of bacteria can be increased up to 12 days, and the CFU maintains the maximum value of 20×10^6/mL of the bacteria culture. The degradation rate of crude oil by "*Bacillus subtilis*" was rapid from first day until ten, which it could achieve the maximum of 28×10^6 CFU/mL and 80% of total degradation of crude oil. This shows the biosurfactant has the ability to degrade a wide range of hydrocarbon present in crude oil. Instead of degradation rate, the efficiency of bioremediation can be determined by Gas Chromatography–Mass Spectrometry (GCMS) on changing the chemical composition of oil spills before and after the growth of bacteria.

A study conducted by Italo et al. (2020) developed *Bacillus cereus* UCP 1615 as a biosurfactant for marine oil spill bioremediation. In bioassays conducted in seawater, this biosurfactant can encourage the development of autochthonous microorganisms without the need for motor oil. It also improved oil solubilization and dispersion, which aided cell development. *Bacillus cereus* UCP 1615 toxicity resulted in greater than 90% and 55% survival of the fish *Poecilia vivipara* and the bivalve *Anomalocardia*, respectively. As a result, these biosurfactants are good in degrading oil pollution in the sea (Italo et al., 2020). Rhamnolipids, a kind of biosurfactant utilized in bioremediation, have been identified to improve petroleum hydrocarbon biodegradation. In general, this biosurfactant can increase the bioavailability of crude oil, diesel, and PAHs in a variety of environments, including wastewater, polluted seawater, and contaminated soil (Whang et al., 2009). In 2013, Chen et al. used a bacterial consortium that had been treated with rhamnolipids. With various alkanes, PAHs, and biomarkers biodegradation, combining rhamnolipids enhances overall oil biodegradation efficiency by about 5.63%. This research shows rhamnolipids played a negative role in the hydrocarbon degradation with relatively volatile properties such as n-alkanes and PAH but a positive role shows toward normal long-chain alkanes and PAHs for the biodegradation (Chen et al., 2013).

On the other hand, bacteria need some support to run efficiently, especially in harsh conditions such as intertidal zones. The failure of bioremediation in intertidal zones may be due to microbes having difficulty adapting to harsh environments with biological and abiotic restrictions and in indigenous microbial competition (Mercer and Trevors, 2011; Suja et al., 2014). Furthermore, the addition of nutrients or biological stimulants becomes insignificant and the adding agents are easily removed by sea current; thus their inhabitation becomes a failure (Xia et al., 2010; Boufadel et al., 2016). Thus, adding a suitable agent such an enzyme to microbes can overcome the problems since an enzyme did not need nutrients, preventing predators and toxic substances (Sharma et al., 2018; Bautista et al., 2015).

Immobilization of microorganisms can speed up the biodegradation process by enhancing the breakdown of particular pollutants. Bacteria can be immobilized to retain their viability and catalytic capabilities, allowing them to withstand harsh environmental conditions and high pollutant concentrations for a prolonged half-life (Dzionek et al., 2016). It is good for organic molecules with high molecular weights that contain hetero-organometallic compounds. As a result of the decreased solubility and enhanced sorption, pollutant transport and redistribution from oil pollutants are reduced. This method can help lower bioremediation expenses by eliminating cell dispersion and dilution in the environment (Bayat et al., 2015). Chemical immobilization also acts as a reactive barrier, preventing pollutants from seeping out of polluted areas (Basta and McGowen, 2004). Through complexation, precipitation, and sorption, immobilization transforms the original soil metals into a more geochemical phase. Microorganisms, cement, zeolite, organic compost phosphate, and clay are the most often used additions (Finžgar et al., 2006). Enzymes can help bacteria grow and thrive without being hampered by contaminants. Dai et al. (2020) report using enzyme laccase in bacteria consortium with the immobilization system on heavy oil pollutants in the intertidal zones. The high degradation efficiency of the immobilized lactase-bacteria consortium on heavy oil was 66.5% for 100 days of remediation. From GCMS analysis, the degradation efficiency was higher than control, in which the saturated hydrocarbon and aromatic hydrocarbon were 79.2% and 78.7%, respectively. This shows that the degradation of long-chain n-alkanes of C26–C35 and polycyclic aromatic hydrocarbons with more than three rings was significant. The biodiversity of heavy oil-degrading bacteria can be increased, and the degradation of heavy oil can be enhanced by using the immobilized lactase-bacteria consortium (Dai et al., 2020).

Apart from enzymes, zeolite can also help microorganisms such as *Bacillus* sp. to function effectively in oil pollution cleanup. With a medium pH, no secondary pollution, and a large specific surface area, zeolite is widely recognized for helping to reduce pollution (Javed et al., 2016). Guoqiang et al. (2018) used in-situ bioremediation on oil-soaked marine sediments with a combination of oil-degrading bacterium *Bacillus* sp. and chitosan as a wrapping agent and found that over 50% of oil spill pollutants degraded within 70 days. Because the bacteria with zeolite and wrapping agent may spread well on the bottom without being washed away, the percentage oil contribution will degrade. Biofilms, in addition to zeolite, have been shown to be effective in mediated biodegradation. On the basis of polylactic acid and polycaprolactone electrospun membranes, Valentina et al. (2020) reported immobilizing hydrocarbon-degrading gammaproteobacteria and actinobacteria as adsorbing carriers. When compared to embolizing live bacteria, the biodegradable efficiency of this immobilizing bacterium exhibits a 23% improvement in hydrocarbon biodegradation. It could also absorb 100% of spilled oil and biodegrade more than 66% in 10 days without harming the environment.

The bioremediation and bioavailability of oil pollutants can be enhanced with the photocatalytic process mediated by the Reactive Oxygen Species (ROS). The photocatalytic pretreatment of TiO_2 under UV irradiation can increase oil's soluble organic carbon content by 60% and enhance the biodegradation process by 37%. Still, it shows no significance when introduced under sunlight illumination (Jonathon et al., 2013). The photocatalytic pretreatment is capable of stimulating the bioremediation process with the generation of ROS. The generation of ROS such as hydroxyl radicals by TiO_2 under UV-radiation (<400 nm) will hydroxylate hydrophobic oil compounds; thus the solubility and bioavailability are enhanced in the microbial community (Keen et al., 2012; Lee et al., 2011). The hydrophobicity of oil donates to its low bioavailability and causes the time for biodegradation to become slower. Therefore, the solubility of recalcitrant hydrocarbon could be enhanced and the rate of biodegradation with a wide range of pollutant degraded due to the generation of ROS (Jonathon et al., 2013).

The removal of crude oil or oil pollutants can be enhanced by combining the electrokinetic transport and bioremediation process known as electro-bioremediation techniques. The electro-bioremediation technologies could enhance the number of microorganisms to effectively degrade the oil contaminant, including pH, using electrodes as virtually inexhaustible terminal electron acceptors in the metabolism (Wang et al., 2015; Modin and Aulenta, 2017). This system also shows the ability to manipulate the redox potential of a contaminated matrix, therefore creating suitable in-situ conditions conducive to biodegradation (Barba et al., 2018; Yan dan Reible, 2015). Based on the report by Cappello et al. (2019), it has been concluded that electro-bioremediation was shown to be a sustainable technology to eradicate hydrocarbon and PAH from polluted sediments. Besides that, electro-bioremediation technology could increase the Oxygen Reduction Potential (ORP) sediment through oxygen generation in electro-bioremediation. From Next Generation Sequencing (NGS) analysis, the concentration of *Alcanivorax borkumensis* cells, known as an aerobic hydrocarbon clastic bacterium, was increased due to consistency with electrolytic oxygen generation. The combination of electroosmosis and the biodegradation process contributed to the exclusion of contaminants from sediment.

4.3 CONCLUSION

The global increase in oil production and usage as an energy source has increased the likelihood and risk of marine oil spills.The sources and causes of oil spills have been studied to prevent the occurrence of oil spill. Since most of the oil spills are accidental and unpredictable, understanding the causes of oil spills is important. Thus, prevention is regarded as the most important factor in all countries, with significant efforts made to keep the potential of a spill as low as possible. From this study, the causes of oil spills in Malaysia occurred from the discharge of oils from the vessels.

On the other hand, oil spills are raising more concerns across the world as the marine ecosystem and human health will suffer substantial negative and long-term consequences. The most effective method of spill containment is to respond as effectively by applying several bioremediations to clean up the marine oil spills. The key to response with future oil spill incidents in the environment is prevention, understanding the impacts of oil, and the remediation of the oil spill to protect human health and the environment. In the future, bioremediation of oil spillage should be given more attention to lower the resultant disaster occasioned by the oil spill since bioremediation is very beneficial as it proved to be more sustainable and economical.

ACKNOWLEDGMENTS

The authors are grateful to Universiti Sains Malaysia for providing them with both practical assistance and financial support (USM).

REFERENCES

Abayomi, O. A., Range, P., Al-Ghouti, M. A., Obbard, J. P., Almeer, S. H., Ben-Hamadou, R., 2017. Microplastics in coastal environments of the Arabian Gulf. *Mari. Pollut. Bull.*, 124(1), 181–188.

Agarry, S. O. K., 2014. Biodegradation of bitumen in soil and its enhancement by inorganic fertilizer and oxygen release compound: Experimental analysis and kinetic modelling. *J. Microb. Biochem. Technol.*, 4(2), 1–8.

Agarry, S., Latinwo, G.K., 2015. Biodegradation of diesel oil in soil and its enhancement by application of bioventing and amendment with brewery waste effluents as biostimulating-bioaugmentation agents. *J. Ecol. Eng.*, 16 (2), 82–91.

Alther, G.R., 2002. Removing oils from water with organo clays. *J. Am. Water Works Assoc.*, 94, 115–121.

Atlas, R.M., 1995. Petroleum biodegradation and oil spill bioremediation. *Mar. Pollut. Bull.*, 31, 178–182.

Atlas, R.M., Cerniglia, C.E., 1995. Bioremediation of petroleum pollutants. *Bioscience*, 45, 332–338.

Banerjee, S.S., Joshi, M.V., Jayaram, R.V., 2006. Treatment of oil spill by sorption technique using fatty acid grafted sawdust. *Chemosphere*, 64, 1026–1031.

Bao, M.T., Wang, L.N., Sun, P.Y., Cao, L.X., Zhou, J., Li, Y.M., 2012. Biodegradation of crude oil using an effificient microbial consortium in a simulated marine environment. *Mar. Pollut. Bull.*, 64, 1117–1185.

Barba, S., Lopez-Vizcaíno, R., Saez, C., Villasenor, J., Canizares, P., Navarro, V., Rodrigo, M.A., 2018. Electro-bioremediation at the prototype scale: What it should be learned for the scale-up. *Chem. Eng. J.*, 334, 2030–2038.

Basta, N.T., McGowen, S.L., 2004. Evaluation of chemical immobilization treatments for reducing heavy metal transport in a smelter-contaminated soil. *Environ. Pollut.*, 127, 73–82.

Bautista, L.F., Morales, G., Sanz, R., 2015. Biodegradation of polycyclic aromatic hydrocarbons (PAHs) by laccase from Trametes versicolor covalently immobilized on amino-functionalized SBA-15. *Chemosphere*, 136, 273–280.

Bayat, Z., Hassanshahian, M., Cappello, S., 2015. Immobilization of microbes for bioremediation of crude oil polluted environments: A mini review. *Open Microbiol. J.*, 9, 48–54.

Boufadel, M.C., Geng, X.L., Short, J., 2016. Bioremediation of the *Exxon Valdez* oil in Prince William Sound beaches. *Mar. Pollut. Bull.*, 113(1–2), 156–164.

Bragg, J.R., Prince, R.C., Harner, E.J., Atlas. R.M., 1994. Effectiveness of bioremediation for the *Exxon Valdex* oil spill. *Nature*, 368, 413–418.

Buist, I., McCourt, J., Potter, S., Ross, S., Trudel, K., 1999. In situ burning. *Pure Appl. Chem.*, 71, 43–65.

Cappello, S., Cruz Viggi, C., Yakimov, M., Rossetti, S., Matturro, B., Molina, L., Segura, A., Marques, S., Yuste, L., Sevilla, E., 2019. Combining electrokinetic transport and bioremediation for enhanced removal of crude oil from contaminated marine sediments: Results of a long-term, mesocosm-scale experiment. *Water Res.*, 157, 381–395.

Chen, Q., Bao, M., Fan, X., Liang, S., Sun, P., 2013. Rhamnolipids enhance marine oil spill bioremediation in laboratory system. *Mar. Pollut. Bull.*, 71(1–2), 269–275.

Chuanyuan, W., Xing, L., Jie, G., Yingchun, L., Yuanwei, L., 2018. Biodegradation of marine oil spill residues using aboriginal bacterial consortium based on Penglai 19-3 oil spill accident, China. *Ecotoxicol. Environ. Saf.*, 159, 20–27.

Dai, X., Lv, J., Yan, G., Chen, C., Guo, S., Fu, P., 2020. Bioremediation of intertidal zones polluted by heavy oil spilling using immobilized lactase-bacteria consortium. *Bioresour. Technol.*, 309, 123305.

Dave, D., Ghaly, A.E., 2011. Remediation technologies for marine oil spills: A critical review and comparative analysis. *Am. J. Environ. Sci.*, 7, 423–440.

Deziel, E. P. G., Villemur, R., Lepine, F., Bisaillon, J., 1996. Biosurfactant production by a soil Pseudomonas strain growing on polycyclic aromatic hydrocarbons. *Appl. Environ. Microbiol.*, 62 (6), 1908–1912.

Dhaka, A., Chattopadhyay, P., 2021. A review on physical remediation techniques for treatment of marine oil spills. *J. Environ. Manage*, 288, 112428.

Díaz Sanz, J., 2015. Bioremediation of urban soils polluted with nonconventional petroleum in the Canadian context. Ph.D. Thesis, Universidad Politecnica de Madrid, Madrid, Spain.

Durval, I.J.B., Mendonça, A.H.R., Rocha, I.V., Luna J.M., Rufino, R. D., Converti, A., Sarubbo, L.A., 2020. Production, characterization, evaluation, and toxicity assessment of a Bacillus cereus UCP 1615 biosurfactant for marine oil spills bioremediation. *Mar. Pollut. Bull.*, 147, 111357.

Dzionek, A., Wojcieszyńska, D., Guzik, U, 2016. Natural carriers in bioremediation: A review. *Electron J Biotechnol.*, 23, 28–36.

EPA, 2016. Emergency Management: The Fate of Spilled Oil. Retrieved from EPA: https://archive.epa.gov/emergencies/content/learning/web/html/oilfate.html.

Fingas, M., 2011. Oil spill dispersants: A technical summary. In: *Oil Spill Science and Technology*, Gulf Professional Publishing, United States, pp. 435–582.

Fingas, M.F., Kyle, D.A., Larouche, N., Fieldhouse, B., Sergy, G., Stoodley, G., 1995. Effectiveness testing of oil spill-treating agents. *ASTM Spec. Tech. Publ.*, 1252, 286–298.

Fingas, M.F., Stoodley, R., Laroche, N., 1990. Effectiveness testing of spill-treating agents. *Oil Chem. Pollut.*, 7,337–348.

Finžgar, N., Kos, B., Lešta, D., 2006. Bioavailability and mobility of Pb after soil treatment with different remediation methods. *Plant Soil Environ.*, 52, 25–34.

Guoqiang, Z., Yanqing, S., Chuanyuan, W., Jian, Y., Qiaoning, W., Lingxin, C., 2018. In situ microbial remediation of crude oil-soaked marine sediments using zeolite carrier with a polymer coating. *Mar. Pollut. Bull.*, 129, 172–178.

Hernández-López, E.L., Perezgasga, L., Huerta-Saquero, A., Mouriño-Pérez, R., Vazquez-Duhalt, R., 2016. Biotransformation of petroleum´ asphaltenes and high molecular weight polycyclic aromatic hydrocarbons. *Environ. Sci. Pollut.*, 23(11), 10773–10784.

Hoang, A.T., Pham, V., Nguyen, D., 2018. A report of oil spill recovery technologies. *Int. J. Appl. Eng. Res.*, 13, 4915–4928.

Holakoo, L., 2001. On the capability of Rhamnolipids for oil spill control of surface water. Unpublished dissertation in partial fulfillment of the requirements for the degree of Master in applid Science, Concordia University, Montreal, Canada.

Hosokawa, R., Nagai, M., Morikawa, M., Okuyama, H., 2009. Autochthonous bioaugmentation and its possible application to oil spills. *World J. Microb. Biotechnol.*, 25, 1519–1528.

International Tanker Owners Pollution Federation. (2021). Number of Oil Spills. Retrieved 6 August 2021, from https://www.itopf.org/knowledge-resources/data-statistics/statistics/.

Ishak, I.C., Arof, A.M., Zoolfakar, M. Z. (2019). The Review of the Oil Spill Incidents between 2014 to 2016 (Conference, University of Kuala Lumpur). Retrieved 31 October 2020, from https://www.researchgate.net/publication/338036690.

Italo, J.B., Durvala, C., Ana, H.R.M., Igor, V.R, Juliana, M.L., Raquel, D. R., Convertie, A., Sarubbo, L.A., 2020. Production, characterization, evaluation and toxicity assessment of a Bacillus cereus UCP 1615 biosurfactant for marine oil spills bioremediation. *Mar. Pollut. Bull.*, 157, 111–357.

Javed, I., Mateen, F., Rafifique, U., Tabassum, N., Balkhair, K.S., Ashraf, M.A., 2016. Synthesis of zeolite from marble powder waste: A greener approach and its application for the removal of inorganic metals from wastewater. *Desalin. Water Treat.*, 57, 10422–10431.

Jensen, H., McClimans, T.A., Johannessen, B.O., 1995. Evaluation of weir skimmers without testing, Eighteenth AMOP Technical Seminar Proceedings, Edmonton, Alberta, Canada, pp. 689–704.

Jha, M., Levy, N., Gao, J.Y., 2008. Advance in remote sensing for oil spill disaster management: State-of-the- art sensor technology for oil spill surveillance. *Sensors*, 20(8), 236–255.

Jonathon, A.B., Seok, W.H., Jae, S.L., Lee, S.H., Alvarez, P.J., 2013. Photocatalytic pre-treatment with food-grade TiO_2 increases the bioavailability and bioremediation potential of weathered oil from the deep water Horizon oil spill in the Gulf of Mexico. *Chemosphere*, 90, 2315–2319.

Kang, J., Zhang, J., Bai, Y., 2016. Modeling and evaluation of the oil-spill emergency response capability based on linguistic variables. *Mar. Pollut. Bull.*, 113(12), 93–301.

Keen, O.S., Baik, S., Linden, K.G., Aga, D.S., Love, N.G., 2012. Enhanced biodegradation of carbamazepine after UV/H2O2 advanced oxidation. *Environ. Sci. Technol.*, 46, 6222–6227.

Kumari, A., Kaur, R., Kaur, R., 2019. A review on fate and remediation techniques of oil spills. *Int. J. Res. Pharm. Sci.*, 10, 111–116.

Lessard, R.R., Demarco, G., 2000. The significance of oil spill dispersants. *Spill Sci. Technol. Bull.*, 6, 59–68.

Lee. K., Li. Z., Robinson, B., Kepkay, P.E., Blouin, M., Doyon, B., 2011. Field trials of in-situ oil spill countermeasures in ice-infested waters. In: *Proceedings of the 2011 International Oil Spill Conference*, pp. 23–26.

Lee, K., Boufadel, M., Chen, B., Foght, J., Hodson, P., Swanson, S., Venosa, A., 2015. Expert panel report on the behavior and environmental impacts of crude oil released into aqueous environments. *Royal Society of Canada*, Ottawa, pp. 102–126.

Li, P., Cai, Q., Lin, W., Chen, B., Zhang, B., 2016. Offshore oil spill response practices and emerging challenges. *Mar. Pollut. Bull.,* 110 (1), 6–27.

Lim, T.T., Huang, X.F., 2007. Evaluation of kapok (*Ceiba pentandra* (L.) Gaertn.) as a natural hollow hydrophobic– oleophilic fibrous sorbent for oil spill cleanup. *Chemosphere*, 66 (5), 955–963.

Lu, X., Zhang, T., Fang, H.H., 2011. Bacteria-mediated PAH degradation in soil and sediment. *Appl. Microbiol. Biotech.*, 89, 1357–1371.

Maletic, S.P., Dalmacija, B.D., Roncevic, S.D., Agbaba, J.R., Perovic, S.D.U., 2011. Impact of hydrocarbon type, concentration and weathering on its biodegradability in soil. *J. Environ. Sci. Health A*, 46, 1042–1049.

Mancera-López, M.E., Esparza-García, F., Chávez-Gómez, B., Rodríguez-Vázquez, R., Saucedo-Castañeda, G., Barrera-Cortés, J., 2008. Bioremediation of an aged hydrocarbon-contaminated soil by a combined system of biostimulation–bioaugmentation with filamentous fungi. *Int. Biodeterior. Biodegrad.*, 61, 151–160.

Mercer, K., Trevors, J. T., 2011. Remediation of oil spills in temperate and tropical coastal marine environments. *Environmentalist*, 31, 338–347.

Modin, O., Aulenta, F., 2017. Three promising applications of microbial electrochemistry for the water sector. *Environ. Sci. Water Res. Technol.*, 3, 391–402.

Mohan, S.V., Kisa, T., Ohkuma, T., Kanaly, R.A., Shimizu, Y., 2006. Bioremediation technologies for treatment of PAH-contaminated soil and strategies to enhance process effificiency. *Rev. Environ. Sci. Biotechnol.*, 5, 347–374.

Natasha L. (2006). Assessment of Ceiba Pentadra (L.) Gaertn. (Kapok) as Absorbent Material for Oil Spill Control, Final Project Report, Universiti Teknologi Petronas.

Nomack, M., Cleveland, C., 2010. Oil spill control technologies. In: *Encyclopedia of Earth*. http://www.eoearth.org/articles/view/158385/?topic=50366.

OSS, 2010. Oil spill solution. Retrieved on 26th February, 2010 from http://www.oilspillsolutions.org/booms.htm.

Ossai, I.C., Fauziah, S.H., Ghufran, R., 2014. The utilization of water hyacinth (*Eichhornia crassipes*) as an aquatic macrophage treatment system (AMATS) in phytoremediation for palm oil mill effluent (POME). *Int. J. Sci.: Basic Appl. Res.*, 13(2), 31–47.

Prince, R.C., 2010. Bioremediation of marine oil spills. In: Timmins, K.N. (ed) *Handbook of Hydrocarbon and Lipid Microbiology*. Springer, Berlin, Heidelberg.

Radwan, S., 2008. Microbiology of oil-contaminated desert soils and coastal areas in the Arabian Gulf region. *Soil Biol.*, 13(3), 275–298.

Sakthipriya, N., Dobleb, M., Sangwaia, J.S., 2015. Bioremediation of coastal and marine pollution due to crude oil using a microorganism *Bacillus subtilis. Procedia Eng.*, 116, 213–220.

Santos, H.F., Carmo, F.L., Paes, J.E.S., Rosado, A.S., Peixoto, R.S., 2011. Bioremediation of mangroves impacted by petroleum. *Water Air Soil Pollut.*, 216(1–4), 329–350.

Schreiber, L., Fortin, N., Tremblay, J., Elias, M., Mason, J., Sanschagrin, S., Cobanli, S., KingT., Lee, K., Greer, C. W., 2019. Evaluation of the natural attenuation potential of diluted bitumen by microbial communities in the Douglas Channel and Hecate Strait, British Columbia. *Appl. Environ. Microbiol.*, 85(1),1–19.

Seyyed, M. D., Saba, M., Mehrdad, T., Satinder, K.B., Rosa, G., Richard, M., 2020. Bioremediation of unconventional oil contaminated ecosystems under natural and assisted conditions: A review. *Environ. Sci. Technol.*, 54, 2054–2067.

Sharma, B., Dangi, A.K., Shukla, P., 2018. Contemporary enzyme based technologies for bioremediation: A review. *J. Environ. Manage.*, 210, 10–22.

Singh, P., Patil, Y., Rale, V., 2019. Biosurfactant production: Emerging trends and promising strategies. *J. Appl. Microbiol.*, 126, 2–13.

Sugai, S.F., Lindstrom, J.E., Braddock, J.F., 1997. Environmental influences on the microbial degradation of *Exxon Valdez* oil on the shorelines of Prince William Sound, Alaska. *Environ. Sci. Technol.*, 31, 1564–1572.

Suja, F., Rahim, F., Taha, M.R., Hambali, N., Razali, M.R., Khalid, A., Hamzah, A., 2014. Effects of local microbial bioaugmentation and biostimulation on the bioremediation of total petroleum hydrocarbons (TPH) in crude oil contaminated soil based on laboratory and field observations. *Int. Biodeterior. Biodegrad.*, 90, 115–122.

Thomé, A., Reddy, K.K., Reginatto, C., Cecchin, I., 2015. Review of nanotechnology for soil and groundwater remediation: Brazilian perspectives. *Water Air Soil Pollut.*, 226, 1–20.

Tyagi, M., Fonseca, M.M.R., Carcalho, C.C.C.R., 2010. Bioaugmentation and biostimulation strategies to improve the effectiveness of bioremediation processes. *Biodegradation*, 22(2), 231–241.

Valentina, C., Francesco, L., Simone, C., Roberto, S., Paola, Q., 2020. Innovative, ecofriendly biosorbent-biodegrading biofifilms for bioremediation of oil- contaminated water. *New Biotechnol.*, 58, 25–31.

Ventikos, N.P., Vergetis, E., Psaraftis, H.N., Triantafyllou, G., 2004. A high-level synthesis of oil spill response equipment and countermeasures. *J. Haz. Mat.*, 107, 1–58.

Wang, H., Luo, H., Fallgren, P.H., Jin, S., Ren, Z.J., 2015. Bioelectrochemical system platform for sustainable environmental remediation and energy generation. *Biotechnol. Adv.*, 33, 317–334.

Whang, L.M., Liu, P.W., Ma, C.C., Cheng, S.S., 2009. Application of rhamnolipid and surfactant for enhanced diesel biodegradation – effects of pH and ammonium addition. *J. Hazard. Mater.*, 164, 1045–1050.

Xia, Y.Q., Li, H.L., Boufadel, M.C., Sharififi, Y., 2010. Hydrodynamic factors affecting the persistence of the Exxon Valdez oil in a shallow bedrock beach. *Water Resour. Res.*, 46(10), 10–28.

Xiang, J.F.K. (2011). Investigation of Oil Spill Absorbents Using Different Materials (Bachelor of Engineering, Universiti Teknologi Petronas). Retrieved 7 November 2020 from http://utpedia.utp.edu.my/10524/1/2011.

Yan, F., Reible, D., 2015. Electro-bioremediation of contaminated sediment by electrode enhanced capping. *J. Environ. Manag.*, 155, 154–161.

Yang, Y.S., Jin, H.J., Wei, Z., He, R., Ji, Y., Li, X.M., Yu, S.P., 2009. Bioremediation of oil spills in cold environments: A review. *Pedosphere*, 19(3), 371–381.

Zahed, M.A., Aziz, H.A., Isa, M.H., Mohajeri, L., 2010. Effect of initial oil concentration and dispersant on crude oil biodegradation in contaminated seawater. *Bull. Environ. Contam. Toxicol.*, 84, 438–442.

Zhang, B., Matchinski, E.J., Chen, B., Ye, X., Jing, L., Lee, K., 2019. Chapter 21 - Marine oil spills—Oil pollution, sources and effects. World Seas: an Environmental Evaluation (Second Edition). *Academic Press,* pp. 391–406.

5 Bioreactor Scale-Up Strategies

Aayush Kumar Choudhary, A. Ayush Kumar, Ojshwi Prakash, Godwin Glivin, N. Kalaiselvan, H. Hareesh Krishnan, Premalatha M, and V. Mariappan
National Institute of Technology Tiruchirappalli

Joseph Sekhar
University of Technology and Applied Sciences

CONTENTS

5.1 INTRODUCTION

The recent period has been a witness to novel bioreactor design concepts. The high shear sensitivity of the reactors has been an ever-present speed bump in the development of bioreactor models, continuing the trend even with state-of-the-art design concepts (Ji et al., 2020). The stirred tank reactors need to be operated at low aeration rates and restrained impeller speed to counteract the shear sensitivity, leading to low mass transfer coefficients, and this adjustment doesn't fall in line for the optimal delivery of the high-density cells. The economic and regulatory considerations drive

DOI: 10.1201/9781003188292-5

the design and the selection of the cell culture bioreactors, keenly influenced by the varied technical aspects, and specific cell requirements. Key strategies for gentle agitation and aeration need to be analysed alongside other specific requirements such as pH-controlled environments, temperature, dissolved carbon dioxide concentration, and low concentration of toxic metabolites. Keeping scalability as a key determinant, high cell and product concentration with optimized media utilization and adherent cell surface area must be considered as well.

Single-use bioreactors have sprung to the horizon in recent years as one of the highly rated design concepts and a new generation utility idea (Rout et al., 2021). The surge of technology aims to address the process development problems in the initial stages, quality and regulatory issues, economic efficiency, and time to market. Bag technology forms the key basis of this concept where bags of hundreds of litres are placed on a tilting apparatus for passing oxygen and effective agitation. These single-use bioreactors include several potential advantages of reduced procedures for cleaning operations, easier adaptation to dynamic process demands, and lower risks of contamination. The stage of setting up a bioprocess from a low to a larger scale is referred to as the scale-up operation. The optimal conditions obtained in the small bioreactors need to be translated proportionately to the large bioreactors (Junne & Neubauer, 2018).

These scale-up studies are regarded to be essential for the development of the fermentation process in an effort to establish adequate criteria to change the scale without impacting the kinetic behaviour of the microorganisms. The kinetics are influenced by local environmental conditions such as temperature, pH value, dissolved oxygen, and nutrient concentration which affect the performance of the process (He et al., 2019). The small-scale trials tend to over-predict the process performance till the variations and the inconsistencies in the design are not eliminated. The adoption of effective strategies and techniques for a proper scale-up operation thus becomes necessary to implement. The environmental conditions that can influence the process need to be restrained and controlled. Physical, chemical, biological, and various process factors are taken into consideration for the same (Teworte et al., 2022).

5.2 FACTORS AFFECTING BIOREACTOR SCALE-UP

5.2.1 Physical Factors

The heat and mass transfer operating conditions, agitation, aeration, shear rate, pH, temperature, and energy consumption are the key parameters which carry the innate potential to influence the scale-up evaluations (Mahdinia et al., 2019). As discussed by Zhou et al. (2018) the scaling strategies are dependent on the oxygen transfer coefficient per unit volume (k_La), tip speed of the impeller (Vs), energy consumption per unit volume (P/V), and mixing time (t_m). The microbial growth and product formation are impacted heavily by the limited oxygen availability, making volumetric oxygen transfer coefficient a necessary criterion for scaling operations (Potumarthi et al., 2007).

The aerobic processes are largely impacted by the agitation and aeration which significantly curtail the formation of the biopolymers like curdlan, gellan, and xanthan to name a few. Agitation is regarded to be instrumental in interphase mass and oxygen transfer alongside its ability to maintain homogeneity with reference to chemical and physical conditions in the medium. The movement owing to the continuous mixing does create shear forces that impact metabolite formation and morphology and lead to variations in the growth. These derived effects from agitation are detrimental to the cell species. Aeration determines the oxygen supply to the fermentation process also contributing to the mixing of fermentation broth at reduced agitation speeds.

Shear stresses are defined for broth viscosity during fermentation process, expressed as a function of rotational speed and geometry of the impeller.

$$\text{For Newtonian fluids } \pi = \mu \upsilon \tag{5.1}$$

$$\upsilon = K * N \tag{5.2}$$

π, μ, υ represent average shear stress between fermenter inner wall and impeller blades, dynamic viscosity, and average shear rate between impeller blades and fermenter inner wall, respectively. K is a constant depending on the system's geometry and the impeller rotational speed (rps) is denoted by N (Yahia et al., 2016). These equations are utilized to estimate the shear rates in any stirred system where the operating fluids exhibit perfect Newtonian behaviours like water. These conventional equations, namely (5.1) and (5.2), are invalid in case of the highly viscous, non-Newtonian broths. To attain robust agitation is the key target when the feedstock is highly viscous. To attain the required robustness, we can use a larger impeller or a higher number of impellers which is easier but isn't energy efficient to be brought into a regular practice. So the engineers can opt to scale up on the basis of equal mixing or blending time. Mixing time can be expressed as t, a function of volume (V, m^3), impeller rotation speed (N_r, rps), and impeller diameter (D_i, m).

$$t = \frac{V}{N_r * D_i^3} \tag{5.3}$$

Mahdinia et al. (2019) described the impacts of the scale up from a pilot scale fermenter of 80 L to a production fermenter of 10,000 L capacity, on the parameters of energy input, impeller rpm, impeller diameter, Reynold's number, and pump rate of impeller. The impacts are studied in terms of folds of the initial value under distributed conditions (Table 5.1).

TABLE 5.1
Impacts of Scale-Up Operations

Scale-Up Criteria	Designation	Constant p/V	Constant N	Constant Re
Energy input	Po	125	3125	0.2
Impeller rpm	N	0.34	1	0.4
Impeller diameter	Di	5	5	5
Pump rate of impeller	Q	0.34	1	0.04
Reynold's number	$\frac{NDi^2\rho}{\mu}$	8.5	25	1

5.2.2 Chemical Factors

To analyse the chemical activity and their subsequent impacts on the performance of the bioreactor, Arshi et al. (2020) discuss the electrocatalytic activity of oxidoreductase. These are a particular class of enzymes which possess the ability to catalyse the redox reactions, namely oxygenation, dehydrogenation, electron transfer operations, and the bond formation by the oxidative interaction. Oxidoreductases are subjected to the transfer of electrons from electrode's surface by mediated and direct electron transfer mechanism. As the redox active centres are located at a great depth in enzymes, the rate of the electron transfers between the redox centre and the electrode can be restricted and only a limited number of these enzymes can undergo the direct electron transfer. The key factors that regulate the direct electron transfer, proper orientation of the enzyme, location and configuration of the active centres within the enzyme, and the distance between the redox centre and the electrode. If the redox centre is not accessible, mediators can be used for the transfer of electrons between the active site of enzymes and electrode surface.

Control of pH is of crucial importance in bioreactor operation and is typically implemented by a two-sided control loop using CO_2 rinsing and addition of base in a media buffered by bicarbonate. While this is a common approach, the addition of bases could impact the culture performance considering the effects of pH variations and increased osmolality in large bioreactors (Hoshan et al., 2019).

The control of the pH is implemented by a bidirectional control circuit in which the injection of CO_2 or the addition of base can be instrumental to increase or decrease the pH value. If the pH is higher than the set point, the CO_2 purge can be used to modulate the CO_2- bicarbonate balance in media buffered by bicarbonate also lowering the pH. Conversely, if the pH value is less than the set point, a pump is activated to deliver the base sodium carbonate, sodium bicarbonate, sodium hydroxide to increase the pH. In case of insufficient mixing, adding a base to control pH might lead to local pH drifts due to localized non-linearity effects.

5.2.3 Biological Parameters

When increased from lab scale to industry scale, there are several biological parameters which affect the performance of the bioreactors. Considering fermentation as an example, the physiological responses of the microbial cells involved are one of the determining constraints for the process intensification model. During the lab scale, the distribution of the nutrients is homogeneous and hence not applicable to the fluctuating conditions of the pilot plant scale or the industrial scale. To better study the biological parameters, several strategies for scale down of the industrial scale equipment to heterogeneous lab-scale bioreactors have been proposed. This helps in determining the cell response to the fluctuating environment and also provides an economical method of studying the cell responses. The main difference between the chemical and biological entities in the biochemical processes is the living nature of the biochemical microorganisms which make them fairly active when compared to the chemical catalysts and reactants. Hence, if the environment is fluctuating, which is a common occurrence in the industrial scale models, there is a heterogeneity induced in the cell population. This oscillating condition decreases the yield and productivity of the process and makes it uneconomical compared to the small-scale bioreactors used in labs and pilot plants.

One of the main causes of the changes to cell metabolism is the exposure to the concentration gradients produced during the huge mass transfer operations. Hence, to study the effect of the chemical parameters on the cell biology and characteristics, scale down models of stirred tank reactors and plug flow reactors are designed. To study their characteristics, the pulse response is analysed with the change of the substrate. Since these living entities have a varied dynamic response, the robustness of the cells with some selective chemical processes and agents can be mapped and suitable cells can be chosen according to the applications. It is shown that *Corynebacterium glutamicum* (Käß et al., 2013) is robust to oxygen and *Escherichia coli* shows a low death rate in a dynamic environment (Enfors et al., 2001). It was also shown that *Aspergillus niger* shows a fast response to the upper glycolysis and flux which leads to lesser efficiency in the industry scale dynamic environments (Li et al., 2018).

Apart from studying the process conditions, a kinetic model should also be developed to efficiently map the behaviour of the microorganisms in scale-up conditions. One of the widely used tools to predict the parameters of the kinetics of enzymatic reactions is the pulse response experiment. In this, a static chemical system is studied by stimulating parameters externally and sampling and quenching techniques are applied. When applied multiple times, valuable in-vivo data can be obtained which can then be studied to determine the stability of cells (Wu et al., 2006). These in-vivo chemical kinetic parameters can be used to conduct several high-precision experiments with different metabolite concentrations.

These studies show that different microorganisms show different responses at different process conditions. Hence, while designing an efficient process, the nature, and characteristics of both the biological and chemical entities should be considered.

5.2.4 Process Parameters

Apart from the physical, chemical, and biological parameters, there are other factors that influence the scale up of bioreactors. Some of the determining factors are the oxygen transfer rate, mass transfer coefficient, and biological enhancement factor. Most of the biochemical processes are aerobic in nature and hence oxygen is the main component that is transported. This process happens via a gas bubble that rises into a liquid film and then to the site of the reaction into the cell. A number of resistances control the process as there are several steps in the process of the oxygen transport, but the strongest factor of all these is the liquid film resistances. The process takes place through seven steps which involve transfer from the gas interior, movement through the interface followed by diffusion through the liquid film, bulk, and stagnant liquid film across the cells. Finally, the liquid-cell movement occurs from the interface to the inside of the cytoplasm.

All the transport rates are determined by the mass transfer coefficient. This is also detrimental in calculating the overall efficiency of the process and studying the effects of the dissolved oxygen. Several process factors like the aeration system, type and design of the biochemical reactor system, intrinsic characteristics of the fermentation system, and the impact of the microbes taken into consideration should be taken into account for the determination of the mass transfer coefficient. The methods like sodium sulphite oxidation, CO_2 absorption, gas phase analysis, and empirical correlations are used for the determination of k_L depending on the biological system. This also varies according to the reactor chosen. For a stirred tank bioreactor, since mechanical agitation is provided, they greatly influence the mass transfer coefficient with the velocity of agitation and the geometric parameters. Similarly, for the bubble column and airlift reactors, the pneumatic agitation parameters are considered and their characteristics depend on the pressure of the system and the bubble coalescence factors (Garcia-Ochoa & Gomez, 2009).

Since the consumption of oxygen by the microorganism changes at different scales, a biological enhancement factor is defined to determine the extent of the enhancement of mass transfer over physical absorption. This can be determined using several theories including the simple film model of mass transfer. The biological enhancement factor E is defined as the ratio of the absorption flux of the oxygen in presence of the microorganism to the absorption flux without the microorganism in the same process conditions. It should be made sure that the driving force of the mass transfer is maintained to be identical in both the processes. The fluxes J and J_0 are defined in Eq. 5.4 in terms of mass transfer coefficients k_L and K_L

$$E = \frac{J}{J_0} = \frac{K_L a}{k_L a}. \tag{5. 4}$$

It was determined that there are three resistances to the mass transfer of this kind: the surfactant film resistance on the interface, the adsorption resistance of the microbes, and the resistance by the liquid films. There are several correlations for the biological enhancement factor defined in terms of the diffusion coefficient, thickness of the layers, concentration of the oxygen, etc.

5.3 BIOREACTOR SCALE-UP STRATEGIES

5.3.1 Continuously Stirred Tank Bioreactors

The operating stirred bioreactors have been categorized on the basis of these different scales. Small spinner flasks (100 Ml–5 L capacity) are operated with conical pendulum or the magnetic paddle stirrers which can be used in warm rooms with a larger volume or in a humidified CO_2 incubator. The impeller speed is kept low around a 300–100 rpm. The headspace probed through open lids is utilized to feed oxygen, and this can be under application only for low oxygen rates (0.1–4/h). Superspinners equipped with microporous hydrophobic polypropylene membrane tube offers improved oxygen transfer rate (Valverde-Pérez et al., 2020). A number of bioreactors which are equipped with additional control and monitoring units are operated for screening purposes and better process development. Bioreactors on a laboratory scale up to 10 L, pilot scale up to 500 L is equipped with the additional media collection and supply facilities, pH control buffer, gas mixing junctions to supply air, carbon dioxide, oxygen, exhaust gas cooler, and sterile filter in the hose to facilitate ventilation.

When designing stirred tank bioreactors, cells are damaged due to stirring and/or aeration shear stresses must primarily be addressed. Stirred tank reactors are regarded to be suitable for floating cells. The current models are built to a capacity of 20,000L. The basic configuration of a ventilated and agitated bioreactor is expressed as a cylindrical vessel loaded with impellers mounted on a rotating shaft driven by an external motor. There is a sprinkler near the ground to supply gas bubbles. Installation of up to four baffles is considered to improve mixing and restrain turbulence (Figure 5.1).

The validated model introduced by Amer et al. (2019) intended to predict the effects on k_La by varying impeller diameter and using different sized pipe collectors. Simulations test if ring sprinklers lead to higher k_La values as compared to tubular sprinklers, with an optimal sprinkler-to-impeller diameter ratio of 0.8. The k_La value can also be improved by enlarging the size of impeller. A relation of k_La is plotted as a function of reactor geometry (i.e., the relationship between the sparger and impeller diameter and the impeller diameter) and operating conditions like flow rate of gas and Reynold's number of the fluid for instance.

A variety of methods are under scrutiny for the scale-up operations which include the basic methods involving microbalances for heat, moment, and mass transfer. The semi-fundamental methods based on the simplified plug flow models and dispersed flow of piston are also under consideration. The thumb rules, dimensionless analysis based on the dimensionless parameter groups and the principle of similarity or the regime analysis, applied widely might lead to erroneous conclusions. However, the complexity involved in solving the microbalances propagates the application of the thumb rule which can be extrapolated to a larger scale.

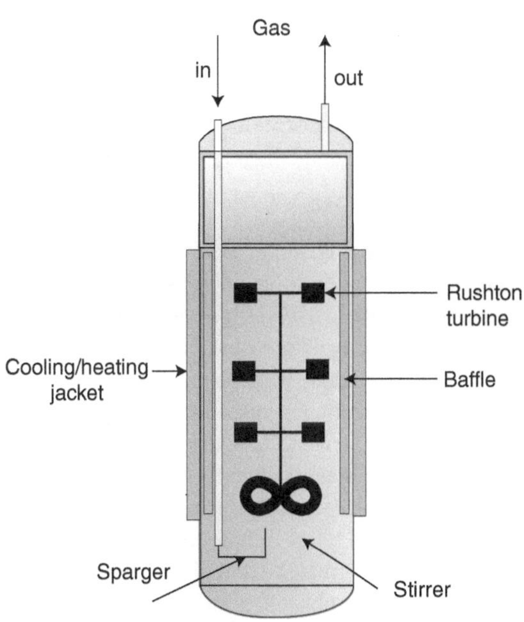

FIGURE 5.1 Schematic representation of continuous stirred tank reactor.

Longer mixing times carry a potential risk of developing carbon dioxide and oxygen concentration gradients, which are detrimental to cell performance. As discussed by Mahdinia et al. (2019) the mean input power by volume (P/V), stirrer diameter *dr* and the container's diameter *Dr* can be utilized to evaluate the mixing time for the radial and the axial flow impellers. Volumetric mean power input can be enhanced given that the mixing time is held constant during the scale-up process. An equation for estimating the mixing time can be stated as given:

$$\theta = 5.9\left(\frac{P}{V}\right)^{-\frac{1}{3}} * \left(\frac{dr}{Dr}\right)^{-\frac{1}{3}} * Dr^{\frac{2}{3}} \tag{5.5}$$

where θ is referred to as the corresponding mixing time (NOW, 1990).

The cell lines are more tolerant to mechanical movements and the shear effects are less pronounced on a larger scale (Bae et al., 2020). The aeration rate must be maintained below 0.1 vvm to avoid cellular damage from the bubbles and the foam generated during the sparging operation. As discussed by Weber et al. (2018) higher aeration rates improve mass transfer through sparging. To tackle the bubbling issue the strategy can be amended by the stirred tank being operated in the flood regime where the gas distribution is poor.

A more recent idea is to equip commercially available bioreactors with internal components comprising a separate chamber with a counter electrode and a membrane window coupled with a working electrode. The stirred tank reactors are primarily used for the setup to gain advantages with regard to aeration and mixing. Unfortunately, these systems restrict the application of the well-known scaling parameters counting the likes of geometric ratio, mixing time, and the specific energy consumption. The variation in the flow regime and the flow rate get altered continuously leading to this inefficiency of the reactor. These variations lead to the unequally distributed electric fields (Enzmann et al., 2019).

5.3.2 Bubble Column Bioreactor

Bubble column bioreactors can be referred to as the multi-phase mass transfer devices that have been designed to rapidly dissolve any gas which has been sparged in the liquid phase. Replenishment of the dissolved gas consumed during the liquid phase reaction is regarded as a top priority. The liquid phase in question can be stationary or flowing, parallel, or counter-current with respect to the injected air. The lack of moving components, ease of maintenance, and low operating costs make them attractive alternatives for fermentation, aerobic industrial operations, and other gas-liquid applications where the equivalent mass transfer is essential (Deshpande et al., 2019).

The mixing of the liquid takes place mainly during the bubbling. The flow is regarded as heterogeneous at higher gas flow rates. Bubbles and liquid have the tendency to rise mainly in the column which in turn creates a downflow of liquid adjacent to the column wall. Apparently, the mixing in the bubble columns is considered inferior to the stirred vessel and the airlift reactors. Biotechnical processes observed in industries include the production of vinegar, yeast, beer, and wastewater treatment (Mahdinia et al., 2019).

Bubble column bioreactors are instrumental to address the impending issues arising from the large-scale usage of the stirred tank reactors. Bubble column reactors can be designed with a working electrode symmetrical in the centre of the setup backed up by the high shear forces which are applicable only for small gas bubbles at high gassing rates (Enzmann et al., 2019). Therefore a bubble column would be preferred for microbial electrosynthesis cells with gaseous substrates or sensitive biofilms (Figure 5.2).

The scale up of the bubble column reactors is characterized by the specification of the vessel primarily referring to batch volume, dimensions, etc., specification of the sparger which may be fine or coarse bubble diffusers, and operating specifications which are the maximum air flow rate, minimum liquid volume; the size and the interaction of the bubbles also affects the optimization and the overall scale up of the reactor (Babanezhad et al., 2020). The scale-up process must be easy to maintain over a large period, must be meaningful on the commercial front, and the process must be reliable.

As explained by (Deshpande et al., 2019) the productivity of a bubble column reactor is dependent on gas-liquid mass transfer coefficient, *kLa*. Bubble column scale up is impacted by the values of *kLa* which can be explained as a function of design and operating conditions. The mass transfer coefficient, *kLa* has been characterized experimentally as a function of superficial gas velocity (*Usg*), using the power law relation:

$$kLa = \alpha * Usg^{\beta} \tag{5.6}$$

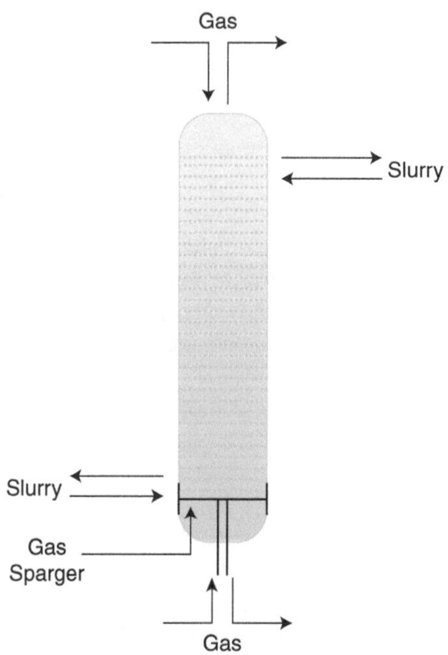

FIGURE 5.2 Schematic representation of the bubble column reactor.

The rate of mass transfer from sparged gas to the target liquid phase is a measure of productivity of the reactor. A mass conservative equation is used to describe the rate of mass transfer:

$$\frac{dVlc}{dT} = kLa * Vl * \left(C - C^*\right) \tag{5.7}$$

C: Dissolved gas concentration; C^*: saturation concentration; Vl: liquid volume; kLa: kinetic parameter representing the gas-liquid mass transfer coefficient.

The scale-up strategy of bioreactors as explained by Wilkinson et al. (1992) and the criteria which can be suitable guides to scale from laboratory to the commercial scale bubble column have been discussed as follows:

1. To prevent the bubble column reactor from operating in the slug regime under all conditions, the bubble column diameter should be $D_c > 0.2\,\text{m}$. This condition is essential to enforce as the industrial scale operations are not performed in the slug regime.
2. The ratio of liquid height (H) to bubble column reactor diameter (D_c), also known as the aspect ratio (AR) must be greater than 5. This condition states that the 'end effects' are not highly prioritized.
3. Orifice diameter of sparger must be greater than 1–2 mm. The coarse spargers under robust operation in the heterogeneous flow regime are characterized by a large distribution of the bubble sizes. The hydrodynamics and mass transfer are regarded to be unimpacted by the varying details of the sparger design.

5.3.3 Airlift Bioreactors

For cost-efficient applications where the microorganisms used are resistant to shear, airlift bioreactors (ALRs) are used. They are pneumatically agitated with a gas stream leading to circulation of broth between the downcomer and riser. Especially known for the efficient mass and heat transfer, they are energy efficient and are easy to scale up. They are generally used for the culturing of plant cells, algae, and mammalian cells. The vertical circulating flow generated provides efficient oxygen transfer and since they have no means of mechanical agitation, they rely on the transfer of air (Bai et al., 2011).

ALRs are briefly divided into three zones: riser, downcomer, and disengagement zone. The design is made to promote the gas-liquid mass transfer with the driving force provided by the sparger at the bottom of the reactor. The operation of ALRs is dependent on the density difference between the riser and the downcomer. Only the riser has the gas sparging and this decreased density due to the gas hold-up causes the liquid to move upwards. The heavier liquid is recirculated using the downcomer as the gaseous bubbles disengage (Doran, 2013; Guieysse et al., 2011). Figure 5.1 shows a split-cylinder ALR (Zhang et al., 2017) (Figure 5.3).

To model ALRs and analyse the scale-up technologies, there are two methods predominantly used. They are the Axial Dispersion Model (ADM) and the Tanks

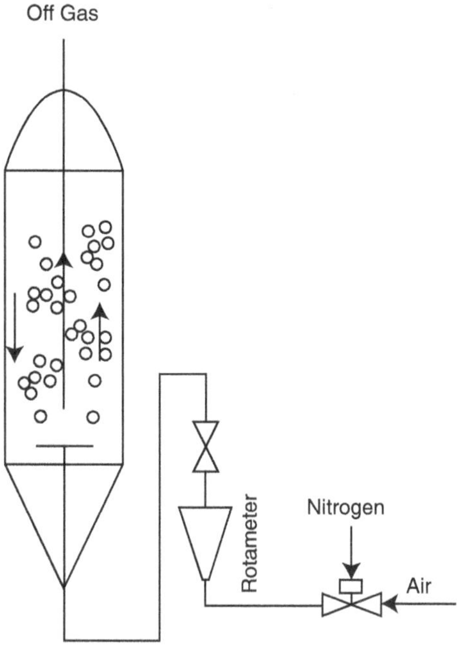

FIGURE 5.3 Schematic representation of airlift bioreactors.

in-Series Model (TSM). ADM describes only the mixing where there are slight deviations from the plug flow mode whereas TSM can be applied to both perfect mixing and plug flow mixing. ADM considers only one parameter, the dispersion coefficient, but TSM considers both the number of tanks and backflow (Znad et al., 2004).

Scaling up of ALRs should consider kinetic parameters which are dependent on the mass transfer coefficient and the resistance offered which is expected to increase with the increasing scale. The factors which should be primarily considered during the scale-up modelling are mixing characteristics, stress and growth kinetics of the microbes, oxygen transfer during the biochemical reaction, etc. The major design parameters of ALRs include the gas hold-up, residence time, and the mass transfer coefficient. Due to the slow energy requirements and exceptionally low shear which is suitable for sensitive microorganisms, ALRs have relatively less construction and operational costs. Instead of a pneumatically agitated design, a mechanically agitated ALR can be used to increase the oxygen transfer.

For a reactor with an inverse fluidized downcomer, the model formula for the liquid circulation velocity is shown in Eq. 8 (Han et al., 2000). To evaluate the performance of the bioreactor, the hydrodynamic and performance characteristics are used. Since there are complex inter-relationships between the process operating parameters, scaling up is not limited just to the geometrical parameters. Instead, the superficial gas velocity, liquid level, and other fluid properties like the gas hold-up, bubble coalescence properties, and gas hold-up are to be considered.

$$v^2 = \frac{2g\left(\varepsilon_g H_r - \left(1 - \frac{\rho_s}{\rho_l}\right)\varepsilon_{s0} H_p\right.}{\frac{K_t}{\left(1-\varepsilon_g\right)^2} + K_b\left(\frac{S_r}{S_d}\right)^2} \tag{5.8}$$

To achieve the high energy efficiency aimed at the ALRs, the energy optimization of the influent material should be carried out. When the gas superficial velocity is increased five times, the mass transfer rate increases by 3.9 times (Guo et al., 1997). Experimental results have also shown that the liquid level influences the gas holdup and gas superficial velocity. There is an inverse relationship between the holdup in the riser and the unaerated liquid level. Also, the circulation and mixing time decrease but with an increased circulation of liquid velocity.

5.3.4 Fluidized Bed Bioreactors

Fluidized Bed Bioreactors (FBBs) have enormous applications in the domain of environmental engineering. They are the prospective alternatives to settling tanks because of their easy integration characteristics, minimal bed clogging, and high surface area for biofilms. Since they are resistant to changes and system failures, these reactors are more suitable for biological applications. They are environmentally sustainable with a smaller reactor footprint and are non-toxic. They can be readily used in place of fixed bed reactors in wastewater treatment (Aslam et al., 2017), pharmaceutical industries (Naghdi et al., 2018), advanced oxidation processes, and chemical recovery in process industries (Özkaya et al., 2019) (Figure 5.4).

Providing one of the best heat and mass transfer characteristics, fluidized beds are used in a variety of chemical process industries. If a proper scaling-up methodology is developed for FBBs, the processes can be made even more efficient and economical. One of the most difficult challenges in scaling up bioreactors is the hydrodynamics of the bed which influences the mass transfer and heat transfer characteristics. Especially the parameters like bubble growth, mixing characteristics, gas compression, and interparticulate forces should be taken care of while designing an effective scale-up strategy.

Scaling up of fluidized reactors requires constant monitoring and optimization of the bed density characteristics, entrainment inside the column, pressure and hydrodynamic profiles, and other intrinsic particle properties. Even micro-level interactions like the van der Waals force or the coulombic forces should be considered for an efficient intensification algorithm. Along the lines of Werther (1992), scaling up deals not only with the drastic changes in the dimensions of the bed but also the design characteristics and physical parameters.

Dimensional analysis is one of the earliest methods ever to be used for developing scaling-up strategies. The dimensionless parameters which are frequently used in fluidized bed modelling are shown in Eq. 5.9 (Maurer et al., 2013)

$$\frac{u\rho_g D}{\eta}, \frac{u^2}{gD}, \frac{\rho_g}{\rho_p}, \frac{D}{H}, \frac{d_p}{D}, \phi, psd \tag{5.9}$$

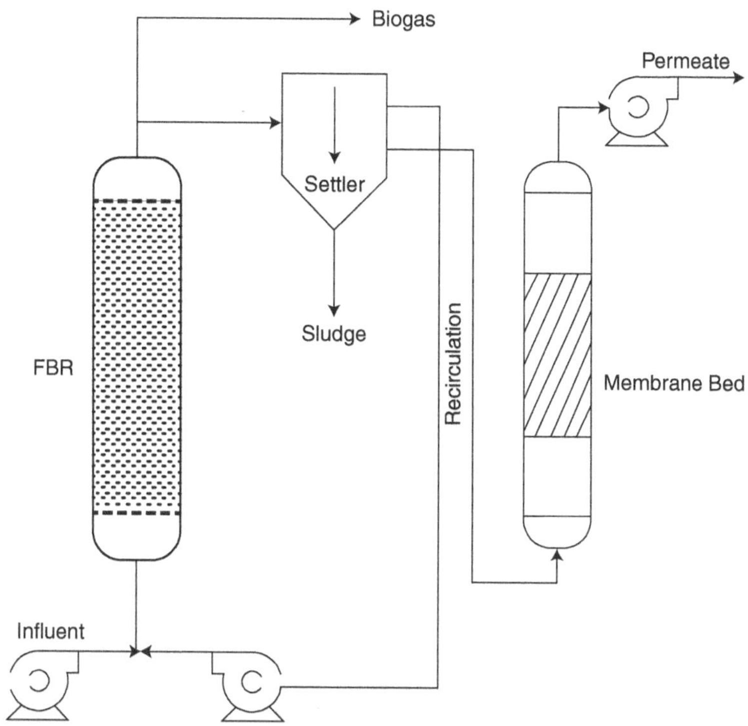

FIGURE 5.4 Schematic representation of fluidized bed reactors.

To scale up a system, data on the physicochemical parameters like Reynold's number, pressure drop, and velocity profile is required. These are then used to determine the number of scale independent factors which remain the same at all scales. From the computational fluid dynamics data, the required parameters are obtained which are then used to scale up through the Buckingham Pi Theorem. A hydrodynamic identicality is aimed for all the independent parameters which infer that the dependent variables should also be identical at all points of the bed. Both the operational and physical parameters are taken into consideration in this type of modelling and then the value of the dimensionless numbers for a reactor ε times the size of the baseline reactor is obtained. The relationship between the gas superficial velocity and the minimum fluidization velocity is shown in Eq. 5.10 (Tisa et al., 2014).

$$\sqrt{m} = \frac{U_{mf}^{l}}{U_{mf}^{s}} = \frac{(U_F - U_{mf})^l}{(U_F - U_{mf})^s} \tag{5.10}$$

These correlations can be safely used to determine the scale-up characteristics of FBBs. But when the bed is catalysed and the impact of the external mass transfer around every particle of the catalyst is observed, Ergun's equation experiences some deviation. Hence, to calculate the mass transfer characteristics of these beds, the particle Reynolds number should be considered with the Schmidt number, void fraction, and the gas superficial velocity. All these might change during the scale-up process as these are strong functions of the particle diameter. Another method to analyse this behaviour is by tracking the selectivity and the activity of the particles. For the beds with vertical internals, a sectoral method is followed which changes the absolute diameter to the hydraulic diameter. When other factors like interchange coefficient, reaction number, and selectivity are considered, a case-specific scale-up methodology can be adopted based on the variation of the dimensionless parameters.

5.3.5 Packed Bed Bioreactor

Packed bed bioreactors have a packed bed supporting the cells and a reservoir for recirculating the oxygen medium. They are a traditional type of bioreactors which use forced aeration. The recirculation medium can be either internal or external. There are two types of PBBs: conventional and Zymotis. The traditional PBBs do not have an internal heat transfer plates for heat removal. The Zymotis type of PBBs has internal plates which use a moist solid medium for controlling the temperature.

The design and development of PBBs start with modelling a lab-scale model to analyse the packing matrix which depends on the nature and use of the reactor. Post selection of the matrix, the geometrical and operational parameters like dimensions, velocity, and perfusion rates are determined. The scale-up experiments should be conducted in different conditions like isothermal and non-isothermal conditions. Also, the reactor can be made jacketed with an aim to study the different thermal characteristics for similar kinetic behaviour.

The main limitation to the scale-up of PBBs is the axial concentration gradients arising during the operation. Also, the geometry of the bed cannot be increased to any scale as a bed diameter of more than 2 m affects the mixing and does not provide uniform distribution of the process nutrient fluid. But, for small-scale applications, PBBs are highly efficient because of their high volumetric productivity. The maximum volume of the PBBs is calculated to be around 0.2–0.9 m^3 due to the aforementioned difficulties (Meuwly et al., 2007).

There are several hydrodynamic and transport characteristics that affect the performance of the PBBs and hinder efficient scale-up. There are primarily two modes of operation: upflow and downflow which show different kinetic and hydrodynamic parameters. The kinetic parameters considered should be suitable enough to agree to experiments in different operating conditions. During the operation of the PBBs in co-current nature, the axial dispersion and external mass transfer characteristics are important and they should be thoroughly studied.

It has been shown that the upflow mode of operation gives a lower outlet conversion because of the fully wetted catalysts. This causes limited mass transport among the phases in the lab-scale model (Somsaluay Suwanprasop et al., 2005). In the strategy shown by Finkler et al. (2021), it is shown that the first step in reactor scaling up should be the characterization of growth in optimal conditions and study of the temporal profile of oxygen uptake. This phase involves the kinetic modelling and analysis of the reaction and process. This should be followed by the scaling up to a pilot plant mimicking the industry scale reactors. The dimensions and heat transfer characteristics should be studied and the model should be validated with its ability to predict the axial temperature gradients. Finally, this can be scaled up to a full-scale model and the operation of the bioreactor can be studied.

5.3.6 Photobioreactors

Photobioreactors are most widely used for microalgal cultivation. An airlift PBR provides an enhanced residence time and better mixing conditions while being energy efficient.

Numerical model simulations should be performed before the actual implementation of the reactor to study the hydrodynamic, mixing, mass transfer, and heat transfer characteristics. The optimization of parameters like mixing efficiency, gas hold-up, overall process efficiency and yield, and liquid circulation should be performed. These reactors are highly energy efficient and the power input is shown in Eq. 5.11 (AslanbayGuler et al., 2020).

$$\frac{P_G}{V_L} = \frac{\rho_L g U_{Gr}}{1 + \frac{A_d}{A_r}} \tag{5.11}$$

The conventional large-scale system does not have high cell densities which cause the growth rate to decline and hence give a lower yield. In the photobioreactors, upscaling should consider several limitations like self-shading of the reactor. This drastically reduces the growth rate and hence the heterogeneous intensity reduces the process efficiency. But, a flat panel photoreactor provides this homogeneity and stops the adverse effects (Socher et al., 2016).

Enhanced mixing and scaled-up operation give a higher efficiency to the process. The transfer ability of the upgradation of the PBRs with an airlift setup gives a high local and average mass transfer coefficient values and increases the driving force. Computational fluid dynamics achieves a precise simulation of the interphase mass transfer between the gas and liquid layers (Ndiaye et al., 2018).

5.4 CONCLUSION

In this chapter, the scaling and setting up of continuous stirred tank, bubble column, airlift, fluidized bed, packed bed, and photo bioreactors have been examined. The key physical, chemical, and biological factors which influence the scale-up strategies including the factors of the shear rate, pH, reactor temperature, and physiological factors impacting the cell culture are realized. The process conditions counting oxygen transfer rate, mass transfer coefficient, and biological enhancement factor have been regarded as the principal parameters to fixate the scale-up methodology.

The key takeaway from the work points out that a successful scaled-up operation needs to maintain the productivity and the quality of a process. The larger volume operation needs to uphold the robustness of the similar smaller volume process. Cell density, viability, and expression rates can be rated as key metrics for performing evaluations. Effective expressions for evaluation of mixing time in stirred tank reactor scale up, rate of mass transfer from the sparged gas to the liquid phase, and biological enhancement factors have been stated which give the impression of the impact of the scale up from a more theoretical point of view.

REFERENCES

Amer, M., Feng, Y., & Ramsey, J. D. (2019). Using CFD simulations and statistical analysis to correlate oxygen mass transfer coefficient to both geometrical parameters and operating conditions in a stirred-tank bioreactor. *Biotechnology Progress*, *35*(3), e2785. https://doi.org/10.1002/BTPR.2785

Arshi, S., Nozari-Asbemarz, M., & Magner, E. (2020). Enzymatic Bioreactors: An electrochemical perspective. *Catalysts*, *10*(11), 1232. https://doi.org/10.3390/CATAL10111232

Aslam, M., McCarty, P. L., Shin, C., Bae, J., & Kim, J. (2017). Low energy single-staged anaerobic fluidized bed ceramic membrane bioreactor (AFCMBR) for wastewater treatment. *Bioresource Technology*, *240*, 33–41. https://doi.org/10.1016/J.BIORTECH.2017.03.017

AslanbayGuler, B., Deniz, I., Demirel, Z., & Imamoglu, E. (2020). Computational fluid dynamics simulation in scaling-up of airlift photobioreactor for astaxanthin production. *Journal of Bioscience and Bioengineering*, *129*(1), 86–92. https://doi.org/10.1016/J.JBIOSC.2019.06.010

Babanezhad, M., Marjani, A., & Shirazian, S. (2020). Multidimensional machine learning algorithms to learn liquid velocity inside a cylindrical bubble column reactor. *Scientific Reports*, *10*(1), 1–14. https://doi.org/10.1038/s41598-020-78388-x

Bae, S., de Sotto, R., Lee, W., & Ho, J. (2020). Energy efficiency and biofouling control in a pilot-scale membrane bioreactor using low-frequency reciprocating motion and the succession of biofilm communities resistant to mechanical shear. *Bioresource Technology Reports*, *11*, 100523. https://doi.org/10.1016/J.BITEB.2020.100523

Bai, F. W., Zhao, X. Q., & Xu, J. (2011). Immobilization technology: Cells. *Comprehensive Biotechnology, Second Edition*, *2*, 477–489. https://doi.org/10.1016/B97-0-08-088504-9.00115-X

Deshpande, S. S., Kar, K., Pressler, J., Tebeka, I., Martins, B., Rosenfeld, D., & Biggs, J. (2019). Mass transfer estimation for bubble column scale up. *Chemical Engineering Science*, *205*, 350–357. https://doi.org/10.1016/J.CES.2019.05.011

Doran, P. M. (2013). Reactor engineering. In *Bioprocess Engineering Principles*, pp. 761–852. https://doi.org/10.1016/B978-0-12-220851-5.00014-9

Enfors, S. O., Jahic, M., Rozkov, A., Xu, B., Hecker, M., Jürgen, B., Krüger, E., Schweder, T., Hamer, G., O'Beirne, D., Noisommit-Rizzi, N., Reuss, M., Boone, L., Hewitt, C., McFarlane, C., Nienow, A., Kovacs, T., Trägårdh, C., Fuchs, L., … & Manelius, Å. (2001). Physiological responses to mixing in large scale bioreactors. *Journal of Biotechnology*, *85*(2), 175–185. https://doi.org/10.1016/S0168-1656(00)00365-5

Enzmann, F., Mayer, F., Stöckl, M., Mangold, K. M., Hommel, R., & Holtmann, D. (2019). Transferring bioelectrochemical processes from H-cells to a scalable bubble column reactor. *Chemical Engineering Science*, *193*, 133–143. https://doi.org/10.1016/J.CES.2018.08.056

Finkler, A. T. J., de Lima Luz, L. F., Krieger, N., Mitchell, D. A., & Jorge, L. M. (2021). A model-based strategy for scaling-up traditional packed-bed bioreactors for solid-state fermentation based on measurement of O_2 uptake rates. *Biochemical Engineering Journal*, *166*, 107854. https://doi.org/10.1016/J.BEJ.2020.107854

Garcia-Ochoa, F., & Gomez, E. (2009). Bioreactor scale-up and oxygen transfer rate in microbial processes: An overview. *Biotechnology Advances*, *27*(2), 153–176. https://doi.org/10.1016/J.BIOTECHADV.2008.10.006

Guieysse, B., Quijano, G., & Muñoz, R. (2011). Airlift bioreactors. In *Comprehensive Biotechnology*, Second Edition, *Vol.* 2, pp. 199–212. https://doi.org/10.1016/B978-0-08-2088504-9.00095-7

Guo, Y. X., Rathor, M. N., & Ti, H. C. (1997). Hydrodynamics and mass transfer studies in a novel external-loop airlift reactor. *Chemical Engineering Journal*, *67*(3), 205–214. https://doi.org/10.1016/S1385-8947(97)00043-0

Han, S. J., Tan, R. B. H., & Loh, K. C. (2000). Hydrodynamic behaviour in a new gas-liquid-solid inverse fluidization airlift bioreactor. *Food and Bioproducts Processing*, *78*(4), 207–215. https://doi.org/10.1205/096030800051065313

He, C., Ye, P., Wang, H., Liu, X., & Li, F. (2019). A systematic mass-transfer modeling approach for mammalian cell culture bioreactor scale-up. *Biochemical Engineering Journal*, *141*, 173–181. https://doi.org/10.1016/J.BEJ.2018.09.019

Hoshan, L., Jiang, R., Moroney, J., Bui, A., Zhang, X., Hang, T.-C., & Xu, S. (2019). Effective bioreactor pH control using only sparging gases. *Biotechnology Progress*, *35*(1), e2743. https://doi.org/10.1002/BTPR.2743

Ji, J., Kakade, A., Yu, Z., Khan, A., Liu, P., & Li, X. (2020). Anaerobic membrane bioreactors for treatment of emerging contaminants: A review. *Journal of Environmental Management*, *270*, 110913. https://doi.org/10.1016/J.JENVMAN.2020.110913

Junne, S., & Neubauer, P. (2018). How scalable and suitable are single-use bioreactors? *Current Opinion in Biotechnology*, *53*, 240–247. https://doi.org/10.1016/J.COPBIO.2018.04.003

Käß, F., Hariskos, I., Michel, A., Brandt, H.-J., Spann, R., Junne, S., Wiechert, W., Neubauer, P., & Oldiges, M. (2013). Assessment of robustness against dissolved oxygen/substrate oscillations for *C. glutamicum* DM1933 in two-compartment bioreactor. *Bioprocess and Biosystems Engineering*, *37*(6), 1151–1162. https://doi.org/10.1007/S00449-013-1086-0

Li, C., Shu, W., Wang, S., Liu, P., Zhuang, Y., Zhang, S., & Xia, J. (2018). Dynamic metabolic response of *Aspergillus niger* to glucose perturbation: Evidence of regulatory mechanism for reduced glucoamylase production. *Journal of Biotechnology*, *287*, 28–40. https://doi.org/10.1016/J.JBIOTEC.2018.08.005

Mahdinia, E., Cekmecelioglu, D., & Demirci, A. (2019). *Bioreactor Scale-Up*, pp. 213–236. https://doi.org/10.1007/978-3-030-16230-6_7

Maurer, S., Rüdisüli, M., Schildhauer, T. J., Biollaz, S., & van Ommen, J. R. (2013). Scale-up of bubbling fluidized bed reactors with vertical internals: A new approach accounting for chemistry and hydrodynamics. In *The 14th International Conference on Fluidization - From Fundamentals to Products.*

Meuwly, F., Ruffieux, P. A., Kadouri, A., & von Stockar, U. (2007). Packed-bed bioreactors for mammalian cell culture: Bioprocess and biomedical applications. *Biotechnology Advances*, *25*(1), 45–56. https://doi.org/10.1016/J.BIOTECHADV.2006.08.004

Naghdi, M., Taheran, M., Brar, S. K., Kermanshahi-pour, A., Verma, M., & Surampalli, R. Y. (2018). Removal of pharmaceutical compounds in water and wastewater using fungal oxidoreductase enzymes. *Environmental Pollution*, *234*, 190–213. https://doi.org/10.1016/J.ENVPOL.2017.11.060

Ndiaye, M., Gadoin, E., & Gentric, C. (2018). CO_2 gas–liquid mass transfer and kLa estimation: Numerical investigation in the context of airlift photobioreactor scale-up. *Chemical Engineering Research and Design*, *133*, 90–102. https://doi.org/10.1016/J.CHERD.2018.03.001

NOW, A. W. N. (1990). Gas dispersion performance in fermenter operation. *Chemical Engineering Progress*, *86*(2), 61–71.

Özkaya, B., Kaksonen, A. H., Sahinkaya, E., & Puhakka, J. A. (2019). Fluidized bed bioreactor for multiple environmental engineering solutions. *Water Research*, *150*, 452–465. https://doi.org/10.1016/J.WATRES.2018.11.061

Potumarthi, R., Ch, S., & Jetty, A. (2007). Alkaline protease production by submerged fermentation in stirred tank reactor using *Bacillus licheniformis* NCIM-2042: Effect of aeration and agitation regimes. *Biochemical Engineering Journal*, *34*(2), 185–192. https://doi.org/10.1016/J.BEJ.2006.12.003

Rout, P. R., Dash, R. R., Bhunia, P., Lee, E., & Bae, J. (2021). Comparison between a single unit bioreactor and an integrated bioreactor for nutrient removal from domestic wastewater. *Sustainable Energy Technologies and Assessments*, *48*, 101620. https://doi.org/10.1016/J.SETA.2021.101620

Socher, M. L., Löser, C., Schott, C., Bley, T., & Steingroewer, J. (2016). The challenge of scaling up photobioreactors: Modeling and approaches in small scale. *Engineering in Life Sciences*, *16*(7), 598–609. https://doi.org/10.1002/ELSC.201500134

Suwanprasop, S., Eftaxias, A., Stüber, F., Polaert, I., Julcour-Lebigue, C. and Delmas, H. (2005). Scale-up and modeling of fixed-bed reactors for catalytic phenol oxidation over adsorptive active carbon. *Industrial and Engineering Chemistry Research*, *44*(25), 9513–9523. https://doi.org/10.1021/IE050242D

Teworte, S., Malcı, K., Walls, L. E., Halim, M., & Rios-Solis, L. (2022). Recent advances in fed-batch microscale bioreactor design. *Biotechnology Advances*, *55*, 107888. https://doi.org/10.1016/J.BIOTECHADV.2021.107888

Tisa, F., Abdul Raman, A. A., & Daud, W. M. A. W. (2014). Simulation for supporting scale-up of a fluidized bed reactor for advanced water oxidation. *Scientific World Journal*, *2014*. https://doi.org/10.1155/2014/348974

Valverde-Pérez, B., Xing, W., Zachariae, A. A., Skadborg, M. M., Kjeldgaard, A. F., Palomo, A., & Smets, B. F. (2020). Cultivation of methanotrophic bacteria in a novel bubble-free membrane bioreactor for microbial protein production. *Bioresource Technology*, *310*, 123388. https://doi.org/10.1016/J.BIORTECH.2020.123388

Weber, S., Schaepe, S., Freyer, S., Kopf, M. H., & Dietzsch, C. (2018). Impact of nozzle operation on mass transfer in jet aerated loop reactors. Characterization and comparison to an aerated stirred tank reactor. *Engineering in Life Sciences*, *18*(8), 579–588. https://doi.org/10.1002/ELSC.201800008

Werther, J. (1992). Scale-up modeling for fluidized bed reactors. *Chemical Engineering Science*, *47*(9–11), 2457–2462. https://doi.org/10.1016/0009-2509(92)87076-3

Wilkinson, P. M., Spek, A. P., &Dierendonck, L. L. van. (1992). Design parameters estimation for scale-up of high-pressure bubble columns. *AIChE Journal*, *38*(4), 544–554. https://doi.org/10.1002/AIC.690380408

Wu, L., Mashego, M. R., Proell, A. M., Vinke, J. L., Ras, C., Van Dam, J., Van Winden, W. A., Van Gulik, W. M., & Heijnen, J. J. (2006). In vivo kinetics of primary metabolism in Saccharomyces cerevisiae studied through prolonged chemostat cultivation. *Metabolic Engineering*, *8*(2), 160–171. https://doi.org/10.1016/J.YMBEN.2005.09.005

Yahia, A., Mantellato, S., & Flatt, R. J. (2016). Concrete rheology: A basis for understanding chemical admixtures. *Science and Technology of Concrete Admixtures*, 97–127. https://doi.org/10.1016/B978-0-08-100693-1.00007-2

Zhang, T., We, C., Ren, Y., Feng, C., & Wu, H. (2017). Advances in airlift reactors: Modified design and optimization of operation conditions. *Reviews in Chemical Engineering*, *33*(2), 163–182. https://doi.org/10.1515/REVCE-2016-0005

Zhou, Y., Han, L.-R., He, H.-W., Sang, B., Yu, D.-L., Feng, J.-T., & Zhang, X. (2018). Effects of agitation, aeration and temperature on production of a novel glycoprotein GP-1 by *Streptomyces kanasenisi* ZX01 and scale-up based on volumetric oxygen transfer coefficient. *Molecules*, *23*(1), 125. https://doi.org/10.3390/MOLECULES23010125

Znad, H., Báleš, V., & Kawase, Y. (2004). Modeling and scale up of airlift bioreactor. *Computers & Chemical Engineering*, *28*(12), 2765–2777. https://doi.org/10.1016/J.COMPCHEMENG.2004.08.024

6 Biotechnological Advancements in the Treatment of Plastic Wastes

Daniel Joe Dailin, Luo Zaini Mohd Izwan Low, Nurul Zahidah Nordin, Nur Izyan Wan Azelee, Shanmugaprakasham Selvamani, Vasantha M. Nayagam, and Dayang Norulfairuz Abang Zaidel
Universiti Teknologi Malaysia (UTM)

Hesham Ali El Enshasy
Universiti Teknologi Malaysia (UTM) City of Scientific Research and Technology Applications (SRTA)

CONTENTS

DOI: 10.1201/9781003188292-6

6.1 INTRODUCTION

Plasticos, the Greek word from which the word plastic is derived, implies materials that can be shaped or moulded when the temperature changes (Ncube et al., 2021; Kehinde et al., 2020). Plastic was originally well-known as pliable, inexpensive, lightweight, and can adapt with high thermal, most used material and synthetic compounds made from polymers (Venkatesh et al., 2021; Muthukumar and Veerappapillai, 2015). It is defined as a type of synthetic organic polymer made by polymerizing monomers to form a chain-like structure (Paço et al., 2019). Plastic production began in the 1860s, and in the 1940s it was one of the world's fastest-growing industries. After World War II, widespread use of plastic outside of the military began, even though the first synthetic plastics, such as Bakelite, appeared in the early 20th century (Zaman and Newman, 2021; Geyer et al., 2017).

Plastic materials present several properties, such as lightweight, technically sophisticated, heat resistance, tensile strength, colour, transparency, versatility, ease of processing making plastics, and needed for a variety of applications (Thompson et al., 2009). In many industrial applications, polymers like plastic are preferred due to their resistivity to organic solvents, oxidation, and ionizing radiation. Plastics are used in a broad array of applications, including packaging, film production, coating, as well as sealant production for consumer goods such as single-use products, electronic pipe and cable coatings, automotive manufacturing and construction, and furniture making. Examples include acrylonitrile butadiene styrene (ABS), polyamide, polyethylene (PE), polyimide (PI), poly-methyl methacrylate (PMMA), polypropylene (PP), polystyrene (PS), polytetrafluoroethylene (PTFE), polyvinyl chloride (PVC), and polyvinylidene chloride (PVDC) (Bassi, 2017; Geyer et al., 2017). As per United Nations Environment Programme (UNEP), roughly 80% of plastic wrapping is single-use plastic, including shopping bags, containers, and bottles. Plastic packaging makes up 33% of total plastic production (Zaman and Newman, 2021; Maurya et al., 2020).

In 2018, 359 million metric tons of polymer/plastic were manufactured internationally; in 1950, only 1.5 million metric tons were produced (Shanmugam et al., 2020; Garside, 2019). There are around 8,300 metric tons of plastic that have been produced between 1950 and 2015. Only 500 million tons of those plastics have been recycled (Shanmugam et al., 2020; Geyer et al. 2017). The amount of plastic that had already been deposited in terrestrial waters is estimated to be between 4 and 12 million metric tons, and it has a damaging effect on marine life (Shanmugam et al., 2020; Jambeck et al. 2015). If present patterns in plastic usage continue, there will be 12,000 million metric tonnes of plastic pollution on the globe by 2050 (Geyer et al, 2017). This wide consumption of plastics has led to a rise in plastic trash in diverse ecosystems since the late 20th century. In nature, plastic is extremely resistant to degradation and takes 1,000 years to degrade. When plastic waste is disposed of, not only does it contribute to global warming and pollution but also releases carbon dioxide and other gases as it burns (Venkatesh et al., 2021; Kale et al., 2015). When plastic and waste accumulate in the environment, it poses several threats to living organisms. Plastic waste was identified as the accumulation of plastic objects or material in the Earth's environments that adversely affects wildlife, wildlife habitat, and humans (Kehinde et al., 2020). According to the study, 100,000 tonnes of plastic items are tossed into oceans, seas, and aquatic ecosystems each year, killing numerous creatures (Venkatesh et al., 2021; Thompson et al., 2009).

According to U.N. Environment Programme statistics, only 21% of plastic waste is recycled, and 12% and 9% of plastic waste are incinerated and recycled, respectively (Chen et al., 2021; Zaman and Newman, 2021). The balance is disposed of in landfills. A significant amount of plastic is not recycled and ends up in landfills or, in developing countries, unregulated dumpsites.

Plastics' biodegradability in the environment is typically poor and takes a long time to degrade. Plastic waste can be recycled, burnt for energy recovery, or buried in landfills (Ncube et al., 2021). However, for the management of plastic trash, feasible reduction solutions based on biotechnology breakthroughs are being evaluated by using microorganisms and the mechanism of microbial degradation will be discussed deeply in this chapter. The microorganism is being used in the synthesis of bioplastics as well as the degradation of plastics (Bassi, 2017). Furthermore, besides encouraging and educating the public to use plastic more efficiently, it is necessary to develop sustainable solutions to handle plastic waste both in the future and today, as plastic waste management is a complex task. Table 6.1 summarizes the different types of plastics and their properties and applications.

6.2 IMPACT OF PLASTIC WASTES ACCUMULATION

Generally, plastics can be defined as a synthetic material made from a wide range of organic polymers that consist of monomeric building blocks such as PE, PVC, and nylon. Due to that, plastics tend to secrete several toxic materials that could be harmful to human health and the environment. Bisphenol A (BPA) is the main type of additive on plastic components that could lead to the secretion of these toxic materials. BPA is a chemical that is usually added with other compounds into plastic containers such as food containers and baby bottles to obtain strong and resilient plastics. However, BPA could be harmful to human health because it mimics the structure and function of the oestrogen hormone (Konieczna et al., 2015). Due to its oestrogen-like structure, BPA can bind to oestrogen receptors and alter body processes like reproductive, endocrine functions, and immune toxicity (Ohore and Zhang, 2019).

Marine animals are the most affected by the issue of plastic dumping. Plastic pellets that polluted the deep sea cause marine animals to ingest them indirectly which blocks their respiratory system and leads them to death (Thushari and Senevirathna, 2020). Other than that, the breakdown of plastics that were used, recycled, or disposed of, or left in the environment as litter causes the release of harmful chemicals such as phthalates and BPA. These pollutants include heavy metals such as cadmium and lead, and chemicals such as benzene, dioxins, and other pollutants, which all release harmful toxins to the environment (Pavani and Rajeswari, 2014). In addition, the structure of plastics that consist of synthetic polymers causes them to have slow degradation which imposes a hazardous effect on the environment (mainly water pollution), wildlife, and human food chain (Aganguly, 2018). The release of chemicals into the soil makes the soil infertile, hence plants could not grow well and lower the fruit production.

TABLE 6.1
Plastic Types, Properties, and Applications

Plastic Types	Properties	Applications	References
Acrylonitrile butadiene styrene (ABS)	• High toughness • Good shock durability, even at low temperatures • Good insulation properties • Good mechanical properties • Good corrosion and wear resistance • High ductility (mechanically strong and long-lasting) • Weatherproofing • Weight reduction	• Automotive • Electrical & electronics applications • Household appliances (shavers, vacuum cleaners, food processors, refrigerator liners) • Pipes, hoses, and fittings	Olivera et al. (2016)
Polyamide a) Polyamide 6 b) Polyamide 11 c) Polyamide 12 d) Polyamide 6-10 e) Polyamide 46	**a) Polyamide 6** • High durability at extreme heat • High rigidity and strength even at low temperatures • Great flow for simplicity of use • Good corrosion and wear resistance • Highly resistant to oil and gasoline • High electrical insulating qualities • High water absorption **b) Polyamide 11** • Lowest water absorption • Exceptional hardness value, even at temperatures below zero • Chemically resistant • Strain cracking, ageing, and corrosion-resistant • Low friction coefficient • Noise and vibration cushioning properties • Tolerance to high filler loading • High protection to ionization ray	• Act as thermoplastics • Metal's substitute in a broad variety of uses • Used In Processing Technologies (extrusion, extrusion blow-moulding, injection moulding, and rotomoulding) • Sterilized films and bags for pharmaceutical and medical sectors, as well as films for wrapping in the food industry • Insulators for the electronic industry Manufacture several automotive/ transportation parts • Manufacture electrical and electronics appliances • Industrial and consumer products, safety controls in devices such as kettles and ovens	Neis et al. (2017)

(Continued)

TABLE 6.1
Plastic Types, Properties, and Applications

Plastic Types	Properties	Applications	References
	c) Polyamide 12 • Low water absorption • Good shock durability, even at very low temperature • Chemically resistant • Tension break resistant • Good corrosion and wear resistant • Minimal friction coefficient • Vibration and noise absorption capabilities • Fatigue resistance when subjected to high-frequency cyclical loading **d) Polyamide 6-10** • Low water absorbency • Low breaking temperature • Corrosion and chemical resistant • Low strength and rigidity • Low friction coefficient • Good electrical insulation • Very resistant to dangerous radiation (gamma and X-rays) **e) Polyamide 46** • Good heat performance • Good mechanical properties • Good corrosion resistance • Good chemical resistance • Good electrical resistance		
Polyethylene (PE) a) HDPE b) LDPE c) LLDPE d) UHMWPE e) PEX or XLPE	**a) High Density Polyethylene (HDPE)** • HDPE Melting point: 120–140°C • Density of HDPE: 0.93 to 0.97 g/cm³ • Chemically resistant (most solvents, alcohols, dilute acids, alkalis, oils, and greases) • Higher tensile strength • Good low temperature resistance • Weather resistance • Great electrically resistant • Very low water absorption	• Used in several packaging applications and household/consumer goods • Used in fibres and textiles production • Used in pipes and fittings • Used in automotive • Used in wiring and cables • Used in packaging industry	Padhan and Sreeram (2018); Liang et al. (2019)

(*Continued*)

TABLE 6.1
Plastic Types, Properties, and Applications

Plastic Types	Properties	Applications	References
	b) Low Density Polyethylene (LDPE) • LDPE Melting point: 105 to 115°C • Density of LDPE: 0.910–0.940 g/cm^3 • Chemically resistant (alcohols, dilute alkalis, acids) • High impact strength at low temperature, good weather ability • Great electrically resistant • Very low water absorption **c) Linear Low Density Polyethylene (LLDPE)** • Very flexible with high impact strength • Translucent and natural milky colour • Excellent for mild and strong buffers, good chemical resistance • Good water vapour and alcohol barrier properties • Good stress crack and impact resistance **d) Ultrahigh-Molecular-Weight Polyethylene (UHMWPE)** • High abrasion resistance and impact strength • Low coefficient of friction • Resistant to several solvents except for aromatic, halogenated hydrocarbons and strong oxidizing materials **e) Cross-linked Polyethylene (PEX or XLPE)** • Suitable used in high and low temperature • Hydrolysis resistance • High electrical and insulation properties • High abrasion resistance • High extrusion speed on standard lines	• Water pipes and hoses for the pipes and fittings industry • Consumer goods • Wiring and cables • Used in film applications such as general purpose film, stretch film, garment packaging, agricultural film • Used in high wear applications such as tubes, liners, silos, containers, and other equipment • Used for critical applications like chemical storage pipework systems, hydronic radiant heating and cooling systems, and insulation for high voltage electrical cables	

(Continued)

TABLE 6.1
Plastic Types, Properties, and Applications

Plastic Types	Properties	Applications	References
Polyimide (PI)	• High mechanical performance • Superior temperature adaptability • Excellent tensile and compressive strength • Chemical and radiation resistance • Superior bearing and wear properties	• Use as plastics, films, laminating resins, insulating coatings and high temperature structural adhesives	Yi et al. (2020)
Poly-methylmethacrylate (PMMA)	• High resistance to UV light and weathering • Excellent light transmission • Chemical Resistance	• Used for applications in various markets from car windows, smartphone screens to aquariums	Khan et al. (2018)
Polypropylene (PP)	• Chemical resistance to diluted and concentrated acids, alcohols, and bases • Highly flammable material • Stress cracking resistance • Good resistance to steam sterilization	• Automotive industry • Industrial applications • Consumer goods and furniture market	Wang et al. (2019)
Polystyrene (PS)	• Insoluble in water • Good chemical resistance to diluted acids and bases • Good electrical insulator • Low impact strength • Non-biodegradable	• Automotive • Household appliances • Electronics appliances • Food packaging • Construction of buildings, roofing, and cold storages • Medical instruments (Petri dishes, test tubes, and culture trays)	Hirschberg et al. (2018)
Polytetrafluoroethylene (PTFE)	• Good resistance to heat and low temperature • Good electrical insulating power • Good resistance to light, UV, and weathering • Low coefficient of friction • Strong anti-adhesion properties • Low water absorption	• Act as a non-stick coating in kitchen cookware (pans, baking trays, etc.) • Used in the oil & gas industry • Used in the electrical/electronic industry	Huang et al. (2018)
Polyvinyl chloride (PVC) & Polyvinylidene chloride (PVDC)	• Good insulation material for electrical properties • Resistant to weathering, chemical rotting, corrosion, shock, and abrasion • Chemical resistance to all inorganic chemicals	• Household purposes • Used for food packaging	Choi et al. (2017)

6.3 FACTORS AFFECTING DEGRADATION RATE OF PLASTICS

The fast and complete degradation of plastic in fully natural environments is seen to be almost impossible. Chemical structures building up the plastics have made them invulnerable and resistant to degradation. This phenomenon has put a loud siren for immediate actions to be taken. Factors determining the degradation rate of plastics can be categorized into two which are environmental factors and physicochemical characteristics.

6.3.1 Environmental Factors

As generally known, plastic waste has become a crisis to the whole world due to its resistance characteristic towards degradation. This resistance was influenced by the additives used in synthesizing the commercial plastics such as antioxidants and light stabilizers which have delayed the degradation process (Hahladakis et al., 2018). However, the dynamic environmental conditions such as the intensity of sun rays, UV radiation, oxygen level, the wind blows, seawater (level of alkalinity and presence of hydroxide ions) and wave movements, and the action of microorganisms have indirectly helped in the degradation of the plastic wastes (Marion et al. 2011). All these abiotic and biotic factors have contributed towards the cracking, erosion of the plastic surfaces, abrasion, and the breakdown of the plastic into smaller-sized plastic such as mesoplastic, large microplastic, small microplastic, and nanoplastic with the size range of approximately 5–20 mm, 1–5 mm, 20–999 μm, and <1 μm, respectively (Min et al., 2020). Plastic wastes can also be biodegraded with the assistance of certain microbes such as bacteria (biotic factors). Biotic and abiotic factors usually work in synergy with each other. The mechanisms for the environmental degradation of plastics can be classified under two categories namely physical (bulk structure changes, e.g., cracking, embrittlement, flaking) and chemical (molecular changes, e.g., bond cleavage, hydrolysis, oxidation) (Chamas et al., 2020). Both mechanisms accelerate the degradation by microbes, heat, and light. Table 6.2 shows the contribution of biotic and abiotic factors in plastic degradation.

Naturally, certain plastics such as polyethylene terephthalate (PET) can be degraded by thermal oxidation. However, the factor of UV radiation is much more dominant under ambient conditions where it initiates photo-oxidation and hydrolytic cleavage (Suits and Hsuan, 2003). The rate of hydrolytic cleavage is strongly influenced by acidic conditions. The introduction of polar groups and surface area enhancement by UV radiation has slightly assisted the degradation of plastics that is reachable by the sun rays (Chamas et al., 2020). The synergistic effect of UV radiation and oxygen has proven to increase the photodegradation of plastics into microplastics by cracking to a depth of 50–100 μm (Gewert et al., 2018).

6.3.2 Physicochemical Characteristics of Plastics

A huge investigation has been performed to evaluate the degree of plastic degradation. The reduction in the plastic molecular weight, density, surface roughness, and mass was recorded as an indicator of plastic degradation. The existence of

TABLE 6.2
Contribution of Biotic and Abiotic Factors in Plastic Degradation

Factor		Description	Reference
Biotic	Bacteria	• *Acinetobacter* bacterium (degrade polystyrene) • Isolated from *Tribolium castaneum* larvae	Wang et al. (2020)
		• *Pseudomonas* (*aeruginosa* and *putida*), *Sphingobacterium moltivorum*, *Delftia tsuruhatansis*, *Stentrophomonas* (*humi* and *maltophilia*), *Ochrobacterum* (*oryzae* and *humi*), *Micrococcus uteus*, *Acinetobacter pitti*, and *Citrobacter amalonaticus*	Montazer et al. (2018)
	Fungi	• *Trichoderma viride* and *Aspergillus nomius* • Isolated from landfill soil	Munir et al. (2018)
		• *Cladosporium cladosporioides*, *Xepiculopsis graminea*, and *Penicillium griseofulvum*, *Agaricus bisporus*, and *Marasmius oreades* able to degrade polyurethane	Brunner et al. (2018)
	Biofilm	• *Burkholderiales*, *Acidovorax*, and *Undibacterium* genera • Most prevalent genera in biofilms	Morohoshi et al. (2018)
Abiotic	UV radiation/sun rays	• Triggers photodegradation • Introduce polar groups • Increase surface area • Increase enzyme accessibility for degradation	Ranjan and Goel (2019)
	Oxygen level	• Reactive oxygen species simulated sun rays' radiation	Zhu et al. (2020)
	Mechanical forces (Wind/waves)	• Selectively transport heavier and denser plastic offshore	Ho and Not (2019)
	Seawater salinity	• High salinity seawater imposes higher degradation polycaprolactone	Lu et al. (2018)
	Temperature	• High temperature increases degradation rate • Pyrolysis of low density polyethylene (LDPE), polypropylene (PP), and polyvinyl chloride (PVC)	Xu et al. (2018)
	Location (depth, lake/sea/soil)	• Increasing depth in seawater decreases the biofilm formation on the PE	Tu et al. (2020)
	pH	• A combination effect of low pH and low temperature favours microplastic degradation	Ariza-Tarazona et al. (2020)

different functional groups in plastic wastes such as esters, amides, carbonates, and urethanes will assist in enhancing the degradation rate. The type of plastic materials is one of the contributors to the degradation rate of plastic as different types of plastics undergo different degradation rates. Moreover, the degree of plastic crystallinity, enthalpy of melting, and hydrophobicity influence the degradation rate (Min et al., 2020). The decrease in hydrophobicity will increase the probability of surface erosion while the degradation by surface erosion decreases with the increase in hydrophobicity, especially for PVC, Polycarbonate (PC), PS, PE, and PP. High hydrophobicity also corresponds to low density which would cause plastic floating problems on the ocean's surface. Even worse, PE and PP types are among the highest volume of plastic being produced worldwide and the addition of additives in polyolefins such as antioxidants and light stabilizers has, even more, reduce the degradation of the PE and PP. Nevertheless, most of the plastics with high hydrophobic contain a large C-H bond percentage which is susceptible to photodegradation even though they may not have any functional groups (e.g., polyolefins) to assist abiotic hydrolysis. Additionally, the plastic's particle size (surface-volume ratio) and time of exposure to degradation factors also contribute to the degradation rate of the plastic. Smaller particle sizes with prolonged exposure time will fasten the degradation of plastics.

As we are moving towards sustainable development, several strategies have been implemented to overcome all the factors which delay the degradation rate of plastics. Reuse and recycling of plastic wastes are the simplest way to minimize the global carbon footprint and can be implemented directly by all parties. Moreover, some plastic manufacturers have incorporated photosensitizers, photoacid generators, and 'weak links' in the polymers, mixing with water-soluble polymers and green additives which can promote photo-initiated oxidation (Hosono et al., 2007, 2008). All these initiatives enable a faster degradation rate compared to conventional plastic manufacturing (Martin et al., 2014). Additional plasticizers are reported to influence the degradability of plastic. Besides producing flexible plastic, blending with hydrophilic plasticizers enhanced plastic susceptibility towards hydrolysis (Boulven et al., 2019). A low degree of acetylation increases the degradation possibility of plastic (Yadav and Hakkarainen, 2020).

6.4 MICROBIAL PLASTIC DEGRADATION

Degradation of plastics involves complex processes that depend on multiple communities of microorganisms, and the intricacies of plastic breakdown have been widely discussed over the last few decades (Lucas et al., 2008; Ru et al., 2020; Shah et al., 2008; Venkatesh et al., 2021). The large varieties and diverse mechanisms of these microbes have recently been extensively reviewed by Ru et.al. (Ru et al., 2020) and these authors have clearly illustrated that plastic degradation is multifaceted. Plastic is a collective term that describes long-chain polymers which are lightweight yet strong, corrosion-resistant, and durable. They can encompass distinctly different forms such as PE, PVC, and polyurethane (PU). Thus, it is not too difficult to grasp that each of these polymer types may require different sets of microbes and conditions for their degradation.

The microbes involved can range from single-cell bacteria such as *Bacillus* and *Pseudomonas* to more complex mushrooms and fungi. Table 6.3 shows a compilation of microorganisms involved in plastic degradation. Also shown, the plastic degradation can take from a week to nearly a year, raising concerns especially since the rate of plastic waste production annually can amount to trillions of tonnes (Venkatesh et al., 2021). Besides this, based on weight loss of the plastic, which is the indicator of degradation, very few studies show significant weight loss, i.e. beyond 75%. However, it is interesting to note that for PET, where specific enzymes were utilized, the rate of degradation was more promising. This may indicate that enzymes can

TABLE 6.3
List of Microorganisms Tested for Plastics Degradations

Tested Source	Strain	Microbial Source	Degradation Conditions	Performance Result (Plastic Weight Loss %)	Reference
Polystyrene (PS)	• *Pseudomonas* sp. • *Actinomycetes* sp. • *Penicillium* sp.	Soil buried expanded PS film	Inoculation of cultures on PS foam (cultivation media and incubation T not mentioned)	FTIR assays showed formation of ether and ester group resulted from PS degradation by isolates after 30 days	Murali and Umamaheswari (2019)
	• *P. aeruginosa* DSM 50071	Superworms, *Zophobas atratus*	Cultivation in Liquid C Free Basal Medium plate with PS film	2.6% without Serine hydrolase (SH) inhibitor, 1.3% with SH inhibitor	Kim et al. (2020)
	• *Microbacterium* sp. NA23 • *Paenibacillus urinalis* NA26 • *Bacillus* sp. NB6 • *P. aeruginosa* NB26	Soil buried expanded PS film	Cultivation in mineral salt medium (MSM) with PS at 30°C, 120 rpm	HPLC analysis showed no significant chemical changes on the surface of PE through the isolates able to extract some C from the PE	Naima et al. (2010)
Polyethylene (PE)	• *Alcanivorax borkumensis*	Mediterranean Sea	Formation of biofilm degrading bacteria on PE at 30°C	3.5% ± 0.34% after 80 days	Delacuvellerie et al. (2019)
	• *Phomidium lucidum* • *Oscilatoria subbrevis*	Domestic sewage water	Incubation of the culture in BG-1 media with PE strips (incubation T not mentioned)	30% after 42 days	Sarmah and Rout (2018)
	• *Achromobacter xylosoxidans*	Soil	Incubation of the culture in Davis Minimal Broth Medium at 27°C	9% after 150 days	Kowalczyk et al. (2016)

(*Continued*)

TABLE 6.3 (*Continued*)
List of Microorganisms Tested for Plastics Degradations

Tested Source	Strain	Microbial Source	Degradation Conditions	Performance Result (Plastic Weight Loss %)	Reference
Polypropylene (PP)	• *Bacillus* sp. Strain 27 • *Rhodococcus* sp. Strain 36	Mangrove environments	Incubation of the culture in Bushnell Haas medium (incubation T not mentioned)	6.4% by *Rhodococcus* sp. strain 36% and 4.0% by *Bacillus* sp. strain 27 after 40 days	Auta et al. (2018)
	• *Aneurinibacillus aneurinilyticus* btDSCE01 • *Brevibacillus agri* btDSCE02	Sewage treatment plants and waste management landfills	Incubation of the culture in minimal media (MM) broth with plastic strips and pellets at 50°C	26.21% ± 3% by *Aneurinibacillus* and 28.27% ± 2% by *Brevibacillus* after 140 days	Skariyachan et al. (2018)
	• *Stenotrophomonas panacihumi* PA3-2	Soil of waste storage yard	Inoculation of culture into compost blended with PP powder at 37°C	28.7± 1.4% (LMWPE-1, Mw: 1,700) and 19.7± 1.43% (LMWPE-2, Mw: 23,700) by 90 days	Jeon and Kim (2016)
Polyvinyl chloride (PVC)	• *Bacillus* sp. AIIW2	Marine microbial culture repository	Incubation of culture in Bushnell Haas medium at 30°C, 180 rpm	0.26% ± 0.02% after 90 days	Kumari et al. (2018)
	• *Phanerocheate chrysosporium* NK-1	Plastic and wood waste disposal site	Incubation of culture in MSM with plastic film at 25°C, 150 rpm	31% after 60 days	Khatoon et al. (2019)
	• *Pseudomonas citronellolis*	Soil	Incubation of culture in MSM with plastic film at 30°C or 37°C	19% after 30 days	Giacomucci et al. (2019)
Polyurethane (PUR)	• *Penicillium section Lanata-divaricata*	PUR wastes	Incubation of culture in MM broth with thermoplastic PUR pieces at 30°C	8.9% for polycaprolactone-based thermoplastic PUR after 60 days	Magnin et al. (2019)
	• *B. subtilis* MZA-75 • *P. aeruginosa* MZA-85	Soil	Incubation of culture in MSM with PUR film pieces at 37°C at 150 rpm	30%–40% after 30 days	Shah et al. (2013)
	• *P. denitrificans* ATCC 19244 • *P. fluorescens* ATCC 13525 • *B. subtilis* • *Yaworria lipolytica* CBS 224	-	Incubation of culture in NB medium (bacteria) and SB medium (yeast) with PUR (Tecoflex®, EG/ Tecothane®, TT) samples at 30°C	No weight lost for PUR TT). 2.8%–10.5% lost for EG	Stepien et al. (2017)

exert better efficiency in the degradation process, especially as the final indicated crystallinity was below 10%, but it is also important to consider if there was prior processing of the substrate.

Pre-processing of plastics before microbial degradation can involve photodegradation, where the substrate is treated with UV irradiation, and thermo-oxidation, where heat (and sometimes chemicals) is applied, to weaken the structure of the polymer. Mechanical action such as pulverizing to increase surface area and deteriorate surface integrity also aids in enhancing the plastic degradation process by a microbe as this allows for wider access to the substrate (Han et al., 2020).

Curiously also, there have been no reports which quantitatively document the effects of different compositions of microbes or related enzymes, on plastic degradation. Based on the compilation of data from work carried out over three decades (Ru et al., 2020), certain combinations of microbes may prove to be advantageous in accelerating the plastic degradation process. Basically, the breakdown of plastics involves four steps which include bio-deterioration, bio-fragmentation, assimilation, and mineralization (Dussud and JF, 2014);

1. **Bio-deterioration**: This is caused by microbial (usually bacteria) growth over the surface of the plastic which can enlarge any disruptions in the surface integrity (such as cracks). The proliferation of bacteria eventually produces biofilms which can further unsettle structural integrity by producing degrading chemicals.
2. **Bio-fragmentation**: This process involves the action of extracellular enzymes produced by the adherent microbes which act on the plastic polymers, cleaving them into smaller subunits. The types of products formed are highly dependent on enzymes produced by the microorganisms growing on the plastic. Water-soluble products, for example, are produced from the action of oxygenases, while short peptide molecules are produced by endopeptidases.
3. **Assimilation**: At this stage, the products formed in the first two stages are absorbed and integrated into the microbes. Usually, these are small molecules that are less than 600Da and they are transformed within the microbes into cellular material.
4. **Mineralization**: At this stage, the plastic moiety would have been completely degraded into simple molecules like CO_2, N_2, water, and methane.

6.5 ALTERNATIVE APPROACHES

Alternative approaches to minimize the impact of plastic wastes are by having genetically engineered plastic-eating bacteria, effective enzyme tool technology, and by inventing new materials to substitute plastics.

6.5.1 Genetically Engineered Plastic-Eating Bacteria

As the race to isolate 'plastic-eating' continued to be exploited globally, some scientists also induced this ability in other microorganisms through gene editing.

The heterologous expression of genes from a native plastic-degrading bacterium into another compatible recombinant cell enhances an effective production of the desired enzymes. Yoon et al. (2012) evaluated a recombinant alkane hydrolase gene in *Escherichia coli* host. This heterologous enzyme which is capable of mineralizing low-molecular PS was isolated from *Pseudomonas* sp. strain E4. Recombinant technology helped scientists to solve certain lacking points found in the native hosts. Similarly, Lee et al. (2016) evaluated polycyclic aromatic hydrocarbon degradation potentials in the white-rot fungus, *Peniophora incarnata* KUC8836. The heterologous expression of the fungal manganese-dependent peroxidase gene into *Saccharomyces cerevisiae* BY4741 had improved anthracene degradation (Lee et al. 2016). Overexpression of genes also improves the functional characteristic of the plastic-degrading enzymes. A study by Lo Piccolo et al. (2011) demonstrated plastic-degrading ability in Gram-positive bacterium, *Gordonia* sp. The bacterium was able to grow on n-alkanes from C12 to C36. However, the long-chain and solid n-alkanes are insoluble and ubiquities. Recombinant of *Gordonia* sp. alkB (alkane 1-monooxygenase) gene into *Streptomyces coelicolor* M145 had proven to degrade the long-chain n-triacontane as the sole carbon source (Lo Piccolo et al., 2011).

The production of plastic-degrading enzymes is often reported at a minimal level by the native bacterium, in the natural environment. Recombinant DNA technology is used to overexpress the enzyme genes in another well-known cell, such as *E. coli*. This helped to evaluate the stability of the production of the enzyme. The shelf-life, substrate range, and physical parameters such as temperature and pH could be improved by the genetic engineering approach. Recombinant technology is also cost-effective as the purification of the enzymes is much easier compared to a native bacterium (Soe et al., 2019). The PET-degrading activity by *Ideonella sakaiensis* is well known and extensively studied since its discovery. Various recombinant studies involving PET hydrolases from *I. sakaiensis* have also been reported recently. Joo et al. (2018) performed pioneer works on heterologous expression of PET-ase in *E. coli*, to evaluate the molecular mechanism of plastic degradation. The recombinant study by Seo et al. (2019) improved several problems encountered during PET-ase expression in the native bacterium. Expression of *Ideonella* origin PET-ase gene into *E. coli* BL21 (DE3)-T1R improved the structural stability and solubility of the enzyme. The natural secretion of the enzymes by *I. sakaiensis* was found to have a limitation as the PET polymers were unable to penetrate membranes of Gram-negative bacteria. The study evaluated the fusion of *E. coli* Sec-dependent signal peptides with PET-ase gene to express the enzyme extracellularly. This study also had overcome the loss of enzyme activity which is often reported in continuous secretory production of recombinant enzymes (Soe et al., 2019).

Isolation and recombinant study of the novel PET-ase from *I. sakaiensis* had drawn interest to find PETase-like genes. Almeida et al. (2019) performed a computational screening for PETase-like genes among marine origin actinobacterium isolates. A PETase-like gene labelled as SM14est was identified from a marine sponge-associated *Streptomyces* sp. The SM14est gene was expressed in *E. coli* to evaluate plastic-degrading capabilities.

Heterologous expression of the gene is not sufficient to solve plastic degradation problems. Gene editing is also required to alter the protein sequence of the enzymes to improve the catalytic activity of the enzymes. Genome editing tools including CRISPR and TALEN help to 'customize' the biosynthesis of desired enzymes and secondary metabolites in the bacterium (Purohit et al., 2020). A study by Friello et al. (2001) is among the earliest reports on genetic manipulation. The study demonstrated the hydrocarbon degradation of *Pseudomonas* strains was improved by the transfer of multiple degradative plasmids into a single culture. The gene edition enabled a single bacterium able to oxidize various hydrocarbons including aromatic, aliphatic, polyaromatics, and terpenoids (Friello et al., 2001). The genera *Pseudomonas* are extensively cited as plastic degraders. Thus, modification of the genes towards improved catalytic efficiency and stability on plastic degradation is a possible and promising approach. Although the *Ideonella* origin PET-ase is the most efficient enzyme described so far, it is still a slow process in the context of plastic degradation. Plastic is denser and has a high crystalline structure compared to PET or PE. The PET-ase degradation of plastics would be a very slow process. Therefore, extensive studies are required on protein engineering of plastic-degrading enzymes including the *Ideonella* origin PET-ase systems, to speed up the enzyme activity (Austin et al., 2018).

6.5.2 Effective Enzyme Tools Technology

Although numerous plastic-eating microorganisms and their respective recombinants had been reported frequently, the practical applications of their plastic-degrading enzymes still face several problems in terms of efficiency, stability, and productivity. Perturbation in the physical and chemical conditions at the treatment site often results in the loss of enzyme activity. Thus, efficient and practical enzyme tools are required to overcome this limitation. The enzyme immobilization technology involves a free or soluble attachment of enzymes to several types of support materials (Kumari et al., 2017; Nikolaivits et al., 2017). This will reduce the enzyme mobilization but has enhanced enzymatic activity and their stability, in turn. There are several different methods to immobilize enzymes into the supportive materials, including adsorption on alginate beads, affinity-tag binding, and covalently bound to a matrix or insoluble support like silica gel (Basso and Serban, 2019). Method of immobilization would have impacted the enzymatic properties; however, these methods should not affect the enzymatic activity. The use of immobilized enzymes is to allow for high recovery and reusability. The enzymatic activity of immobilized enzymes must be retained for a longer time period as compared to the free enzymes (Basso and Serban, 2019; Samak et al., 2020).

To date, immobilization of plastic-degrading enzymes is very limited. Hitherto immobilization of microbial cutinases with PET-hydrolysing abilities has been reported (Table 6.4). The major aim of immobilizing the cutinases was to enhance thermostability of PET-hydrolyses. High temperature as 70°C was found to enhance better degradation of PET as the high temperature favours easy accessibility of the ester bonds in the crystalline structures of PET (Austin et al., 2018). Microbial cutinases are immobilized on different types of immobilization matrixes including Fe_3O_4 nanoparticles, reduced or non-reduced graphene oxide nanosheets. A study by Nikolaivits et al. (2017) demonstrated immobilization of *Fusarium*-origin cutinase in

TABLE 6.4
Immobilization of PET-Hydrolysing Microbial Cutinase

Origin of Enzyme	Immobilization Method	Improvement of Catalytic Performance	Reference
Thermobifida fusca	Covalently bonded into SulfoLink™ coupling resins	Achieved 94% of activity at 60°C and pH of 8.	Barth et al. (2016)
Thermobifida cellulosilytica	Covalently bonded to Opal	Relative activity achieved at 57% at 21°C and pH of 7. Activity decreased to 42% after 24 h.	Pellis et al. (2017)
	Covalently bonded to Amber	Relative activity achieved at 78% at 21°C and pH of 7. Activity decreased to 58% after 24 h.	
	Covalently bonded to Coral	Relative activity achieved at 76% at 21°C and pH of 7. Activity decreased to 58% after 24 h.	
Aspergillus oryzae *Humicola insolens*	Physically bonded to weak-basic anion exchange resins (Lewatit VP OC 1065)	Achieved 100% of activity at 80°C and pH of 5–9. 100% of relative activity sustained for 1 h and decreased to 50% after 2 h.	Su et al. (2018)
Thielavia terrestris		77% of enzyme activity retained for 2 h at 80°C and pH of 5–9.	

cross-linked enzyme aggregates (CLEAs). Similarly, Barth et al. (2016) immobilized *Thermobifida fusca*-based cutinases on SulfoLink™ coupling resins. The immobilized cutinase systems demonstrated successful improvement over thermostability (Barth et al., 2016; Nikolaivits et al., 2017). Yet, the reported immobilized systems were mostly emphasizing the synthesis of the system rather than evaluating the PET-hydrolysis mechanisms (Su et al., 2018).

6.5.3 Plastic Substitute Materials

As the demand for synthetic plastics has not decreased as well as the concern on the significant impacts of accumulating plastic wastes, the bio-based plastic materials have been given much attention. These biodegradable plastics are made from various renewable biomasses such as starch, cellulose, chitosan, and protein. The biodegradable characteristic has drawn a positive impact and increased public awareness. About 50% of the available biodegradable plastic materials were starch-based materials. Starch is abundant and cheap polymer, extracted from various renewable sources such as roots and stalks of agricultural wastes (Marichelvam et al., 2019). In the last decades, numerous biodegradable plastic products were developed from different types of starches (Xie et al., 2014; Dai et al., 2015; Maulida and Tarigan, 2016; Edhirej et al., 2017). Starch is the best biopolymer with great potential and is extensively used in various fields including food and medicine packaging, agriculture, as well as in engineering. Starch-based membranes are used in food packaging for their good barrier properties against oxidations, besides the edible and good mechanical properties (Galgano et al., 2015). In agriculture and medical fields, starch-based biodegradable plastics are used for the controlled release of pesticides or drugs (Shafqat et al., 2020). Besides biodegradability and edible, starch-based plastic materials are also characterized as consumer acceptable biopolymers as it is odourless, non-toxic, and tasteless characteristics. However, starch-based bioplastics also had several disadvantages such as soft and poor mechanical properties, lower water vapour barriers, and low tolerance in freezing (Marichelvam et al., 2019; Shafqat et al., 2020). Various mechanisms such as physical, chemical, enzymatic, and genetic modification have been employed nowadays to improve the qualities of starch-based bioplastics (Khan et al., 2017).

Besides carbohydrate-polymers, poly(lactic acids) (PLA) also developed successfully as biodegradable plastic materials. PLA is made up of monomer lactic acid which is derived from the fermentation process of renewable carbohydrates (Jem and Tan, 2020; Yusoff et al., 2021). The PLA-based bioplastics have better durability, mechanical strength, and transparency. This thermo-polyester can be stretched into rigid films and can be used as thermoformed packaging materials (Lim et al., 2008; Jem and Tan, 2020). Another component that shares similar properties with PLA would be the poly(glycolic acid) (PGA). Both PLA and PGA have similar chemical structures and can be degraded quickly in the natural environment (Jem and Tan, 2020). The combination of both materials had improved the properties of PLA as it is well-known for poor heat stabilities and water barrier properties. The combination of PLA and PGA is investigated in various fields including medical, packaging, automobile engineering, and electronics (Takayama et al., 2014). However, large-scale production of PGA in a cost-effective way is still a major challenge. In a recent study, a combination of PLA with starch polymers was evaluated in the synthesis of bioplastics for packaging. The composite material had shown a significant improvement over tensile strength (Yusoff et al., 2021).

Although bioplastics are promising alternatives for conventional plastic materials, there are several challenging points that hindered the complete enforcement of this alternative. Major challenging point would be the production of bioplastics must not interfere with food sources. This challenge could be solved by utilizing agricultural wastes as renewable sources for biopolymers. However, processing agricultural wastes for polymer extractions could be more expensive and cost-effective methods are completely investigated (Mostafa et al., 2018). Recent trends had shown the demand for biodegradable plastics has raised significantly compared to conventional plastics. Assimilation of biodegradable plastics had been recognized as a promising solution for environmental pollution issues. Thus, sustainable production of biodegradable plastic materials requires further research to improve the manufacturing processes, reduce production costs, and enhance a healthy environment.

6.6 CONCLUSIONS

Biotechnology can offer many different approaches for the controlled management, utilization, and disposal of plastic wastes. The advances in biotechnology are creating exciting possibilities to design novel pathways to known biodegradable polymers. The areas of plastic waste management continue to pose significant challenges and offer opportunities for new research and discovery in the future. The environment provided a variety of source for plastic-degrading bacteria and enzymes. However, knowledge of the depolymerases involved in the breakdown of plastics is limited. Therefore, further investigation on biodegradation mechanism and identification of additional depolymerases from plastic-degrading microbes should be conducted in the future.

ACKNOWLEDGEMENT

The authors would like to thank Research Management Center at UTM, Malaysia, and Ministry of Higher Education, Malaysia, through Fundamental Research Grant Scheme (FRGS/1/2020/TK0/UTM/02/16) grant No. R.J130000.7851.5F339.

REFERENCES

Almeida, E. L., Carrillo Rincón, A.F., Jackson, S.A., and Dobson, A.D. 2019. In silico screening and heterologous expression of a polyethylene terephthalate hydrolase (PETase)-like enzyme (SM14est) with polycaprolactone (PCL)-degrading activity, from the marine sponge-derived strain *Streptomyces sp.* SM14. *Front. Microbiol.* 10: 2187.

Aganguly, S. 2018. Plastic pollution and its adverse impact on environment and ecosystem. In *International Conference on Recent Trends in Arts, Science, Engineering and Technology*.

Ariza-Tarazona, M. C., Villarreal-Chiu, J. F., Hernández-López, J. M., De la Rosa, J. R., Barbieri, V., Siligardi, C., and Cedillo-González, E. I. 2020. Microplastic pollution reduction by a carbon and nitrogen-doped TiO2: Effect of pH and temperature in the photocatalytic degradation process. *J. Hazard. Mater.* 395: 122632.

Austin, H.P., Allen, M.D., Donohoe, B.S., Rorrer, N.A., Kearns, F.L., Silveira, R.L., Pollard, B.C., Dominick, G., Duman, R., El Omari, K., and Mykhaylyk, V., 2018. Characterization and engineering of a plastic-degrading aromatic polyesterase. *Proc. Natl. Acad. Sci. U.S.A.* 115(19): E4350–E4357.

Auta, H. S., Emenike, C. U., Jayanthi, B., and Fauziah, S. H. 2018. Growth kinetics and biodeterioration of polypropylene microplastics by *Bacillus* sp. and *Rhodococcus* sp. isolated from mangrove sediment. *Mar. Pollut. Bull.* 127: 15–21.

Bae, S., Kim, J. H., Lim, Y.-H., Park, H. Y., and Hong, Y.-C. 2012. Associations of bisphenol A exposure with heart rate variability and blood pressure. *Hypertension* 60(3): 786–793.

Barth, M., Honak, A., Oeser, T., Wei, R., Belisário-Ferrari, M.R., Then, J., Schmidt, J., and Zimmermann, W. 2016. A dual enzyme system composed of a polyester hydrolase and a carboxylesterase enhances the biocatalytic degradation of polyethylene terephthalate films. *Biotechnol. J.* 11(8): 1082–1087.

Bassi, A. 2017. Biotechnology for the management of plastic wastes. In *Current Developments in Biotechnology and Bioengineering*. Elsevier, pp. 293–310.

Basso, A. and Serban, S., 2019. Industrial applications of immobilized enzymes—A review. *Mol. Catal.* 479: 110607.

Boulven, M., Quintard, G., Cottaz, A., Joly, C., Charlot, A., and Fleury, E. 2019. Homogeneous acylation of cellulose diacetate: Towards bioplastics with tuneable thermal and water transport properties. *Carbohydr. Polym.* 206: 674–684.

Brunner, I., Fischer, M., Rüthi, J., Stierli, B., and Frey, B. 2018. Ability of fungi isolated from plastic debris floating in the shoreline of a lake to degrade plastics. *PLoS One* 13(8): 0202047.

Chamas, A., Moon, H., Zheng, J., Qiu, Y., Tabassum, T., Jang, J.H., Abu-Omar, M., Scott, S.L., and Suh, S. 2020. Degradation rates of plastics in the environment. *ACS Sustain. Chem. Eng.* 8(9): 3494–3511.

Chen, H.L., Nath, T.K., Chong, S., Foo, V., Gibbins, C., and Lechner, A.M. 2021. The plastic waste problem in Malaysia: Management, recycling and disposal of local and global plastic waste. *SN Appl. Sci.* 3(4): 1–15.

Choi, M. S., Rehman, S. U., Kim, H., Han, S. B., Lee, J., Hong, J., and Yoo, H. H. 2017. Migration of epoxidized soybean oil from polyvinyl chloride/polyvinylidene chloride food packaging wraps into food simulants. *Environ. Sci. Pollut. Res.* 25(5): 5033–5039.

Dai, L., Qiu, C., Xiong, L., and Sun, Q. 2015. Characterisation of corn starch-based films reinforced with taro starch nanoparticles. *Food Chem.* 174: 82–88.

Delacuvellerie, A., Cyriaque, V., Gobert, S., Benali, S., and Wattiez, R. 2019. The plastisphere in marine ecosystem hosts potential specific microbial degraders including *Alcanivorax borkumensis* as a key player for the low-density polyethylene degradation. *J. Hazard. Mater.* 380: 120899.

Dussud, C. and JF, G. 2014. R63 Degradation of plastics at sea. Retrieved from French Society of Ecology (SFE).

Edhirej, A., Sapuan, S.M., Jawaid, M., and Zahari, N.I. 2017. Effect of various plasticizers and concentration on the physical, thermal, mechanical, and structural properties of cassava-starch-based films. *Starch-Stärke* 69(1–2): 1500366.

Friello, D.A., Mylroie, J.R., and Chakrabarty, A.M. 2001. Use of genetically engineered multi-plasmid microorganisms for rapid degradation of fuel hydrocarbons. *Int. Biodeterior. Biodegradation* 48(1–4): 233–242.

Galgano, F., Condeli, N., Favati, F., Di Bianco, V., Peretti, G., and Caruso, M.C. 2015. Biodegradable packaging and edible coating for fresh-cut fruits and vegetables. *Ital J Food Sci.* 27(1): 1–20.

Gewert, B., Plassmann, M., Sandblom, O., and MacLeod, M. 2018. Identification of chain scission products released to water by plastic exposed to ultraviolet light. *Environ. Sci. Technol. Lett.* 5: 272–276.

Geyer, R., Jambeck, J.R., and Law, K.L. 2017. Production, use, and fate of all plastics ever made. *Sci. Adv.* 3(7): 1700782.

Giacomucci, L., Raddadi, N., Soccio, M., Lotti, N., and Fava, F. 2019. Polyvinyl chloride biodegradation by *Pseudomonas citronellolis* and *Bacillus flexus*. *N. Biotechnol.* 52: 35–41.

Hahladakis, J. N., Velis, C. A., Weber, R., Iacovidou, E., and Purnell, P. 2018. An overview of chemical additives present in plastics: Migration, release, fate and environmental impact during their use, disposal and recycling. *J. Hazard. Mat.* 344: 179–199.

Han, Y. N., Wei, M., Han, F., Fang, C., Wang, D., Zhong, Y. J., and Li, F. M. 2020. Greater biofilm formation and increased biodegradation of polyethylene film by a microbial consortium of *Arthrobacter sp.* and *Streptomyces sp. Microorganisms* 8(12): 1–15.

Hirschberg, V., Schwab, L., Cziep, M., Wilhelm, M., and Rodrigue, D. 2018. Influence of molecular properties on the mechanical fatigue of polystyrene (PS) analyzed via Wöhler curves and Fourier Transform rheology. *Polymer* 138: 1–7.

Ho, B. T., Roberts, T. K., and Lucas, S. 2017. An overview on biodegradation of polystyrene and modified polystyrene: The microbial approach. *Crit. Rev. Biotechnol.* 38(2): 308–320.

Ho, N. H. E. and Not, C. 2019. Selective accumulation of plastic debris at the breaking wave area of coastal waters. *Environ. Pollut.* 245: 702–710.

Hosono, K., Kanazawa, A., Mori, H., and Endo, T., 2007. Photodegradation of cellulose acetate film in the presence of benzophenone as a photosensitizer. *J. Appl. Polym. Sci.* 105(6): 3235–3239.

Hosono, K., Kanazawa, A., Mori, H., and Endo, T., 2008. Enhanced degradation of cellulose acetate films in the copresence of triphenylsulfonium salt and benzophenone. *J. Appl. Polym. Sci.* 109(5): 3157–3164.

Huang, A., Peng, X., and Turng, L.-S. 2018. In-situ fibrillated polytetrafluoroethylene (PTFE) in thermoplastic polyurethane (TPU) via melt blending: Effect on rheological behavior, mechanical properties, and microcellular foamability. *Polymer.* 134: 263–274.

Jeon, H. J. and Kim, M. N. 2016. Isolation of mesophilic bacterium for biodegradation of polypropylene. *Int. Biodeterior. Biodegrad.* 115: 244–249.

Jem, K.J. and Tan, B., 2020. The development and challenges of poly (lactic acid) and poly (glycolic acid). *Polym. Adv. Technol.* 3(2): 60–70.

Joo, S., Cho, I.J., Seo, H., Son, H.F., Sagong, H.Y., Shin, T.J., Choi, S.Y., Lee, S.Y., and Kim, K.J., 2018. Structural insight into molecular mechanism of poly (ethylene terephthalate) degradation. *Nat. Commun.* 9(1): 1–12.

Kehinde, O., Ramonu, O.J., Babaremu, K.O., and Justin, L.D., 2020. Plastic wastes: Environmental hazard and instrument for wealth creation in Nigeria. *Heliyon* 6(10): 05131.

Khan, A. A., Mirza, E. H., Mohamed, B. A., Alharthi, N. H., Abdo, H. S., Javed, R., and Vallittu, P. K. 2018. Physical, mechanical, chemical and thermal properties of nanoscale graphene oxide-poly methylmethacrylate composites. *J. Compos. Mater.* 52(20): 2803–2813.

Khan, B., Bilal Khan Niazi, M., Samin, G., and Jahan, Z., 2017. Thermoplastic starch: A possible biodegradable food packaging material-a review. *J. Food Process Eng.* 40(3): 12447.

Khatoon, N., Jamal, A., and Ali, M. 2019. Lignin peroxidase isoenzyme: A novel approach to biodegrade the toxic synthetic polymer waste. *Environ. Technol.* 40: 1366–1375.

Kim, H. R., Lee, H. M., Yu, H. C., Jeon, E., Lee, S., Li, J., and Kim, D.-H. 2020. Biodegradation of polystyrene by *Pseudomonas* sp. Isolated from the Gut of Superworms (Larvae of *Zophobas atratus*). *Environ. Sci. Technol.* 54(11): 6987–6996.

Konieczna, A., Rutkowska, A., and Rachon, D. (2015). Health risk of exposure to Bisphenol A (BPA). *Roczniki Państwowego Zakładu Higieny*, 66(1).

Kowalczyk, A., Chyc, M., Ryszka, P., and Latowski, D. 2016. *Achromobacter xylosoxidans* as a new microorganism strain colonizing high-density polyethylene as a key step to its biodegradation. *Environ. Sci. Pollut. Res. Int.* 23(11): 11349–11356.

Kumari, A., Chaudhary, D. R., and Jha, B. 2018. Destabilization of polyethylene and polyvinylchloride structure by marine bacterial strain. *Environ. Sci. Pollut. Res. Int.* 26(2): 1507–1516.

Kumari, V., Kumar, S., Kaur, I., and Bhalla, T.C., 2017. Graft copolymerization of acrylamide on chitosan-co-chitin and its application for immobilization of *Aspergillus sp.* RL2Ct cutinase. *Bioorg. Chem.* 70: 34–43.

Lee, A.H., Kang, C.M., Lee, Y.M., Lee, H., Yun, C.W., Kim, G.H., and Kim, J.J., 2016. Heterologous expression of a new manganese-dependent peroxidase gene from *Peniophora incarnata* KUC8836 and its ability to remove anthracene in *Saccharomyces cerevisiae*. *J. Biosci. Bioeng.* 122(6): 716–721.

Liang, M., Xin, X., Fan, W., Zhang, J., Jiang, H., and Yao, Z. 2019. Comparison of rheological properties and compatibility of asphalt modified with various polyethylene. *Int. J. Pavement Eng.* 22(1): 11–20.

Lim, L.T., Auras, R. and Rubino, M., 2008. Processing technologies for poly (lactic acid). *Prog. Polym. Sci.* 33(8): 820–852.

Lo Piccolo, L., De Pasquale, C., Fodale, R., Puglia, A.M., and Quatrini, P., 2011. Involvement of an alkane hydroxylase system of *Gordonia sp.* strain SoCg in degradation of solid n-alkanes. *Appl. Environ. Microbiol.* 77(4): 1204–1213.

Lu, B., Wang, G. X., Huang, D., Ren, Z. L., Wang, X. W., Wang, P. L., and Ji, J. H. 2018. Comparison of PCL degradation in different aquatic environments: Effects of bacteria and inorganic salts. *Polym. Degrad. Stab.* 150, 133–139.

Lucas, N., Bienaime, C., Belloy, C., Queneudec, M., Silvestre, F., and Nava-Saucedo, J. E. 2008. Polymer biodegradation: Mechanisms and estimation techniques - A review. *Chemosphere* 73(4): 429–442.

Magnin, A., Hoornaert, L., Pollet, E., Laurichesse, S., Phalip, V., and Avérous, L. 2019. Isolation and characterization of different promising fungi for biological waste management of polyurethanes. *Microb Biotechnol.* 12(3): 544–555.

Marichelvam, M.K., Jawaid, M., and Asim, M., 2019. Corn and rice starch-based bio-plastics as alternative packaging materials. *Fibers* 7(4): 32.

Marion, G. M., Millero, F. J., Camões, M. F., Spitzer, P., Feistel, R., and Chen, C. T. 2011. pH of seawater. *Mar. Chem.* 126(1–4): 89–96.

Martin, R. T., Camargo, L. P., and Miller, S. A. 2014. Marine-degradable polylactic acid. *Green Chem.* 16(4): 1768–1773.

Maulida, M.S. and Tarigan, P., 2016. Production of starch based bioplastic from cassava peel reinforced with microcrystalline celllulose avicel PH101 using sorbitol as plasticizer. *In J. Phys. Conf. Ser.* 710: 12012.

Maurya, A., Bhattacharya, A., and Khare, S.K., 2020. Enzymatic remediation of polyethylene terephthalate (PET)–based polymers for effective management of plastic wastes: An overview. *Front. Bioeng. Biotechnol.* 8: 1332.

Min, K., Cuiffi, J. D., and Mathers, R. T. 2020. Ranking environmental degradation trends of plastic marine debris based on physical properties and molecular structure. *Nat. Commun.* 11(1): 1–11.

Montazer, Z., Habibi-Najafi, M. B., Mohebbi, M., and Oromiehei, A. 2018. Microbial degradation of UV-pretreated low-density polyethylene films by novel polyethylene-degrading bacteria isolated from plastic-dump soil. *J. Polym. Environ.* 26(9): 3613–3625.

Mostafa, N.A., Farag, A.A., Abo-dief, H.M., and Tayeb, A.M., 2018. Production of biodegradable plastic from agricultural wastes. *Arab. J. Chem.* 11(4): 546–553.

Munir, E., Harefa, R. S. M., Priyani, N., and Suryanto, D. 2018. Plastic degrading fungi *Trichoderma viride* and *Aspergillus nomius* isolated from local landfill soil in Medan. In *IOP Conference Series: Earth and Environmental Science*, IOP Publishing. Vol. 126, No. 1, p. 012145.

Murali, M and Umamaheswari, S. 2019. Potential of soil microbes in degrading polystyrene foam. *Int. J. Adv. Sci. Res. Manag.* 4(4):109–117.

Muthukumar, A. and Veerappapillai, S., 2015. Biodegradation of plastics: A brief review. *Int. J. Pharm. Sci. Rev. Res.* 31(2): 204–209.

Ncube, L.K., Ude, A.U., Ogunmuyiwa, E.N., Zulkifli, R., and Beas, I.N., 2021. An overview of plastic waste generation and management in food packaging industries. *Recycling*, 6(1): 12.

Neis, P. D., Ferreira, N. F., Poletto, J. C., Sukumaran, J., Andó, M., and Zhang, Y. 2017. Tribological behavior of polyamide-6 plastics and their potential use in industrial applications. *Wear*, 376–377: 1391–1398.

Nikolaivits, E., Makris, G., and Topakas, E., 2017. Immobilization of a cutinase from *Fusarium oxysporum* and application in pineapple flavor synthesis. *J. Agric. Food Chem.* 65(17): 3505–3511.

Ohore, O. E., and Zhang, S. (2019). Endocrine disrupting effects of bisphenol A exposure and recent advances on its removal by water treatment systems. A review. *Scientific African*, 5, e00135.

Olivera, S., Muralidhara, H. B., Venkatesh, K., Gopalakrishna, K., and Vivek, C. S. 2016. Plating on acrylonitrile–butadiene–styrene (ABS) plastic: A review. *J. Mater. Sci.* 51(8): 3657–3674.

Pavani, P. and Rajeswari, T.R. 2014. Impact of plastics on environmental pollution. *J. Chem. Pharm. Sci.* 3: 87–93.

Paço, A., Jacinto, J., da Costa, J.P., Santos, P.S., Vitorino, R., Duarte, A.C., and Rocha-Santos, T., 2019. Biotechnological tools for the effective management of plastics in the environment. *Crit. Rev. Environ. Sci. Technol.* 49(5): 410–441.

Padhan, R. K. and Sreeram, A. 2018. Enhancement of storage stability and rheological properties of polyethylene (PE) modified asphalt using cross linking and reactive polymer based additives. *Constr. Build Mater.* 188: 772–780.

Pellis, A., Vastano, M., Quartinello, F., Herrero Acero, E., and Guebitz, G.M. 2017. His-tag immobilization of Cutinase 1 From *Thermobifida cellulosilytica* for solvent-free synthesis of polyesters. *Biotechnol. J.* 12(10): 1700322.

Purohit, J., Chattopadhyay, A., and Teli, B., 2020. Metagenomic exploration of plastic degrading microbes for biotechnological application. *Curr. Genomics.* 21(4): 253–270.

Ranjan, V. P. and Goel, S. 2019. Degradation of Low-density polyethylene film exposed to UV radiation in four environments. *J. Hazard. Toxic Radioact. Waste* 23(4): 04019015.

Ru, J., Huo, Y., and Yang, Y. 2020. Microbial Degradation and Valorization of Plastic Wastes. *Front. Microbiol.* 11: 1–20.

Samak, N.A., Jia, Y., Sharshar, M.M., Mu, T., Yang, M., Peh, S., and Xing, J. 2020. Recent advances in biocatalysts engineering for polyethylene terephthalate plastic waste green recycling. *Environ. Int.* 145: 106144.

Sarmah, P. and Rout, J. 2018. Efficient biodegradation of low-density polyethylene by cyanobacteria isolated from submerged polyethylene surface in domestic sewage water. *Environ. Sci. Pollut. Res Int.* 25(33): 33508–33520.

Shah, A. A., Hasan, F., Hameed, A., and Ahmed, S. 2008. Biological degradation of plastics: A comprehensive review. *Biotechnol. Adv.* 26(3): 246–265.

Shah, Z., Krumholz, L., Aktas, D. F., Hasan, F., Khattak, M., and Shah, A. A. 2013. Degradation of polyester polyurethane by a newly isolated soil bacterium, *Bacillus subtilis* strain MZA-75. *Biodegradation* 24(6): 865–77.

Seo, H., Kim, S., Son, H.F., Sagong, H.Y., Joo, S., and Kim, K.J. 2019. Production of extracellular PETase from *Ideonella sakaiensis* using sec-dependent signal peptides in *E. coli. Biochem. Biophys. Res. Commun.* 508(1): 250–255.

Shafqat, A., Tahir, A., Mahmood, A., Tabinda, A.B., Yasar, A., and Pugazhendhi, A. 2020. A review on environmental significance carbon foot prints of starch based bio-plastic: A substitute of conventional plastics. *Biocatal. Agric. Biotechnol.* 27: 101540.

Shanmugam, V., Das, O., Neisiany, R.E., Babu, K., Singh, S., Hedenqvist, M.S., Berto, F., and Ramakrishna, S. 2020. Polymer recycling in additive manufacturing: An opportunity for the circular economy. *Mater. Circ. Econ.* 2(1): 1–11.

Stepien, A. E., Zebrowski, J., Piszczyk, Ł., Boyko, V. V., Riabov, S. V., Dmitrieva, T., and Ryszkowska, J. 2017. Assessment of the impact of bacteria *Pseudomonas denitrificans, Pseudomonas fluorescens, Bacillus subtilis* and yeast *Yarrowia lipolytica* on commercial poly (ether urethanes). *Polym. Test.* 63: 484–493.

Su, A., Shirke, A., Baik, J., Zou, Y., and Gross, R. 2018. Immobilized cutinases: Preparation, solvent tolerance and thermal stability. *Enzyme Microb. Technol.* 116: 33–40.

Suits, L. D. and Hsuan, Y. G. 2003. Assessing the photo-degradation of geosynthetics by outdoor exposure and laboratory weatherometer. *Geotext. Geomembr.* 21(2): 111–122.

Takayama, T., Daigaku, Y., Ito, H., and Takamori, H. 2014. Mechanical properties of bioabsorbable PLA/PGA fiber-reinforced composites. *J. Mech. Sci. Technol.* 28(10): 4151–4154.

Thompson, R.C., Moore, C.J., Vom Saal, F.S., and Swan, S.H. 2009. Plastics, the environment and human health: Current consensus and future trends. *Philos. Trans. R. Soc. Lond., B, Biol. Sci.* 364(1526): 2153–2166.

Thushari, G. G. N. and Senevirathna, J. D. M. 2020. Plastic pollution in the marine environment. *Heliyon* 6(8): 04709.

Tu, C., Chen, T., Zhou, Q., Liu, Y., Wei, J., Waniek, J. J., and Luo, Y. 2020. Biofilm formation and its influences on the properties of microplastics as affected by exposure time and depth in the seawater. *Sci. Total Environ.* 734: 139237.

Venkatesh, S., Mahboob, S., Govindarajan, M., Al-Ghanim, K.A., Ahmed, Z., Al-Mulhm, N., Gayathri, R., and Vijayalakshmi, S. 2021. Microbial degradation of plastics: A sustainable approach to tackling environmental threats facing big cities of the future. *J. King Saud. Univ. Sci.* 33: 101362.

Wang, J., Dai, Q., Si, R., and Guo, S. 2019. Mechanical, durability, and microstructural properties of macro synthetic Polypropylene (PP) fiber-reinforced rubber concrete. *J. Clean. Prod.* 234: 1351–1364.

Wang, Z., Xin, X., Shi, X., and Zhang, Y. 2020. A polystyrene-degrading *Acinetobacter* bacterium isolated from the larvae of *Tribolium castaneum*. *Sci. Total Environ.* 726: 138564.

Xie, F., Flanagan, B.M., Li, M., Sangwan, P., Truss, R.W., Halley, P.J., Strounina, E.V., Whittaker, A.K., Gidley, M.J., Dean, K.M., and Shamshina, J.L. 2014. Characteristics of starch-based films plasticised by glycerol and by the ionic liquid 1-ethyl-3-methylimidazolium acetate: A comparative study. *Carbohydr. Polym.* 111: 841–848.

Xu, F., Wang, B., Yang, D., Hao, J., Qiao, Y., and Tian, Y. 2018. Thermal degradation of typical plastics under high heating rate conditions by TG-FTIR: Pyrolysis behaviors and kinetic analysis. *Energy Convers. Manag.* 171: 1106–1115.

Yadav, N. and Hakkarainen, M. 2020. Degradable or not? Cellulose acetate as a model for complicated interplay between structure, environment and degradation. *Chemosphere* 265: 128731.

Yi, C., Li, W., Shi, S., He, K., Ma, P., Chen, M., and Yang, C. 2020. High-temperature-resistant and colorless polyimide: Preparations, properties, and applications. *Solar Energy* 195: 340–354.

Yoon, M.G., Jeon, H.J., and Kim, M.N. 2012. Biodegradation of polyethylene by a soil bacterium and AlkB cloned recombinant cell. *J. Bioremed. Biodegrad.* 3(4): 1–8.

Yusoff, N.H., Pal, K., Narayanan, T., and de Souza, F.G. 2021. Recent trends on bioplastics synthesis and characterizations: Polylactic acid (PLA) incorporated with tapioca starch for packaging applications. *J. Mol. Struct.* 1232: 129954.

Zaman, A. and Newman, P. 2021. Plastics: Are they part of the zero-waste agenda or the toxic-waste agenda? *Sustain. Earth* 4(1): 1–16.

Zhu, K., Jia, H., Sun, Y., Dai, Y., Zhang, C., Guo, X., and Zhu, L. 2020. Long-term phototransformation of microplastics under simulated sunlight irradiation in aquatic environments: Roles of reactive oxygen species. *Water Res.* 173: 115564.

7 Production of Biopolymer from Waste Materials as the Suitable Alternative for Plastics

Rohaida Che Man, Nur Nadia Binti Mohd Zakaria, and Nurul Nabila Huda Baharudin
Universiti Malaysia Pahang

CONTENTS

DOI: 10.1201/9781003188292-7

7.1 INTRODUCTION

An increase in the use of plastic materials, especially in industry and domestic purposes, has outpaced global production, imposing serious problems such as toxicity to human health, environmental contamination, and disposal process (Li and Wilkins, 2020). Plastics comprise a huge portion of landfill waste. They are also classified as hazardous contaminants that substantially impact the environment due to extensive spreading, non-biodegradability, and high concentration. Presently, the severe accumulation of waste from synthetic plastic has contributed to serious pollution problems. These conditions led to strict rules on the management of landfill waste, recycling procedure, and the reusability of materials, thus the suggestion for the application of bioplastic for daily use was raised (Kourmentza et al., 2017).

The polyhydroxyalkanoates (PHA) as a promising eco-friendly biopolymer have garnered more attention to replace synthetic plastics for daily use (Sohn et al., 2020). This is due to its biocompatibility, good thermal stability, nontoxicity, and biodegradability. These promising characteristics of PHA prompt its use in a wide variety of applications such as in electronics, biomedical devices, automotive, packaging, agricultural sectors, and construction (Anjum et al., 2016; Sirohi et al., 2020a).

PHA is a macromolecular biopolymer produced by pure isolated microorganisms and genetically modified microorganisms, which use this compound as an energy and carbon store (Alias and Tan, 2005). Even though PHA can significantly reduce the environmental problem, the global market of PHA is still small (Aeschelmann and Carus, 2015). The production of PHA at large scale still faces problems due to the high production cost of PHA compared to synthetic plastics. Recently, the commercial price of PHA and polypropylene plastic is about €2.2–5.0/kg and €1.0/kg, respectively (Ong et al., 2018). Substrates such as fatty acids and sugars play a significant role in the production of biopolymer, making up around 50% of the final cost. Therefore, cheaper and broadly accessible substrates need to be used in the production of biopolymer, and the process must give high total yield and productivity.

The synthesis of PHA by microbes has gained attention in the global view due to its unique characteristics. It can be produced by subjecting certain bacteria to an excess of carbon sources and limited nutritional starvation such as nitrogen, oxygen, and phosphorous (Le Meur et al., 2012). More than 30% of bacteria living in soil and sludge in extreme conditions could produce PHA polymers (Chen, 2010). Different microorganisms would synthesize different amounts and sizes of PHA (Choi et al., 2020).

Gram-positive and Gram-negative bacteria produce PHA in their cytoplasm under an excess of carbon source, severe environmental conditions, and limited nutritional sources. These important parameters are considered in cost-competitive PHA production. The carbon sources affect cell metabolism, cell growth, productivity, and biopolymer characteristics (Saratale et al. 2021; Favaro et al., 2019). Many factors need to be taken into consideration for effective and sustainable synthesis of PHA, such as cost, availability of feedstock with suitable composition, transportation, storage, and more significantly there must be no competition with feed and food.

Poly-3-hydroxybutyrate (PHB) is another type of biopolymer produced by starch or glucose metabolizing microorganisms (Sirohi et al., 2020b). PHB is also a promising biopolymer for the substitution of synthetic plastics and could reduce the pollution problem. Nevertheless, the cost for the synthesis of PHB is high, making it less attractive for use as a commercial biopolymer. To overcome this limitation, many investigators proposed using cheaper substrates and energy-efficient processes to produce PHB. Therefore, fruit waste is recommended to be processed and fermented to efficiently generate PHB.

Alginates, β-glucans, cellulose, and xanthan are also among the popular biopolymers produced by microorganisms. The availability of renewable and inexpensive carbon sources such as milk waste, sugarcane molasses, glycerol, and fruit wastes can be exploited in the synthesis of biopolymer.

PHA is used in a wide variety of applications. Because of its good biocompatibility, PHA can be used in the medical industry. It is non-carcinogenic and can support the development of a wide range of tissues and organs. PHA materials have a lot of capability as medical implant tools, for example as anti-adhesion membranes, surgical sutures, and various stents applied in medical procedures, including heart valve scaffold and vessel stent (Sodian et al., 2000; Ray and Kalia, 2017). PHA can also be used to load drugs into a variety of forms, including gels, microspheres, nanoparticles, and porous scaffolds (Nigmatullin et al., 2015). PHA has also attracted the attention of researchers as a biodegradable carrier for controlled and targeted release of medication and hormone (Li et al., 2018).

The use of a PHA biopolymer combined with antimicrobial materials could lead to the development of new versatile nanocomposites with noticeable antibacterial activity and needed small nanoparticle concentrations. PHB/chitosan nanofiber was developed by some researchers and was efficiently used in wound dressing and cartilage tissue engineering (Sadeghi et al., 2016). PHB/chitosan was combined with a polyvinylidene fluoride (PVDF) nanofibrous membrane containing antibacterial drugs as wound dressing in another study (Amini et al., 2019).

Because of its mechanical strength, biocompatibility, nontoxicity, and significant elasticity, PHB can be employed broadly as a drug transporter. Peng et al. (2012) produced PHB/PEG nanoparticles for the immobilization of insulin and its release, which could be a realistic selection in the future and opens up new methods to treat diabetes. Using PHB cast films, Sabarinathan et al. (2018) studied the key results for cancer cell diagnosis. They discovered that cancer cells adhered effectively to PHB on the sheet, while normal cells did not. In comparison to a biopsy, which is time-consuming and excruciating, this could be a viable alternative for cancer detection. PHA nanofiber scaffold was studied for the germination of neural stem cells, artificial blood vessels, and heart valves by several researchers (Zaharia et al., 2014; Wang et al., 2010). PHA could be a better choice for stimulating spinal cord repair due to its porous structure (Novikova et al., 2008). Table 7.1 shows other applications of different types of biopolymers in various industries.

This chapter highlights the current progress in addressing the production of PHA by utilizing various cheap waste materials generated from multiple sources. This review also discusses the fermentation process and the optimization of process parameters for cost-effective and eco-friendly biopolymer production. Applications of biopolymer in industries are included as well. Moreover, limitations and future prospects of eco-friendly and cost-effective biopolymer production are addressed.

TABLE 7.1
Application of Different Type of Biopolymers in Various Industries

Biopolymer	Application	References
PHA and PHB	Medical implants	Udayakumar et al. (2021); Bhatt and Jaffe (2015)
PHA and PHB	Food packaging materials	Fabra et al., (2014); Rhim and Ng (2007)
Alginate films crosslinked with cerium (III) and chitosan	Wound healing material	Kaygusuz et al. (2017)
Poly lactic acid (PLA), poly glycolic acid (PGA), poly caprolactone (PCL)	Tissue engineering	Okamoto and John (2013)
Dextrin	Drug delivery system	Das and Pal (2015)
PHA	Source of biofuels	Reddy et al. (2003)
[R]-3-hydroxyalkanoates,	Antimicrobial agents	Chen and Wu (2005)

7.2 ADVANTAGES AND DISADVANTAGES OF BIOPOLYMERS

Biopolymers have identical properties to synthetic plastics, except that they can be produced from inexpensive and renewable resources. Biopolymers are biodegradable and biocompatible and can be totally degraded into safe cycles (Jendrossek and Handrick, 2002; Israni et al., 2020). Biopolymers can also be degraded quickly by microorganisms in the soil, which is an advantage in terms of economic and ecological performance (Gobi and Vadivelu, 2013). In comparison, the duration cycle of synthetic plastics in soil is about 100–200 years. Life cycle assessment proved that biopolymers have great returns compared to synthetic plastics, especially with the use of substrates from ecological and natural waste.

Nevertheless, the rise in industries related to biopolymer production has posed major problems, because PHA is being produced using edible substrates such as food crops, vegetable oils, and purified sugars, which creates competition between the usage of substrate for biopolymer production and food supply. Moreover, about 50% of the overall production cost is just for carbon sources. One of the challenging problems in the commercialization of biopolymers is the high production cost compared with synthetic plastics. With all these factors considered, there is a crucial need to develop a sustainable biopolymer production process using biomass waste as a carbon source (Kourmentza et al., 2017; Sirohi et al., 2020a).

7.3 WASTE MATERIALS FOR BIOPOLYMER PRODUCTION

Figure 7.1 shows the waste materials such as lipid and oil waste, spent coffee waste, glycerol, and sugarcane molasses that can be used for biopolymer production.

7.3.1 Lipid and Oil Wastes

Plant oils, when used as a carbon source, have the advantage of giving a high biopolymer production yield at low price. The main compound in plant oils is triacylglycerols

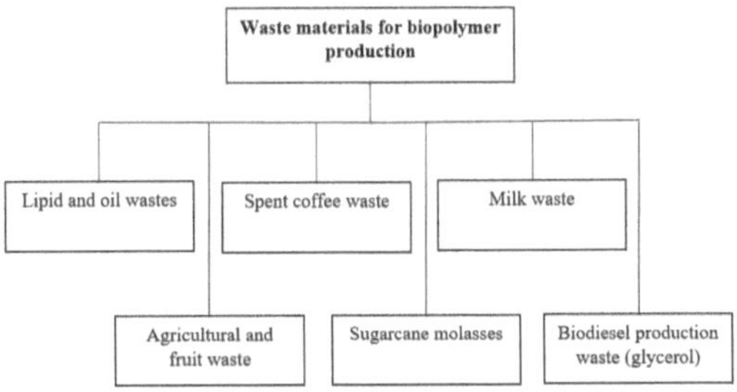

FIGURE 7.1 Waste materials for biopolymer production.

(TAG). In a bioreactor, the lipases secreted by microorganisms hydrolyzed TAG into fatty acids, which are further converted into PHA via the β-oxidation pathway (Talan et al., 2020). Food processing plants, oil mills, slaughterhouses, and edible oil industry produce large amounts of lipid wastes (Jiang et al., 2016). The cheap oily wastes are practical options for a substrate in PHA production to reduce production costs and to maintain the eco-friendliness of the process.

Saturated fatty acids (SFAs) in solid form are found in high quantities in waste animal fats and they have high melting temperature. Inexpensive waste animal fats can be used for PHA production through microbes, although it does present some challenges such as its high melting temperature, which necessitates some pre-treatment and pre-emulsification with gum Arabic (0.5% w/v) (Riedel et al., 2015).

It is not necessary to pre-treat the oil waste before it is used in PHA production, regardless of its origin, whether from households or industries. The production of PHA using *Pseudomonas* sp. and *Cupriavidus necator* was performed using the wastes from corn oil, frying palm oil, frying sunflower oil, and rapeseed oil. The reported range of PHA productivity was between 35% and 68% cell density weight (CDW) (Obruca et al., 2015). Sangkharak et al. (Sangkharak and Prasertsan, 2013) utilized waste cooking oil for the synthesis of PHA with 87% CDW by using *Bacillus thermoamylovorans.* Furthermore, the production of PHA by utilizing rapeseed oil with the addition of propanol and *Cupriavidus necator* H16 resulted in 80% CDW (Obruca et al., 2010). A study conducted by Borrero-de Acuña et al. (2019) showed that cultivating the recombinant *P. putida* KT2440, which has had its tctA gene knocked out, is responsible for encoding the major enzyme in the carboxylic acids transport system, on vegetable oil for 72h, resulted in a PHA yield of 1.91 g/L. The volumetric yield of the recombinant *P. putida* KT2440 was almost two times higher compared to the wild-type strain. Nine different *Halomonas* strains were able to produce PHA when using wastes from sunflower oil and frying oil-rapeseed as the substrates (Pernicova et al., 2019). *Halomonas hydrothermalis* showed the highest synthesis of PHB up to 62% CDW.

7.3.2 Milk Waste

In the process of making casein and cheese, a large amount of whey is produced, about 95% of the total amount of processed milk (Koller, 2018). The main compounds in whey are proteins, lactic acid, and lactose. Whey is also extensively used for human and animal feed as well as for pharmaceutical products. However, the management of milk waste is challenging because of its high BOD and COD values.

The production of PHB using *Methylobacterium* sp. strain and whey was 67% when the optimum nitrogen source was applied (Nath et al., 2008). During cultivation, an extreme halophilic microorganism, *Haloferax mediterranei* grows in normal sterile environment. This strain of *Methylobacterium* sp. can be used as the most suitable strain for PHA production by direct usage of whey (Pais et al., 2014). A research performed by Obruca et al. (2011) showed that the highest production of PHB was 1.05 g/L using *B. megaterium* CCM 2037 and cheese whey as a substrate. Interestingly, the production of PHB increased up to 1.48 g/L when 1% ethanol was supplied as a stressing agent.

Pre-treatment process is essential to effectively utilize whey. Whey can be hydrolyzed effectively under harsh chemical pre-treatment, especially when using strong acids, but that would necessitate further processing before proceeding for PHA production. The enzymatic hydrolysis approach is an efficient and effective alternative to overcome this difficulty. Therefore, the development of β-galactosidase formulation is needed for the conversion of whey lactose to its monosaccharides, and it can also operate under modest pH and temperature (M Koller et al., 2016).

7.3.3 Sugarcane Molasses

Molasses contains high amount of sucrose and low quantity of glucose, vitamins, fructose, and trace elements (Raza, Abid, and Banat, 2018). It has been extensively utilized as a suitable substrate for yeast fermentation to produce value-added products and liquid biofuels. PHA production by *Azotobacter vinelandii* using sugarcane molasses with a PHA yield of 7.8 g/L was detected (Page, 1992). Moreover, by using *R. eutropha* and sugarcane molasses hydrolysates (pre-treated with acid), about 11.1 g/L of PHA was produced (Yu and Stahl, 2008). Many *Bacillus* sp. strains were explored for the production of PHA from molasses (Park et al., 2013). Albuquerque et al. (Albuquerque and Malafaia, 2018) showed that, by using the combination of mixed culture and sugarcane molasses, the production of different organic acids was detected, whereby the presence of organic acids affected the PHA production. This correlation is important for producing PHA using sugarcane molasses at commercial scale. To effectively used molasses (sucrose) as a substrate, contaminants such as inorganic salts and polyphenols must be eliminated because they could affect microbial growth. The elimination of contaminants could be achieved using ceramic nanofiltration and ultrafiltration membranes (Sjölin et al., 2020).

7.3.4 Agricultural and Fruit Waste

Apple waste could be used as a suitable substrate to produce biopolymer. It is composed of cellulose, hemicellulose, fermentable sugars (e.g. glucose, galactose, arabinose, fructose, and sucrose), pectin, and lignin (Cargnin and Gnoatto, 2017). High amounts of fibers, polyphenols, and carbohydrates are also found in apple waste (Liu et al., 2021). The advantages of using this residue include the waste conversion to a biodegradable biopolymer and waste management process. This will lower the

TABLE 7.2
PHA Yield by Using Different Microorganisms and Substrates

Microorganism	PHA Yield (g/L)	Substrate	Fermentation Type	Reference
Pseudomonas chlororaphis	49.25	Apple waste	Bioreactor at temperature 30°C and pH 7	Pereira et al. (2021)
Pseudomonas citronellolis	1.20	Apple waste	Bioreactor at temperature 30°C and pH 7	Rebocho et al. (2019)
Pseudomonas resinovorans	1.4	Apricot waste	Bioreactor at temperature 30°C and pH 6.9	Follonier et al. (2014)
P. putida KT2440	5.8	White grapes pomace	2-step fermentation at temperature 30°C and pH 6.85	Follonier et al. (2015)
Defined mixed culture of *Bacillus* spp.	0.1	Hydrolysates pea shells and potato peels	Shake flask at temperature 37°C and 200 rev/min	Kumar et al. (2016)

overall cost of the process. Around 30%–35% of the mass of a raw apple ends up as apple waste after the apple is consumed or processed (Povolo et al., 2010). The waste contains the peels, seeds, and core. The waste is usually used as animal feed and organic fertilizer. In industrial microbiology, the high content of fermentable sugars is usually utilized as a carbon source to produce value-added products (Pratto et al., 2016). In this context, apple waste can be used as an inexpensive carbon feedstock for the production of eco-friendly bioplastics (Pereira et al., 2021).

Winemaking leaves about 60% of the mass of raw grapes as solid wastes, consisting of grape seeds and skin. Usually, the solid grape wastes are utilized as animal feed. It is suitable for use as a carbon substrate because of its high concentration of fructose and glucose. Research performed by Kovalcic et al. (2018) showed that the production of PHB using *C. necator* H16 and sugar extracted from saccharified grape waste and the grape seeds oil was 5.2 g/L. Table 7.2 shows the PHA yield when using different microorganisms and substrates.

Lignin, hemicellulose, and cellulose are the major compounds in lignocellulosic materials. Examples of lignocellulosic agricultural wastes are bagasse, rice straw, wheat straw, and wheat bran. Lignocellulosic wastes contain low amount of carbohydrates compared to other substrates. Generally, carbohydrates are used for the accumulation of glycogen in activated sludge systems instead of for PHA accumulation (Jiang et al., 2009). The disadvantage of using lignocellulosic waste as a substrate is the enzymatic pre-treatment required to hydrolyze the waste before converting it into simple sugars. Moreover, a detoxification process is also required to remove inhibitory compounds generated during the hydrolysis process (Obruca et al., 2015). Taken together, the pre-treatment and detoxification steps pose some challenges to the PHA production process such as imposing environmental problems, increasing the total production cost, and adding difficulty to the process. In order to overcome these limitations, lignocellulosic pre-treatment through the hydrothermal technique has been effectively carried out (Yin et al., 2019). Hydrothermal technique through hot water pre-treatment is environmentally friendly, inexpensive, and requires no chemical reagents.

Waste paper from municipal solid waste contains a large amount of lignocellulosic biomass. *Burkholderia sacchari* was cultivated with waste paper hydrolysate for the production of PHB, and around 44% of PHB was detected (Al-Battashi et al., 2019). Meanwhile, about 63% of PHB accumulation was obtained by using the recombinant *Ralstonia eutropha* NCIMB and wheat bran hydrolysate that was pre-treated with alkali (Annamalai and Sivakumar, 2016).

Lignin is an abundant aromatic polymer of biological origin that is readily available and suitable for use as feedstock. The monomer composition of lignin differs depending on its plant of origin. Centrifugation is used to separate the PHA (produced intracellularly) from lignin waste. The microorganisms *Ralstonia* sp. and *Bacillus* sp. are also used for the production of PHA using lignin as a substrate (Chen and Wan, 2017). Some investigators used lignin waste as a substrate for PHA production. Liu et al. (Liu et al., 2017) detected PHA with a yield of 1.0 g/L when utilizing lignin waste as a carbon source. Some researchers suggested a combination of chemical catalysis process and PHA production to improve the lignin valorization. First, the lignin waste was used to produce PHA. Then, the PHA was transformed to hydrocarbons and alkenoic acid, which are precursors of many important chemicals by catalytic reaction (Linger et al., 2014).

7.3.5 Spent Coffee Waste

A substantial amount of lipids and sugars (e.g. galactose, proteins, and mannose) could be found in spent coffee (Saratale et al., 2020). Using spent coffee oil as a carbon substrate is a good option to reduce the cost of biopolymer production. Obruca et al. (2014) synthesized 10 g/L of PHB by using *C. necator* H16 with spent coffee oil as a carbon source. Moreover, a study conducted by Bhatia et al. (2018) on PHA production showed that about 78 mol% with 69% of dry cell weight was obtained using a modified strain of *R. eutropha* and coffee waste oil as a substrate. Moreover, the production of PHA increased by 25% when using a combination of *Bacillus megaterium* and *Burkholderia cepacia* with the utilization of spent coffee ground hydrolysates (Obruca et al., 2015).

The oil content in coffee grounds is estimated at around 7%–15% (Karmee, 2018). The remainder includes lignocellulosic materials that are used as a substrate for biopolymer or energy production (through combustion) (Nielsen et al., 2017) with regard to its high carbon density (Atabani et al., 2019). Obruca et al. (2014) preferred utilizing the oil extracted from spent coffee grounds over other waste frying oils such as sunflower oil, palm oil, and rapeseed oil. The highest production of PHB was detected at around 49 g/L using the microorganism *Cupriavidus necator* as a result of the large amount of free fatty acids. Furthermore, spent coffee grounds hydrolysate was also utilized for the production of PHA by using a mixture of *Bacillus megaterium* and *Burkholderia cepacia* (Obruca et al., 2014). A study performed by Kovalcik et al. (2018) showed that PHB biopolymer was detected at 27% (wt/wt) as produced by *Halomonas halophila* with spent coffee grounds hydrolysate as a cheap carbon source.

7.3.6 Biodiesel Production Waste (Glycerol)

Crude glycerol is a significant by-product of the biodiesel industry. Glycerol contains fewer carbon atoms compared to typical carbohydrate molecules. Hence, it has become an attractive feedstock for PHA production. Fauzi et al. (2019) loaded activated sludge with crude glycerol at varying organic loading rates. The authors also reported obtaining PHA with a CDW of up to 80%. Other than that, glycerol has also been employed in metabolically modified organisms. Fukui et al. (2014) introduced *Ralstonia eutropha* H16 with aquaglyceroporin (glpF) and glycerol kinase (glpK) from *E. coli* and were able to obtain PHA content up to 68% CDW. In a recent work by de Meneses et al. (2020), glycerol was used as the sole carbon source in the simultaneous microbial synthesis of biopolymer, resulting in increased molecular weight of extracellular polysaccharides and phenazines (antibiotics and anticancer drugs) by *Pseudomonas chlororaphis*. The production of PHA and extracellular polysaccharides were 2.23 and 6.10 g/L, respectively. With only 19% CDW of PHAs, more work needs to be done to improve the operational circumstances. Nonetheless, the results are encouraging for sustainable production of PHA.

7.4 FERMENTATION PROCESS AND OPTIMIZATION OF PROCESS PARAMETERS FOR BIOPOLYMER PRODUCTION

Figure 7.2 shows the factors affecting biopolymer production. The main factors involved are the fermentation process design and the optimization of process parameters.

7.4.1 Fermentation Process

It was discovered that using a fed-batch fermentation technique boosted the chances of increasing PHA accumulation and PHA titer. Feeding carbon source or combined carbon and nitrogen supply with the varied pulse pattern was the most used fed-batch strategy (Wisuthiphaet and Napathorn, 2016). Furthermore, Ryu et al. (1997)

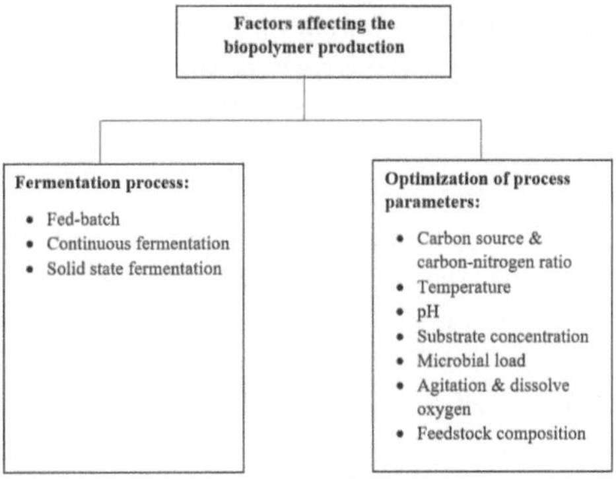

FIGURE 7.2 Factors affecting the biopolymer production.

conducted a study on fed-batch fermentation in a 60 L reactor employing a potential strain of *A. eutrophus*. Maximum cell growth of 281 g/L, PHB titer of 232 g/L, and 3.14 g/L/h production rate were reported when pH was maintained, and phosphate content was limited.

Furthermore, solid-state fermentation (SSF) may be beneficial for the assimilation of various waste biomass resources as well as the production of PHA. Ramadas et al. (2013) used *B. sphaericus* NII 0838 to investigate polyurethane foam (PUF) as a physical inert support in the SSF process for PHB synthesis. They optimized the operating parameters and achieved a maximum PHB production of 0.169 g/g PUF and biomass of 0.4 g/g PUF. An SSF process for PHB production was developed by Oliveira et al. (Oliveira et al., 2007) using soy cake and sugarcane molasses as the substrate and *R. eutropha* as the microbe. After 36 h of fermentation, the highest level of PHB accumulation (39%) was found through this process.

Continuous fermentation is a viable option for lowering production cost and advancing the sustainability of large-scale PHA synthesis with the highest specific growth rate of selected microbial strains (Lopar et al., 2013). However, further research is needed to develop the fermentation strategies that would allow fermenting microorganisms to effectively consume waste stream, thereby leading to a cost-effective and sustainable PHA production.

7.4.2 Optimization of Process Parameters

7.4.2.1 Carbon Source and Carbon-Nitrogen (C/N) Ratio

Generally, in fermentation, lower C/N ratio promotes cell growth, whereas higher C/N ratio promotes PHA yield. Higher PHA levels may be obtained in N-limitation operations because microbial protein synthesis is restricted, and PHA becomes the primary product in the absence of nitrogen (Wen et al., 2010). Johnson et al. (Johnson et al., 2010) investigated the influence of C/N ratio on the biomass generation stage. The authors reported that when the microbial community was exposed to carbon-limited conditions, they accumulated more PHA. This result showed that nitrogen limitation promoted PHA formation. However, carbon limitation is preferred for the enrichment step, and wastewater must be supplemented with nutrients to develop stable PHA storing biomass, according to the researchers. Ince et al. (2012) also investigated the effect of nitrogen content on the ability of activated sludge to store PHA. For the enrichment stage, the experiment was operated under nitrogen-sufficient (C/N:100/12) and nitrogen-deficient (C/N:100/2) conditions. Under nitrogen-sufficient conditions, polymer storage yield increased from 0.43 to 0.61 Cmmol PHA/Cmmol of the substrate. Cui et al. (2017) investigated a wider range of C/N ratios (ranging from 5 to 65) in a pure culture investigation with the archeon *Haloferax mediterranei* and found that the highest PHA cell content (more than 47% CDW) were obtained at a C/N ratio of 35. These findings show that the C/N ratio can alter different stages of PHA formation, while nitrogen limitation is important during PHA development. There must also be enough nitrogen to achieve optimal efficiency. The C/N ratio affects not only the PHA yield but also the product composition.

Silva et al. (2017) investigated the impact of coupled and uncoupled nitrogen feeding on biopolymer formation in order to better control nitrogen levels during feast and famine stages. Nitrogen was fed to the reactors either concurrently with the volatile fatty acid substrate or at the end of the feast phase with a mixture of acetic and propionic acid as substrate. When carbon and nitrogen were fed separately, PHA production increased twofold, and the composition of the polymer product was enriched by an 82% increase in hydroxyvalerate content. When the PHA production was compared at three different C/N ratios of 14.3, 17.9, and 22.3 C mol/N mol, the PHA production was generally consistent at 14.3 and 17.9 but dropped at a higher ratio of 22.3. Meanwhile, raising the C/N ratio from 14.3 to 17.9 3 C mol/ N mol reduced the hydroxyvalerate content in the polymer product from 20% to 12%. Their findings pointed to the possibility of manipulating the properties of polymers by changing the C/N ratio slightly. When nutrient concentrations are limited, the metabolic pathways are driven toward PHA accumulation rather than biomass development.

7.4.2.2 Temperature

The incubation temperature affects the generation of PHB by modifying the enzymes involved in the production process. Mostafa et al. (2020) studied the production of PHB from date syrup by *Pseudodonghicola xiamenensis*, focusing on manipulating the temperature to boost PHB productivity. Incubation temperatures ranging from 25°C to 45°C were examined during the fermentation process. After incubation, it was discovered that 35°C produced the highest amount of biomass, and that temperature had a significant impact on PHB formation and bacterial growth. PHB production was 4.38 g/L, while biomass production was 9.23 g/L, representing 47.45% of total PHB content and 43.8% of total PHB yield, respectively. The *Bacillus dentrensis* strain was inoculated and incubated for 36 hours at temperatures ranging from 25°C to 37°C, with the highest yield and concentration of PHB occurring at 28°C. At temperatures below and above 28°C, the strain was unable to develop (Penkhrue et al., 2020). *Bacillus subtilis* was further exploited to synthesize PHB, utilizing fruit peel extract to maximize biopolymer production. Temperature was identified as a critical element that needed to be optimized among all the characteristics related to the medium. In this investigation, the incubation temperature was raised from 25°C to 50°C, and *B. subtilis* produced the highest amount of PHB (3.35 g/L) at 35°C. Temperatures above 40°C were shown to be lethal to microbial growth and were therefore detrimental for PHB synthesis (Santhi and BalaKumaran, 2018). As the carbon source was added, another *Bacillus subtilis* strain isolated from a sewage sample showed enhanced accumulation of PHB. Physicochemical parameters were monitored during the production process to increase the activity of the bacterial strain to generate PHB. The temperature range tested was 27°C to 45°C, with the highest amount of PHB (336 g/ml) obtained at 37°C (Irsath et al., 2015).

7.4.2.3 pH

pH is also a critical parameter in the biopolymer production process. The pH values were discovered to influence PHB accumulation in bacterial cells. Understanding the activity of the PHB polymerase enzyme is critical for improving PHB production. The concentration of hydrogen ions in the media is evidently a crucial determinant of PHB synthesis since it could obstruct the metabolic machinery of the producing microorganism. Experiments were conducted in which the pH of the fermentation media is altered from 6.5 to 9.0. The highest PHB accumulation of 4.41 g/L and the highest bacterial biomass of 9.26 g/L were achieved at pH 7.5. A significant increase in PHB content and yield was also seen at the same pH range in a report by Mostafa et al. (Mostafa et al., 2020). The pH was adjusted using pineapple juice to achieve the maximum yield of PHB by *B. drentensis*. After 72 hours of incubation, the pH of the fermentation media was varied from 5 to 10, and the concentration of the generated PHB was found to be significantly different in different pH ranges. The highest output of PHB (3.7 g/L) was observed after 36 hours of incubation at pH 6, followed by pH 6.5 and 7.0 (Penkhrue et al., 2020). Santhi and Balakumaran (2018) adjusted the pH of the media during PHB synthesis using fruit peel extract. The maximum yield of 3.21 g/L of PHB was obtained at pH 7. Adjusting the pH of the media from 7 to 8 and 8 to 9 altered PHB production considerably. Furthermore, the optimization technique of changing the pH of the medium resulted in the maximum PHB synthesis by *Bacillus subtilis* at pH 7.5 with a yield of 362 g/mL (Irsath et al., 2015).

Operating the enrichment and accumulation stages at various pH levels significantly impacts the production rate and composition of the biopolymers produced. A broad pH range of 5.5–9.0 is considered suitable for developing most non-extremophilic bacteria during the enrichment stage (Padan et al., 2005). On the other hand, the optimal pH for the accumulation stage is in the range of 7.5–8.5 (Villano et al., 2014). In a previous study, Villano et al. (2014) found that the biomass had a greater polymer content (31%–34% mg PHA/mg VSS) at pH 7.5–8.5, whereas at more alkaline pH values, the biomass had a lower polymer content (21% mg PHA/mg VSS). Furthermore, the authors found that pH management can be an essential tool in managing the 3HV concentration of the final polymer independently of the feedstock composition. The impact of initial pH on the PHA accumulation stage was investigated by Kourmentza and Kornaros (2016). The pH was initially set to 6.4, 6.9, 7.25, and 7.5, but was uncontrolled as the experiment progressed. Setting the initial pH to 6.9 was found to be preferable among the studied conditions, resulting in PHA accumulation of up to 64.5% g PHA/g CDW, compared to just 49% when the initial pH was set to 7.5. Montiel-Jarillo et al. (2017) used activated sludge fed with acetate to investigate the effect of a wider pH range on the accumulation stage. The pH was set and controlled throughout the trials at values of 4, 5.5, 6.5, 7.5, and 8.5, with one uncontrolled pH experiment (varying between 8.9 and 9.2). Under acidic conditions, lower PHA accumulations (17%–23% g PHA/g VSS) were obtained. In the absence of pH control, the highest PHA accumulation capacity of 44% g PHA/g VSS was achieved. This is a promising conclusion since having to regulate fewer operational parameters leads to a less complicated and hence less expensive process.

7.4.2.4 Substrate Concentration

Low substrate cost contributes to improving the economics of the biopolymer synthesis process. The amount of substrate present is a fundamental determinant of bacterial behavior. The nature of the material and the enzymes generated by the microbe play a significant role in using renewable resources for biopolymer synthesis. PHB was produced from *P. xiamenesis* using date syrup as a substrate. To optimize the substrate concentration for PHB synthesis, date syrup, which is high in fermentable sugars, was added to the fermentation media in various concentrations. With 4% date syrup, the highest bacterial biomass (16.40 g/L) and PHB concentration (13.65 g/L) were found. PHB content and productivity were enhanced to 83.23% of total biomass and 0.142 g/(L. h), respectively, at this concentration (Mostafa et al., 2020). The *Bacillus subtilis* was also found to produce PHB from fruit peel waste. Fruit extracts in varying concentrations ranging from 10% to 100% were mixed with the production media for the optimization of the substrate concentration. According to the findings, the maximum concentration of PHB was found at 50% fruit extract concentration, yielding 234 g/mL of PHB (Irsath et al., 2015). Furthermore, Santhi and Balakumaran (2018) also optimized the concentration of sapota and apple fruit extract for PHB manufacturing. Each extract was introduced to the minimal salt media as a carbon and energy source during the production process. It was discovered that the media supplemented with sapota extract yielded more PHB than the media supplemented with apple extract. The best concentrations of sapota and apple extracts were 50% and 60%, yielding 2.68 and 2.46 g/L of PHB, respectively. PHB generation from *Bacillus cereus* was investigated in various fruit pulps, including pineapple, fig, sapota, grape, papaya, and mixed extract. Extracts (individual and mixed) were applied to the production media to replace sugar content at various concentrations, and it was discovered that mixed fruit extract produced the highest yield of PHB in the production media. PHB yields recorded from pineapple, sapota, fig, grape, papaya, and mixed extract were 220, 268, 120, 228, 234, and 298 g/mL, respectively (Paul et al., 2017).

7.4.2.5 Microbial Load

Inoculum concentration in the production media was reported to affect PHB production. PHA synthesis by *Bacillus dentrensis* was examined by Penkhrue et al. (2020) to enhance the proportion of inoculum in media. When five dissimilar seed inoculum with concentrations of 4, 6, 8, 10, and 20% (v/v) were injected into a production vessel, it was shown that a 2% inoculum size generated less biomass and PHB. The PHB value significantly rose from 3.1 to 4.1 g/L when inoculum size was increased from 4% to 10%.

7.4.2.6 Agitation and Dissolved Oxygen

PHB production is recognized to be substantially reliant on the physiological pressure response of the growing cells under restriction or reduction of essential nutrients. Initially, there is a cell growth stage, during which the dissolved oxygen and agitation rate are crucial factors together with other factors. The agitation method might have an impact on PHB crystallinity (McAdam et al., 2020; Rollero et al., 2018; Berwig et al., 2016), whereby cells cultured in a flask on an orbital shaker may produce less crystalline PHB than those in a bioreactor (Berwig et al., 2016). Excitingly, regardless of the agitation method, the carbon source type can also affect PHB crystallinity (Yezza et al., 2007). An appropriate agitation rate is not only required for uniformly dispersing the medium components, but it also dictates the dissolved oxygen (DO) level in the medium (with proper aeration rate).

Microorganisms require oxygen to grow and to carry out their metabolic activity. Garcia-Cabrera et al (García-Cabrera et al., 2020) recently discovered that the oxygen transmission rate influences PHB production. Inadequate DO levels cause oxidative pressure in growing cells, which might negatively impact their growth and metabolic activities. Nevertheless, sustaining an appropriate DO level in large-scale PHB production is difficult because the high density of cell biomass in the medium reduces the solubility of oxygen in it. Hence, great attention must be paid to using an appropriate aeration device. For instance, micro-bubble dispersion provides slighter bubbles and offers greater oxygen transmission surface area (Inan et al., 2016).

7.4.2.7 Feedstock Composition

The PHA production yield is influenced by feedstock composition. Cui et al. (2017) used a variety of substrates such as acetate, glucose, and starch to study the effect of carbon sources on PHA production. The PHA content of the reactors fed with sodium acetate and glucose was 64.7% and 60.5% CDW, respectively, while just 27.3% CDW of PHA was gained from the starch-enriched microbial community. The reason for this is that starch has a more complex structure that cannot be directly exploited by microbes and must be converted to simpler sugars first. Acetate and glucose, on the other hand, can be consumed more effortlessly and quickly in the metabolic pathways. The type and configuration of the polymers formed are also determined by the feedstock characteristics. Jiang et al. (2011) investigated the substrate effect on PHA content and configurations. Dissimilar proportions of acetate and propionate were supplied to the mixed microbial culture with compositions of 100/0, 75/25, 50/50, and 0/100 carbon mol (Cmol) basis. The homopolymer PHB was found in the experiments where acetate was the only substrate, while a copolymer with the composition of 3HB (11 Cmol%) and 3HV (89 Cmol%) was produced when only propionate was fed. Their findings demonstrated that the final polymer composition is highly dependent on the substrate composition. It is of great interest to increase the 3HV fraction in the poly (3-hydroxybutyrate-co-3-hydroxyvalerate) polymer. Higher 3HV content boosts the polymers' flexibility and resistance, broadening their application potential. *Cupriavidus necator* can produce 3HV monomers from odd carbon-number feedstocks, like propionic acid and valeric acid. Solely supplying propionic acid to *cupriavidus necator* resulted in a 50% mol 3HV/mol PHA ratio. Only 32% mol 3HV/mol PHA was acquired while feeding a combination of propionic acid and butyric acid (Grousseau et al., 2014). This showed that by modifying the feedstock characteristics, the configuration and production of PHA may be manipulated. Carvalho et al. (2018) studied the usage of alternating low-priced feedstock for PHA synthesis. Changing the feedstock would change the microbial community's dominant phylum. Moreover, some unknown PHA producer genera (*Paenibacillus* and *Lysinibacillus*) were identified in cheese whey feeding operations on a long-term basis. Despite the changes in the microbial community, the PHA storage performance was quite similar.

7.5 LIMITATIONS AND FUTURE ASPECTS FOR BIOPOLYMER PRODUCTION

Exploiting waste streams as feedstock for PHA production has two advantages: it solves environmental waste disposal issues, and it makes the process more durable and economical. Figure 7.3 summarizes the limitations and future aspects of

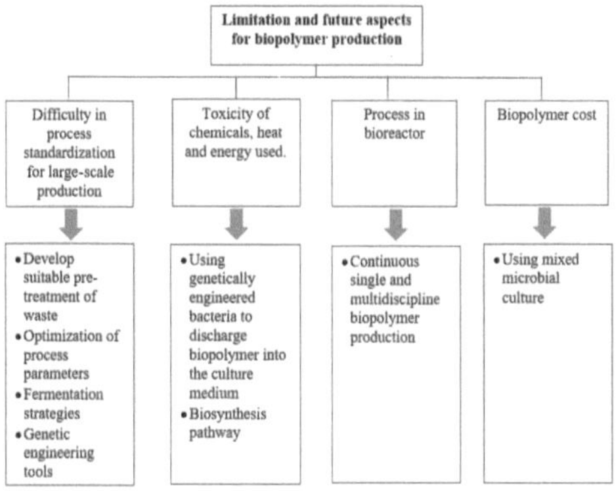

FIGURE 7.3 Limitation and future aspects for biopolymer production.

biopolymer production. According to our literature search, wastes created by various industries are diverse in their chemical configuration, resulting in varying PHA production and cell biomass. This could be due to contaminants in the waste feedstock, as well as variations in the chemical composition of each period. Thus, large-scale applications make standardization of the process impossible. A lesser amount of waste stream utilization by microbes may be overcome by properly pre-treating the waste feedstock, improving operational settings, essential fermentation processes, and nutrient supplementation, as well as using genetic engineering tools.

Even though the process has been progressively improved to increase the size of the cells for high PHA accumulation, there are still issues to be addressed, including the toxicity of the substances used, the environmental impact, sustainability, and the significant contribution of heat and energy consumed. The biggest challenge for PHA synthesis is the downstream process, which requires not only a substantial amount of process energy but also the indirect use of detergents, solvents, and other chemicals. More remarkable scientific research efforts are required to engineer bacteria that would allow PHA granules to be discharged into the medium, making the PHA extraction method more ecologically friendly and economical. Significant efforts are also needed to produce several PHA types with high molecular weight by employing the biosynthesis pathways (Chen et al., 2015).

Nowadays, PHA production on a large scale is reliant on the continuous investment of fed-batch in outsized bioreactors. Many restrictions are imposed by these processes, namely the unusual product grade, the reaction's unproductive response time, the restricted supply possibilities for certain carbon components, and, most importantly, the deficient production. Hence, for the synthesis of various kinds of viral PHAs, continuous single and multidisciplinary PHA biosynthesis is still being explored; this includes thermoplastic PHA homo-polyesters, the very flexible PHA co-polyesters and crystals, together with good structured PHAs containing soft and hard components (Koller and Braunegg, 2015).

PHA's high manufacturing cost, when compared to plastics derived from petroleum, is a major obstacle to its widespread application. The usage of mixed microbial cultures (MMCs) enables the use of a huge quantity of waste, such as food waste apples, as a precursor in the production of PHA (Montiel-Jarillo et al., 2017). Other constraints exist in the selection of microorganisms capable of expressing all types of PHA genes. This polyester's hyper-ester formulation from low-priced biomass-derived ingredients needs further research. To produce PHAs on a large scale, genetically engineered bacteria are required (Muneer et al., 2020).

Improvements in genetic engineering and metabolic biological methods have allowed increased usage of a variety of carbon sources, leading to a greater synthesis yield of PHA with stable monomer compositions. The high amount of fatty acids (FFA) gives an extra chance to be used as a carbon source for PHA production (Surendran et al., 2020). Combining more than one type of bacteria that can utilize a similar substrate to produce variation PHAs types is an alternative strategy for obtaining PHA compounds.

With the shift away from petrochemical plastic, there is some uncertainty about the term "bio-sourced plastic." The misconception about whether all bio-sourced polymers are biodegradable persists today (Mendes and Pedersen, 2021). The distinction between bio-sourced and biodegradable plastics must be understood. Bio-sourced plastics use biomass as feedstock rather than crude oil, whereas biodegradable plastics are formed from the biodegradability point of view (Karan et al., 2019). A plastic's biodegradability is not determined by the feedstock used to produce it, but rather by the composition of the product and the environment in which it must degrade. Furthermore, certain polymers deteriorate quickly, while others take months (Briassoulis et al., 2021). The correct end-of-life management technique would mostly be determined by the quality of the biodegradable substances. Composting is the best last solution for biodegradable plastics in terms of environmental impact. Yet, in order to achieve a desirable output, the process condition must be strictly controlled (Gironi and Piemonte, 2011). Plastics that may be composted should be collected through a separate recycling program and delivered to a commercial composting facility; most countries currently lack such facilities.

Even though PHB research is quite popular among our scientific family, up-scaled PHB production is nearly absent, especially for fruit waste-based PHB. This is due to a lack of process modeling and optimization studies at both the laboratory and pilot scale. The usage of biodegradable conventional plastics (PHB-based) cannot become feasible unless an economic process is established at an industrial scale. The utilization of green and energy-efficient processing technologies, as well as inexpensive substrates, is the main consideration for upscaling PHB synthesis. The substrate, i.e., fruit waste, would be a big asset in this case. Future research should include a life phase assessment of the PHB synthesis process. A circular bioeconomy-based approach could be advantageous and even necessary in lowering the PHB production cost and improving biopolymer generation feasibility.

The extraction step accounts for over a third of the total PHA synthesis cost (Sun et al., 2007). The total cost of PHAs will be significantly reduced if inexpensive and more ecologically friendly methods for extracting the accumulated PHAs are used. Chemical reagents are used extensively in the PHA extraction procedures, including for digestion, solvent extraction, and flotation. A disadvantage is the extra cost of solvent disposal or regeneration. PHA production costs are predicted to be 2–3 times higher than petrochemical plastics when chlorinated solvents or surfactants are used (Yu and Chen, 2006). Moreover, the hazardous wastes generated during extraction are incompatible with the PHA's ecologically friendly nature. The use of cheaper and more ecologically friendly chemical reagents and solvents should be the focus of future research. Moreover, boosting recovery efficiency is an additional feature of extraction that must be addressed. To make downstream processing easier, morphological engineering should be used to change the size and form of the PHA granules. One alternative approach is to knock down certain genes involved in cell wall synthesis (Wang et al., 2014) or promote secretion pathways for extracellular PHA deposition rather than intracellular accumulation. Rahman et al. (2013) studied the feasibility of secreting PHB by pointing binding proteins to the granules' external layer. Establishing the mechanisms for extracellular PHA accumulation opens up novel study opportunities. Extracellular accumulation not only speeds up the process of recovery but also raises accumulation size, because it is not limited by cell volume.

7.6 CONCLUSION

This chapter discusses the importance of numerous wastes such as milk waste, sugarcane molasses, glycerol, and spent coffee waste generated from different processes for biopolymer production, hence at the same time it can manage the serious environmental problem. Recent advances in fermentation strategies and the optimization of process parameters like pH, temperature, and microbial load for cost-effective and eco-friendly biopolymer production are presented. Based on the study and our present perception, this chapter also proposed the technical challenges and future aspects for the sustainable production of biopolymer.

ACKNOWLEDGMENTS

This study was financially supported by the Ministry of Higher Education Malaysia (FRGS/1/2019/TK02/UMP/02/5, Grant No: RDU1901113) and Universiti Malaysia Pahang (RDU190359 and RDU182305).

REFERENCES

Aeschelmann, Florence, and Michael Carus. 2015. "Biobased Building Blocks and Polymers in the World: Capacities, Production, and Applications–Status Quo and Trends towards 2020." *Industrial Biotechnology* 11 (3): 154–59.

Al-Battashi, Huda, Neelamegam Annamalai, Shatha Al-Kindi, Anu Sadasivan Nair, Saif Al-Bahry, Jay Prakash Verma, and Nallusamy Sivakumar. 2019. "Production of Bioplastic (Poly-3-Hydroxybutyrate) Using Waste Paper as a Feedstock: Optimization of Enzymatic Hydrolysis and Fermentation Employing Burkholderia Sacchari." *Journal of Cleaner Production* 214: 236–47.

Albuquerque, Priscilla B S, and Carolina B Malafaia. 2018. "Perspectives on the Production, Structural Characteristics and Potential Applications of Bioplastics Derived from Polyhydroxyalkanoates." *International Journal of Biological Macromolecules* 107: 615–25. https://doi.org/10.1016/j.ijbiomac.2017.09.026.

Alias, Zazali, and Irene K P Tan. 2005. "Isolation of Palm Oil-Utilising, Polyhydroxyalkanoate (PHA)-Producing Bacteria by an Enrichment Technique." *Bioresource Technology* 96 (11): 1229–34. https://doi.org/10.1016/j.biortech.2004.10.012.

Amini, Fatemeh, Dariush Semnani, Saeed Karbasi, and Seyedeh Nooshin Banitaba. 2019. "A Novel Bilayer Drug-Loaded Wound Dressing of PVDF and PHB/Chitosan Nanofibers Applicable for Post-Surgical Ulcers." *International Journal of Polymeric Materials and Polymeric Biomaterials* 68 (13): 772–77.

Anjum, Anbreen, Mohammad Zuber, Khalid Mahmood Zia, Aqdas Noreen, Muhammad Naveed Anjum, and Shazia Tabasum. 2016. "Microbial Production of Polyhydroxyalkanoates (PHAs) and Its Copolymers: A Review of Recent Advancements." *International Journal of Biological Macromolecules* 89: 161–74. https://doi.org/10.1016/j.ijbiomac.2016.04.069.

Annamalai, Neelamegam, and Nallusamy Sivakumar. 2016. "Production of Polyhydroxybutyrate from Wheat Bran Hydrolysate Using Ralstonia Eutropha through Microbial Fermentation." *Journal of Biotechnology* 237: 13–17.

Atabani, A E, Ala'a H Al-Muhtaseb, Gopalakrishnan Kumar, Ganesh Dattatraya Saratale, Muhammad Aslam, Hassnain Abbas Khan, Zafar Said, and Eyas Mahmoud. 2019. "Valorization of Spent Coffee Grounds into Biofuels and Value-Added Products: Pathway towards Integrated Bio-Refinery." *Fuel* 254: 115640. https://doi.org/10.1016/j.fuel.2019.115640.

Berwig, Karina Hammel, Camila Baldasso, and Aline Dettmer. 2016. "Production and Characterization of Poly (3-Hydroxybutyrate) Generated by Alcaligenes Latus Using Lactose and Whey after Acid Protein Precipitation Process." *Bioresource Technology* 218: 31–37.

Bhatia, Shashi Kant, Jung-Ho Kim, Min-Sun Kim, Junyoung Kim, Ju Won Hong, Yoon Gi Hong, Hyun-Joong Kim, Jong-Min Jeon, Sang-Hyoun Kim, and Jungoh Ahn. 2018. "Production of (3-Hydroxybutyrate-Co-3-Hydroxyhexanoate) Copolymer from Coffee Waste Oil Using Engineered Ralstonia Eutropha." *Bioprocess and Biosystems Engineering* 41 (2): 229–35.

Bhatt, Rachana, and Michael Jaffe. 2015. "Biopolymers in Medical Implants." In *Excipient Applications in Formulation Design and Drug Delivery*, 311–48. Springer, Switzerland.

Borrero-de Acuña, José Manuel, Carla Aravena-Carrasco, Izabook Gutierrez-Urrutia, Daniela Duchens, and Ignacio Poblete-Castro. 2019. "Enhanced Synthesis of Medium-Chain-Length Poly (3-Hydroxyalkanoates) by Inactivating the Tricarboxylate Transport System of Pseudomonas Putida KT2440 and Process Development Using Waste Vegetable Oil." *Process Biochemistry* 77: 23–30.

Briassoulis, Demetres, Anastasia Pikasi, and Miltiadis Hiskakis. 2021. "Recirculation Potential of Post-Consumer/Industrial Bio-Based Plastics through Mechanical Recycling-Techno-Economic Sustainability Criteria and Indicators." *Polymer Degradation and Stability* 183: 109217.

Cargnin, Simone Tasca, and Simone Baggio Gnoatto. 2017. "Ursolic Acid from Apple Pomace and Traditional Plants: A Valuable Triterpenoid with Functional Properties." *Food Chemistry* 220: 477–89. https://doi.org/10.1016/j.foodchem.2016.10.029.

Carvalho, Gilda, Inês Pedras, Soren M Karst, Catarina S S Oliveira, Anouk F Duque, Per H Nielsen, and Maria A M Reis. 2018. "Functional Redundancy Ensures Performance Robustness in 3-Stage PHA-Producing Mixed Cultures under Variable Feed Operation." *New Biotechnology* 40: 207–17.

Chen, Guo-Qiang. 2010. "Plastics Completely Synthesized by Bacteria: Polyhydroxyalkanoates." In *Plastics from Bacteria*, 17–37. Springer Berlin, Heidelberg.

Chen, Guo-Qiang, Ivan Hajnal, Hong Wu, Li Lv, and Jianwen Ye. 2015. "Engineering Biosynthesis Mechanisms for Diversifying Polyhydroxyalkanoates." *Trends in Biotechnology* 33 (10): 565–74. https://doi.org/10.1016/j.tibtech.2015.07.007.

Chen, Guo-Qiang, and Qiong Wu. 2005. "Microbial Production and Applications of Chiral Hydroxyalkanoates." *Applied Microbiology and Biotechnology* 67 (5): 592–99.

Chen, Zhu, and Caixia Wan. 2017. "Biological Valorization Strategies for Converting Lignin into Fuels and Chemicals." *Renewable and Sustainable Energy Reviews* 73: 610–21. https://doi.org/10.1016/j.rser.2017.01.166.

Choi, So Young, Mi Na Rhie, Hee Taek Kim, Jeong Chan Joo, In Jin Cho, Jina Son, Seo Young Jo, et al. 2020. "Metabolic Engineering for the Synthesis of Polyesters: A 100-Year Journey from Polyhydroxyalkanoates to Non-Natural Microbial Polyesters." *Metabolic Engineering* 58: 47–81. https://doi.org/10.1016/j.ymben.2019.05.009.

Cui, You-Wei, Yun-Peng Shi, and Xiao-Yu Gong. 2017. "Effects of C/N in the Substrate on the Simultaneous Production of Polyhydroxyalkanoates and Extracellular Polymeric Substances by Haloferax Mediterranei via Kinetic Model Analysis." *RSC Advances* 7 (31): 18953–61.

Das, Dipankar, and Sagar Pal. 2015. "Modified Biopolymer-Dextrin Based Crosslinked Hydrogels: Application in Controlled Drug Delivery." *RSC Advances* 5 (32): 25014–50.

de Meneses, Liane, João Ricardo Pereira, Chantal Sevrin, Christian Grandfils, Alexandre Paiva, Maria A M Reis, and Filomena Freitas. 2020. "Pseudomonas Chlororaphis as a Multiproduct Platform: Conversion of Glycerol into High-Value Biopolymers and Phenazines." *New Biotechnology* 55: 84–90. https://doi.org/10.1016/j.nbt.2019.10.002.

Fabra, M J, A López-Rubio, and J M Lagaron. 2014. "Biopolymers for Food Packaging Applications." In *Smart Polymers and Their Applications*, 476–509. Woodhead Publishing, Cambridge.

Fauzi, Ainil Hawa Mohamad, Adeline Seak May Chua, Li Wan Yoon, Tadashi Nittami, and Hak Koon Yeoh. 2019. "Enrichment of PHA-Accumulators for Sustainable PHA Production from Crude Glycerol." *Process Safety and Environmental Protection* 122: 200–208.

Favaro, Lorenzo, Marina Basaglia, and Sergio Casella. 2019. "Improving Polyhydroxyalkanoate Production from Inexpensive Carbon Sources by Genetic Approaches: A Review." *Biofuels, Bioproducts and Biorefining* 13 (1): 208–27.

Follonier, Stéphanie, Miriam S Goyder, Anne-Claire Silvestri, Simon Crelier, Franka Kalman, Roland Riesen, and Manfred Zinn. 2014. "Fruit Pomace and Waste Frying Oil as Sustainable Resources for the Bioproduction of Medium-Chain-Length Polyhydroxyalkanoates." *International Journal of Biological Macromolecules* 71: 42–52. https://doi.org/10.1016/j.ijbiomac.2014.05.061.

Follonier, Stéphanie, Roland Riesen, and Manfred Zinn. 2015. "Pilot-Scale Production of Functionalized Mcl-PHA from Grape Pomace Supplemented with Fatty Acids." *Chemical and Biochemical Engineering Quarterly* 29 (2): 113–21.

Fukui, Toshiaki, Masaharu Mukoyama, Izumi Orita, and Satoshi Nakamura. 2014. "Enhancement of Glycerol Utilization Ability of Ralstonia Eutropha H16 for Production of Polyhydroxyalkanoates." *Applied Microbiology and Biotechnology* 98 (17): 7559–68.

García-Cabrera, Ramsés I, Norma A Valdez-Cruz, Abel Blancas-Cabrera, and Mauricio A Trujillo-Roldán. 2020. "Oxygen Transfer Rate Affect Polyhydroxybutyrate Production and Oxidative Stress Response in Submerged Cultures of Rhizobium Phaseoli." *Biochemical Engineering Journal* 162: 107721.

Gironi, F, and Vincenzo Piemonte. 2011. "Bioplastics and Petroleum-Based Plastics: Strengths and Weaknesses." *Energy Sources, Part A: Recovery, Utilization, and Environmental Effects* 33 (21): 1949–59.

Gobi, K, and V M Vadivelu. 2013. "By-Products of Palm Oil Mill Effluent Treatment Plant – A Step towards Sustainability." *Renewable and Sustainable Energy Reviews* 28: 788–803. https://doi.org/10.1016/j.rser.2013.08.049.

Grousseau, Estelle, Elise Blanchet, Stéphane Déléris, Maria G E Albuquerque, Etienne Paul, and Jean-Louis Uribelarrea. 2014. "Phosphorus Limitation Strategy to Increase Propionic Acid Flux towards 3-Hydroxyvaleric Acid Monomers in Cupriavidus Necator." *Bioresource Technology* 153: 206–15.

Inan, Kadriye, Fulya Ay Sal, Asif Rahman, Ryan J Putman, Foster A Agblevor, and Charles D Miller. 2016. "Microbubble Assisted Polyhydroxybutyrate Production in Escherichia Coli." *BMC Research Notes* 9 (1): 1–7.

Ince, Orhan, Bertan Basak, Bahar Kasapgil Ince, Zeynep Cetecioglu, Sükriye Celikkol, and Mustafa Kolukirik. 2012. "Effect of Nitrogen Deficiency during SBR Operation on PHA Storage and Microbial Diversity." *Environmental Technology* 33 (16): 1827–37.

Irsath, H, S Santhosh, V Hemalatha, M Vikramathithan, R Dhanasekar, and R Dhandapani. 2015. "Production and Optimization of Polyhydroxybutyrate Using Bacillus Subtilis BP1 Isolated from Sewage Sample." *International Journal of Pure & Applied Bioscience* 3 (1): 158–66.

Israni, Neetu, Prerana Venkatachalam, Bharath Gajaraj, Kilingar Nadumane Varalakshmi, and Srividya Shivakumar. 2020. "Whey Valorization for Sustainable Polyhydroxyalkanoate Production by Bacillus Megaterium: Production, Characterization and in Vitro Biocompatibility Evaluation." *Journal of Environmental Management* 255: 109884. https://doi.org/10.1016/j.jenvman.2019.109884.

Jendrossek, Dieter, and René Handrick. 2002. "Microbial Degradation of Polyhydroxyalkanoates." *Annual Review of Microbiology* 56 (1): 403–32.

Jiang, Guozhan, David J Hill, Marek Kowalczuk, Brian Johnston, Grazyna Adamus, Victor Irorere, and Iza Radecka. 2016. "Carbon Sources for Polyhydroxyalkanoates and an Integrated Biorefinery." *International Journal of Molecular Sciences*. https://doi.org/10.3390/ijms17071157.

Jiang, Yamin, Yinguang Chen, and Xiong Zheng. 2009. "Efficient Polyhydroxyalkanoates Production from a Waste-Activated Sludge Alkaline Fermentation Liquid by Activated Sludge Submitted to the Aerobic Feeding and Discharge Process." *Environmental Science & Technology* 43 (20): 7734–41.

Jiang, Yang, Marit Hebly, Robbert Kleerebezem, Gerard Muyzer, and Mark C M van Loosdrecht. 2011. "Metabolic Modeling of Mixed Substrate Uptake for Polyhydroxyalkanoate (PHA) Production." *Water Research* 45 (3): 1309–21.

Johnson, Katja, Robbert Kleerebezem, and Mark C M van Loosdrecht. 2010. "Influence of the C/N Ratio on the Performance of Polyhydroxybutyrate (PHB) Producing Sequencing Batch Reactors at Short SRTs." *Water Research* 44 (7): 2141–52.

Karan, Hakan, Christiane Funk, Martin Grabert, Melanie Oey, and Ben Hankamer. 2019. "Green Bioplastics as Part of a Circular Bioeconomy." *Trends in Plant Science* 24 (3): 237–49. https://doi.org/10.1016/j.tplants.2018.11.010.

Karmee, Sanjib Kumar. 2018. "A Spent Coffee Grounds Based Biorefinery for the Production of Biofuels, Biopolymers, Antioxidants and Biocomposites." *Waste Management* 72: 240–54.

Kaygusuz, Hakan, Emrah Torlak, Gülşen Akın-Evingür, İlhan Özen, Regine Von Klitzing, and F Bedia Erim. 2017. "Antimicrobial Cerium Ion-Chitosan Crosslinked Alginate Biopolymer Films: A Novel and Potential Wound Dressing." *International Journal of Biological Macromolecules* 105: 1161–65.

Koller, M, D Puppi, F Chiellini, and G Braunegg. 2016. "Comparing Chemical and Enzymatic Hydrolysis of Whey Lactose to Generate Feedstocks for Haloarchaeal Poly (3-Hydroxybutyrate-Co-3-Hydroxyvalerate) Biosynthesis." *International Journal of Pharmaceutical Sciences and Research* 3: 112.

Koller, Martin. 2018. "Advanced Approaches to Produce Polyhydroxyalkanoate (PHA) Biopolyesters in a Sustainable and Economic Fashion." *Journal of Biotechnology* 280: S5.

Koller, Martin, and Gerhart Braunegg. 2015. "Potential and Prospects of Continuous Polyhydroxyalkanoate (PHA) Production." *Bioengineering*. https://doi.org/10.3390/bioengineering2020094.

Kourmentza, C, and M Kornaros. 2016. "Biotransformation of Volatile Fatty Acids to Polyhydroxyalkanoates by Employing Mixed Microbial Consortia: The Effect of PH and Carbon Source." *Bioresource Technology* 222: 388–98.

Kourmentza, Constantina, Jersson Plácido, Nikolaos Venetsaneas, Anna Burniol-Figols, Cristiano Varrone, Hariklia N Gavala, and Maria A M Reis. 2017. "Recent Advances and Challenges towards Sustainable Polyhydroxyalkanoate (PHA) Production." *Bioengineering* 4 (2). https://doi.org/10.3390/bioengineering4020055.

Kovalcik, Adriana, Dan Kucera, Petra Matouskova, Iva Pernicova, Stanislav Obruca, Michal Kalina, Vojtěch Enev, and Ivana Marova. 2018. "Influence of Removal of Microbial Inhibitors on PHA Production from Spent Coffee Grounds Employing Halomonas Halophila." *Journal of Environmental Chemical Engineering* 6 (2): 3495–3501. https://doi.org/10.1016/j.jece.2018.05.028.

Kumar, Prasun, Subhasree Ray, and Vipin C Kalia. 2016. "Production of Co-Polymers of Polyhydroxyalkanoates by Regulating the Hydrolysis of Biowastes." *Bioresource Technology* 200: 413–19. https://doi.org/10.1016/j.biortech.2015.10.045.

Le Meur, Sylvaine, Manfred Zinn, Thomas Egli, Linda Thöny-Meyer, and Qun Ren. 2012. "Production of Medium-Chain-Length Polyhydroxyalkanoates by Sequential Feeding of Xylose and Octanoic Acid in Engineered Pseudomonas Putida KT2440." *BMC Biotechnology* 12 (1): 1–12.

Li, Jifan, Yifeng Hou, Zhe Song, Chunling Liu, Wensheng Dong, Chenghua Zhang, Yong Yang, and Yongwang Li. 2018. "Chemical and Structural Effects of Strontium on Iron-Based Fischer-Tropsch Synthesis Catalysts." *Molecular Catalysis* 449: 1–7. https://doi.org/10.1016/j.mcat.2018.01.037.

Li, Mengxing, and Mark R Wilkins. 2020. "Recent Advances in Polyhydroxyalkanoate Production: Feedstocks, Strains and Process Developments." *International Journal of Biological Macromolecules* 156: 691–703. https://doi.org/10.1016/j.ijbiomac.2020.04.082.

Linger, Jeffrey G, Derek R Vardon, Michael T Guarnieri, Eric M Karp, Glendon B Hunsinger, Mary Ann Franden, Christopher W Johnson, Gina Chupka, Timothy J Strathmann, and Philip T Pienkos. 2014. "Lignin Valorization through Integrated Biological Funneling and Chemical Catalysis." *Proceedings of the National Academy of Sciences* 111 (33): 12013–18.

Liu, Hong, Vinay Kumar, Linjing Jia, Surendra Sarsaiya, Deepak Kumar, Ankita Juneja, Zengqiang Zhang, Raveendran Sindhu, Parameswaran Binod, and Shashi Kant Bhatia. 2021. "Biopolymer Poly-Hydroxyalkanoates (PHA) Production from Apple Industrial Waste Residues: A Review." *Chemosphere* 284, 131427.

Liu, Zhi-Hua, Michelle L Olson, Somnath Shinde, Xin Wang, Naijia Hao, Chang Geun Yoo, Samarthya Bhagia, John R Dunlap, Yunqiao Pu, and Katy C Kao. 2017. "Synergistic Maximization of the Carbohydrate Output and Lignin Processability by Combinatorial Pretreatment." *Green Chemistry* 19 (20): 4939–55.

Lopar, Markan, Ivna Vrana Špoljarić, Aid Atlić, Martin Koller, Gerhart Braunegg, and Predrag Horvat. 2013. "Five-Step Continuous Production of PHB Analyzed by Elementary Flux, Modes, Yield Space Analysis and High Structured Metabolic Model." *Biochemical Engineering Journal* 79: 57–70. https://doi.org/10.1016/j.bej.2013.07.003.

McAdam, Blaithín, Margaret Brennan Fournet, Paul McDonald, and Marija Mojicevic. 2020. "Production of Polyhydroxybutyrate (PHB) and Factors Impacting Its Chemical and Mechanical Characteristics." *Polymers* 12 (12): 2908.

Mendes, Ana C, and Gitte Alsing Pedersen. 2021. "Perspectives on Sustainable Food Packaging:– Is Bio-Based Plastics a Solution?" *Trends in Food Science & Technology* 112: 839–46. https://doi.org/10.1016/j.tifs.2021.03.049.

Montiel-Jarillo, Gabriela, Julián Carrera, and María Eugenia Suárez-Ojeda. 2017. "Enrichment of a Mixed Microbial Culture for Polyhydroxyalkanoates Production: Effect of PH and N and P Concentrations." *Science of the Total Environment* 583: 300–307.

Mostafa, Yasser S, Sulaiman A Alrumman, Saad A Alamri, Kholod A Otaif, Mohamed S Mostafa, and Abdulkhaleg M Alfaify. 2020. "Bioplastic (Poly-3-Hydroxybutyrate) Production by the Marine Bacterium Pseudodonghicola Xiamenensis through Date Syrup Valorization and Structural Assessment of the Biopolymer." *Scientific Reports* 10 (1): 1–13.

Muneer, Faizan, Ijaz Rasul, Farrukh Azeem, Muhammad Hussnain Siddique, Muhammad Zubair, and Habibullah Nadeem. 2020. "Microbial Polyhydroxyalkanoates (PHAs): Efficient Replacement of Synthetic Polymers." *Journal of Polymers and the Environment* 28: 2301–23.

Nath, A, M Dixit, A Bandiya, S Chavda, and A J Desai. 2008. "Enhanced PHB Production and Scale up Studies Using Cheese Whey in Fed Batch Culture of Methylobacterium Sp. ZP24." *Bioresource Technology* 99 (13): 5749–55. https://doi.org/10.1016/j.biortech.2007.10.017.

Nielsen, Chad, Asif Rahman, Asad Ur Rehman, Marie K Walsh, and Charles D Miller. 2017. "Food Waste Conversion to Microbial Polyhydroxyalkanoates." *Microbial Biotechnology* 10 (6): 1338–52.

Nigmatullin, Rinat, Peter Thomas, Barbara Lukasiewicz, Hima Puthussery, and Ipsita Roy. 2015. "Polyhydroxyalkanoates, a Family of Natural Polymers, and Their Applications in Drug Delivery." *Journal of Chemical Technology & Biotechnology* 90 (7): 1209–21.

Novikova, Liudmila N, Jonas Pettersson, Maria Brohlin, Mikael Wiberg, and Lev N Novikov. 2008. "Biodegradable Poly-β-Hydroxybutyrate Scaffold Seeded with Schwann Cells to Promote Spinal Cord Repair." *Biomaterials* 29 (9): 1198–1206. https://doi.org/10.1016/j.biomaterials.2007.11.033.

Obruca, S, P Benesova, L Marsalek, and I Marova. 2015. "Use of Lignocellulosic Materials for PHA Production." *Chemical and Biochemical Engineering Quarterly* 29 (2): 135–44.

Obruca, Stanislav, Pavla Benesova, Dan Kucera, Sinisa Petrik, and Ivana Marova. 2015. "Biotechnological Conversion of Spent Coffee Grounds into Polyhydroxyalkanoates and Carotenoids." *New Biotechnology* 32 (6): 569–74. https://doi.org/10.1016/j.nbt.2015.02.008.

Obruca, Stanislav, Pavla Benesova, Jana Oborna, and Ivana Marova. 2014. "Application of Protease-Hydrolyzed Whey as a Complex Nitrogen Source to Increase Poly (3-Hydroxybutyrate) Production from Oils by Cupriavidus Necator." *Biotechnology Letters* 36 (4): 775–81.

Obruca, Stanislav, Ivana Marova, Sona Melusova, and Ludmila Mravcova. 2011. "Production of Polyhydroxyalkanoates from Cheese Whey Employing Bacillus Megaterium CCM 2037." *Annals of Microbiology* 61 (4): 947–53.

Obruca, Stanislav, Ivana Marova, Ondrej Snajdar, Ludmila Mravcova, and Zdenek Svoboda. 2010. "Production of Poly (3-Hydroxybutyrate-Co-3-Hydroxyvalerate) by Cupriavidus Necator from Waste Rapeseed Oil Using Propanol as a Precursor of 3-Hydroxyvalerate." *Biotechnology Letters* 32 (12): 1925–32.

Okamoto, Masami, and Baiju John. 2013. "Synthetic Biopolymer Nanocomposites for Tissue Engineering Scaffolds." *Progress in Polymer Science* 38 (10–11): 1487–1503.

Oliveira, Fabiane C, Marcos L Dias, Leda R Castilho, and Denise M G Freire. 2007. "Characterization of Poly(3-Hydroxybutyrate) Produced by Cupriavidus Necator in Solid-State Fermentation." *Bioresource Technology* 98 (3): 633–38. https://doi.org/10.1016/j.biortech.2006.02.022.

Ong, Su Yean, Idris Zainab-L, Somarajan Pyary, and Kumar Sudesh. 2018. "A Novel Biological Recovery Approach for PHA Employing Selective Digestion of Bacterial Biomass in Animals." *Applied Microbiology and Biotechnology* 102 (5): 2117–27.

Padan, Etana, Eitan Bibi, Masahiro Ito, and Terry A Krulwich. 2005. "Alkaline PH Homeostasis in Bacteria: New Insights." *Biochimica et Biophysica Acta (BBA)-Biomembranes* 1717 (2): 67–88.

Page, William J. 1992. "Suitability of Commercial Beet Molasses Fractions as Substrates Fro Polyhydroxyalkanoate Production by Azotobacter Vinelandii UWD." *Biotechnology Letters* 14 (5): 385–90.

Pais, Joana, Inês Farinha, Filomena Freitas, Luísa S Serafim, Virginia Martínez, Juan Carlos Martínez, Miguel Arévalo-Rodríguez, M Auxiliadora Prieto, and Maria A M Reis. 2014. "Improvement on the Yield of Polyhydroxyalkanotes Production from Cheese Whey by a Recombinant Escherichia Coli Strain Using the Proton Suicide Methodology." *Enzyme and Microbial Technology* 55: 151–58. https://doi.org/10.1016/j.enzmictec.2013.11.004.

Park, Si Jae, Young-Ah Jang, Hyuk Lee, A-Reum Park, Jung Eun Yang, Jihoon Shin, Young Hoon Oh, et al. 2013. "Metabolic Engineering of Ralstonia Eutropha for the Biosynthesis of 2-Hydroxyacid-Containing Polyhydroxyalkanoates." *Metabolic Engineering* 20: 20–28. https://doi.org/10.1016/j.ymben.2013.08.002.

Paul, Sneha, S C Sasikumar, and M D Balakumaran. 2017. "Optimization, Purification and Characterization of Polyhydroxybutyrate (PHB) Produced by Bacillus Cereus Isolated from Sewage." *International Journal of Chem Tech Research* 10 (7): 884–904.

Peng, Qiang, Zhi-Rong Zhang, Tao Gong, Guo-Qiang Chen, and Xun Sun. 2012. "A Rapid-Acting, Long-Acting Insulin Formulation Based on a Phospholipid Complex Loaded PHBHHx Nanoparticles." *Biomaterials* 33 (5): 1583–88. https://doi.org/10.1016/j.biomaterials.2011.10.072.

Penkhrue, Watsana, Dieter Jendrossek, Chartchai Khanongnuch, Wasu Pathom-Aree, Tomoyasu Aizawa, Rachel L Behrens, and S Lumyong. 2020. "Response Surface Method for Polyhydroxybutyrate (PHB) Bioplastic Accumulation in Bacillus Drentensis BP17 Using Pineapple Peel." *PloS One* 15 (3): e0230443.

Pereira, João R, Diana Araújo, Patrícia Freitas, Ana C Marques, Vítor D Alves, Chantal Sevrin, Christian Grandfils, Elvira Fortunato, Maria A M Reis, and Filomena Freitas. 2021. "Production of Medium-Chain-Length Polyhydroxyalkanoates by Pseudomonas Chlororaphis Subsp. Aurantiaca: Cultivation on Fruit Pulp Waste and Polymer Characterization." *International Journal of Biological Macromolecules* 167: 85–92. https://doi.org/10.1016/j.ijbiomac.2020.11.162.

Pernicova, Iva, Dan Kucera, Jana Nebesarova, Michal Kalina, Ivana Novackova, Martin Koller, and Stanislav Obruca. 2019. "Production of Polyhydroxyalkanoates on Waste Frying Oil Employing Selected Halomonas Strains." *Bioresource Technology* 292: 122028. https://doi.org/10.1016/j.biortech.2019.122028.

Povolo, Silvana, Paolo Toffano, Marina Basaglia, and Sergio Casella. 2010. "Polyhydroxyalkanoates Production by Engineered Cupriavidus Necator from Waste Material Containing Lactose." *Bioresource Technology* 101 (20): 7902–7. https://doi.org/10.1016/j.biortech.2010.05.029.

Pratto, Bruna, Renata Beraldo Alencar de Souza, Ruy Sousa, and Antonio Jose Gonçalves da Cruz. 2016. "Enzymatic Hydrolysis of Pretreated Sugarcane Straw: Kinetic Study and Semi-Mechanistic Modeling." *Applied Biochemistry and Biotechnology* 178 (7): 1430–44.

Rahman, Asif, Elisabeth Linton, Alex D Hatch, Ronald C Sims, and Charles D Miller. 2013. "Secretion of Polyhydroxybutyrate in Escherichia Coli Using a Synthetic Biological Engineering Approach." *Journal of Biological Engineering* 7 (1): 1–9.

Ramadas, Nisha V, Raveendran Sindhu, Parameswaran Binod, and Ashok Pandey. 2013. "Development of a Novel Solid-State Fermentation Strategy for the Production of Poly-3-Hydroxybutyrate Using Polyurethane Foams by Bacillus Sphaericus NII 0838." *Annals of Microbiology* 63 (4): 1265–74.

Ray, Subhasree, and Vipin Chandra Kalia. 2017. "Biomedical Applications of Polyhydroxyalkanoates." *Indian Journal of Microbiology* 57 (3): 261–69.

Raza, Zulfiqar Ali, Sharjeel Abid, and Ibrahim M Banat. 2018. "Polyhydroxyalkanoates: Characteristics, Production, Recent Developments and Applications." *International Biodeterioration & Biodegradation* 126: 45–56. https://doi.org/10.1016/j.ibiod.2017.10.001.

Rebocho, Ana Teresa, Joao Ricardo Pereira, Filomena Freitas, Luisa Alexandra Neves, Vitor Delgado Alves, Chantal Sevrin, Christian Grandfils, and Maria A M Reis. 2019. "Production of Medium-Chain Length Polyhydroxyalkanoates by Pseudomonas Citronellolis Grown in Apple Pulp Waste." *Applied Food Biotechnology* 6 (1): 71–82.

Reddy, C S K, Rashmi Ghai, and V_C Kalia. 2003. "Polyhydroxyalkanoates: An Overview." *Bioresource Technology* 87 (2): 137–46.

Rhim, Jong-Whan, and Perry K W Ng. 2007. "Natural Biopolymer-Based Nanocomposite Films for Packaging Applications." *Critical Reviews in Food Science and Nutrition* 47 (4): 411–33.

Riedel, Sebastian L, Stefan Jahns, Steven Koenig, Martina C E Bock, Christopher J Brigham, Johannes Bader, and Ulf Stahl. 2015. "Polyhydroxyalkanoates Production with Ralstonia Eutropha from Low Quality Waste Animal Fats." *Journal of Biotechnology* 214: 119–27. https://doi.org/10.1016/j.jbiotec.2015.09.002.

Rollero, Stéfhanie, S Roberts, F F Bauer, and Benoit Divol. 2018. "Agitation Impacts Fermentation Performance as Well as Carbon and Nitrogen Metabolism in Saccharomyces Cerevisiae under Winemaking Conditions." *Australian Journal of Grape and Wine Research* 24 (3): 360–67.

Ryu, Hee Wook, Sei Kwang Hahn, Yong Keun Chang, and Ho Nam Chang. 1997. "Production of Poly (3-hydroxybutyrate) by High Cell Density Fed-batch Culture of Alcaligenes Eutrophus with Phospate Limitation." *Biotechnology and Bioengineering* 55 (1): 28–32.

Sabarinathan, Devaraj, Sabapathy Poorna Chandrika, Pitchaikannu Venkatraman, Murugesh Easwaran, Chandrasekaran Senbagavadivoo Sureka, and Kathirvel Preethi. 2018. "Production of Polyhydroxybutyrate (PHB) from Pseudomonas Plecoglossicida and Its Application towards Cancer Detection." *Informatics in Medicine Unlocked* 11: 61–67. https://doi.org/10.1016/j.imu.2018.04.009.

Sadeghi, Davoud, Saeed Karbasi, Shahnaz Razavi, Sajjad Mohammadi, Mohammad Ali Shokrgozar, and Shahin Bonakdar. 2016. "Electrospun Poly (Hydroxybutyrate)/Chitosan Blend Fibrous Scaffolds for Cartilage Tissue Engineering." *Journal of Applied Polymer Science* 133 (47): 44171.

Sangkharak, Kanokphorn, and Poonsuk Prasertsan. 2013. "The Production of Polyhydroxyalkanoate by Bacillus Licheniformis Using Sequential Mutagenesis and Optimization." *Biotechnology and Bioprocess Engineering* 18 (2): 272–79.

Santhi, R, and M D BalaKumaran. 2018. "Studies on Utilization of Fruit Peel Extracts for the Production of Polyhydroxybutyrate Using Bacillus Subtilis." *International Journal of Pharmaceutical Sciences and Research* 8 (3): 379–83.

Saratale, Ganesh Dattatraya, Rahul Bhosale, Arivalgan Pugazendhi, Eyas Mahmoud, Ranjna Sirohi, Shashi Kant Bhatia, A E Atabani, Vincenzo Mulone, Jeong-Jun Yoon, and Han Seung Shin. 2020. "A Review on Valorization of Spent Coffee Grounds (SCG) towards Biopolymers and Biocatalysts Production." *Bioresource Technology*, 314: 123800.

Saratale, Rijuta Ganesh, Si-Kyung Cho, Ganesh Dattatraya Saratale, Avinash A Kadam, Gajanan S Ghodake, Manu Kumar, Ram Naresh Bharagava, Gopalakrishnan Kumar, Dong Su Kim, and Sikandar I Mulla. 2021. "A Comprehensive Overview and Recent Advances on Polyhydroxyalkanoates (PHA) Production Using Various Organic Waste Streams." *Bioresource Technology*, 325: 124685.

Silva, Fernando, Sabrina Campanari, Stefania Matteo, Francesco Valentino, Mauro Majone, and Marianna Villano. 2017. "Impact of Nitrogen Feeding Regulation on Polyhydroxyalkanoates Production by Mixed Microbial Cultures." *New Biotechnology* 37: 90–98.

Sirohi, Ranjna, Jai Prakash Pandey, Anupama Singh, Raveendran Sindhu, Umesh Chandra Lohani, Reeta Goel, and Anil Kumar. 2020a. "Acid Hydrolysis of Damaged Wheat Grains: Modeling the Formation of Reducing Sugars by a Neural Network Approach." *Industrial Crops and Products* 149: 112351. https://doi.org/10.1016/j.indcrop.2020.112351.

Sirohi, Ranjna, Jai Prakash Pandey, Vivek Kumar Gaur, Edgard Gnansounou, and Raveendran Sindhu. 2020b. "Critical Overview of Biomass Feedstocks as Sustainable Substrates for the Production of Polyhydroxybutyrate (PHB)." *Bioresource Technology* 311: 123536. https://doi.org/10.1016/j.biortech.2020.123536.

Sjölin, Mikael, Johan Thuvander, Ola Wallberg, and Frank Lipnizki. 2020. "Purification of Sucrose in Sugar Beet Molasses by Utilizing Ceramic Nanofiltration and Ultrafiltration Membranes." *Membranes* 10 (1): 5.

Sodian, Ralf, Simon P Hoerstrup, Jason S Sperling, Sabine Daebritz, David P Martin, Adrian M Moran, Byung S Kim, Frederick J Schoen, Joseph P Vacanti, and John E Mayer Jr. 2000. "Early in Vivo Experience with Tissue-Engineered Trileaflet Heart Valves." *Circulation* 102 (suppl_3): Iii–22.

Sohn, Yu Jung, Hee Taek Kim, Kei-Anne Baritugo, Seo Young Jo, Hye Min Song, Se Young Park, Su Kyeong Park, Jiwon Pyo, Hyun Gil Cha, and Hoyong Kim. 2020. "Recent Advances in Sustainable Plastic Upcycling and Biopolymers." *Biotechnology Journal* 15 (6): 1900489.

Sun, Zhiyong, Juliana A Ramsay, Martin Guay, and Bruce A Ramsay. 2007. "Fermentation Process Development for the Production of Medium-Chain-Length Poly-3-Hyroxyalkanoates." *Applied Microbiology and Biotechnology* 75 (3): 475–85.

Surendran, Arthy, Manoj Lakshmanan, Jiun Yee Chee, Azlinah Mohd Sulaiman, Doan Van Thuoc, and Kumar Sudesh. 2020. "Can Polyhydroxyalkanoates Be Produced Efficiently from Waste Plant and Animal Oils?" *Frontiers in Bioengineering and Biotechnology* 8: 169.

Talan, Anita, Rajwinder Kaur, Rajeshwar D Tyagi, and P Drogui. 2020. "Bioconversion of Oily Waste to Polyhydroxyalkanoates: Sustainable Technology with Circular Bioeconomy Approach and Multidimensional Impacts." *Bioresource Technology Reports* 11: 100496. https://doi.org/10.1016/j.biteb.2020.100496.

Udayakumar, Gowthama Prabu, Subbulakshmi Muthusamy, Bharathi Selvaganesh, N Sivarajasekar, Krishnamoorthy Rambabu, Fawzi Banat, Selvaraju Sivamani, Nallusamy Sivakumar, Ahmad Hosseini-Bandegharaei, and Pau Loke Show. 2021. "Biopolymers and Composites: Properties, Characterization and Their Applications in Food, Medical and Pharmaceutical Industries." *Journal of Environmental Chemical Engineering* 9 (4): 105322.

Villano, Marianna, Francesco Valentino, Andrea Barbetta, Lucrezia Martino, Mariastella Scandola, and Mauro Majone. 2014. "Polyhydroxyalkanoates Production with Mixed Microbial Cultures: From Culture Selection to Polymer Recovery in a High-Rate Continuous Process." *New Biotechnology* 31 (4): 289–96.

Wang, Lei, Zhi-Hui Wang, Chong-Yang Shen, Ming-Liang You, Jian-Feng Xiao, and Guo-Qiang Chen. 2010. "Differentiation of Human Bone Marrow Mesenchymal Stem Cells Grown in Terpolyesters of 3-Hydroxyalkanoates Scaffolds into Nerve Cells." *Biomaterials* 31 (7): 1691–98. https://doi.org/10.1016/j.biomaterials.2009.11.053.

Wang, Ying, Jin Yin, and Guo-Qiang Chen. 2014. "Polyhydroxyalkanoates, Challenges and Opportunities." *Current Opinion in Biotechnology* 30: 59–65.

Wen, Qinxue, Zhiqiang Chen, Ting Tian, and Wei Chen. 2010. "Effects of Phosphorus and Nitrogen Limitation on PHA Production in Activated Sludge." *Journal of Environmental Sciences* 22 (10): 1602–7.

Wisuthiphaet, Nicharee, and Suchada Chanprateep Napathorn. 2016. "Optimisation of the Use of Products from the Cane Sugar Industry for Poly(3-Hydroxybutyrate) Production by Azohydromonas Lata DSM 1123 in Fed-Batch Cultivation." *Process Biochemistry* 51 (3): 352–61. https://doi.org/10.1016/j.procbio.2015.12.009.

Yezza, Abdessalem, Annamaria Halasz, Wayne Levadoux, and Jalal Hawari. 2007. "Production of Poly-β-Hydroxybutyrate (PHB) by Alcaligenes Latus from Maple Sap." *Applied Microbiology and Biotechnology* 77 (2): 269–74.

Yin, Fen, Dongna Li, Xiaojun Ma, and Chong Zhang. 2019. "Pretreatment of Lignocellulosic Feedstock to Produce Fermentable Sugars for Poly (3-Hydroxybutyrate-Co-3-Hydroxyvalerate) Production Using Activated Sludge." *Bioresource Technology* 290: 121773.

Yu, Jian, and Lilian X L Chen. 2006. "Cost-effective Recovery and Purification of Polyhydroxyalkanoates by Selective Dissolution of Cell Mass." *Biotechnology Progress* 22 (2): 547–53.

Yu, Jian, and Heiko Stahl. 2008. "Microbial Utilization and Biopolyester Synthesis of Bagasse Hydrolysates." *Bioresource Technology* 99 (17): 8042–48. https://doi.org/10.1016/j.biortech.2008.03.071.

Zaharia, Catalin, Eugeniu Vasile, Bianca Galateanu, Mihaela-Cristina Bunea, Angela Casarica, and Paul Octavian Stanescu. 2014. "Bacterial Cellulose-Polyhydroxyalkanoates Composites." *Materiale Plastice* 51: 1–5.

8 Microbial Pigments Production Using Agricultural Biomass Residues

Ganesh Babu Malli Mohan and
Sam Aldrin Chandran
SASTRA Deemed to be University

CONTENTS

8.1 INTRODUCTION

Rapid increase in the global population and economic growth are tremendous stimuli in improving and investing on the food and agriculture industries. With increasing globalization and industrialization of the agriculture division results in generation of one-third of the food, which is lost or wasted every year. The waste products arising due to agriculture and the food processing industries are a substantial environmental challenge (Ravindran et al., 2018). Residues collected from agricultural waste are straws, stems, stalks, leaves, husk, stubble, and bagasse. Wastes generated from food industries are fruit and vegetable juice, seeds, peels, pulps, chips, and so on. Most of these wastes are underutilized and untreated, hence reports to discard either by dumping, burning, or unplanned landfilling (Sadh et al., 2018). Agro-based wastes are rich in nutrients including carbohydrates, fibers, proteins, minerals, vitamins,

DOI: 10.1201/9781003188292-8

and so on depending upon the abovementioned plant-based materials. These biochemical ingredients have the biotechnological potentials to be digested into efficient value-added products like the production of pigments, enzymes, bio-gas, and bio-ethanol which are essential to heading toward zero waste (Carrillo-Nieves et al., 2020; Panesar et al., 2015; Ravindran et al., 2018). Notably, the high nutritional composition present in the residues serves as a rich medium for microbial growth and effectively cuts down the production cost of pigments and other value-added compounds (Babitha, 2009; Sadh et al., 2018).

Pigment delivers a wide variety of colors which are the most attractive and first noticeable parameter mostly employed by the food and cosmetic industries. In general, synthetic dyes and pigments have been extensively utilized which are reliable, and economically feasible when compared to natural colorants and/or pigments. However, many of these pigments show hyper allergenicity, toxicological nature, and carcinogenicity, and have been banned from being used as colorants in the food industry. To overcome these adverse effects of synthetic pigment, recent awareness in safety and environmental conservation has made global investigators and investors toward the use of natural pigments, which are certainly safe due to being non-carcinogenic, non-toxic, non-allergic, and biodegradable (Abdulkadir, 2017). In addition to safety concern, it is a prerequisite to develop natural and economically cost-effective pigments. Natural pigments are regularly obtained from plants, insects, microorganisms, and minerals. Not surprisingly, microbial pigments are best compared to other natural pigments due to their availability throughout the season, scalability, and downstream processing (Sen et al., 2019). Notably, microbial-based pigment production is gaining much importance by employing biotechnological tools and delivers the following advantages and benefits:

1. simple, rapid, high, and predictable yield of pigment under cheaper rate
2. stability and produce color intensity
3. easy to employ genetic engineering and structural complexity for industrial needs
4. easy to propagate with wide range of selection strains
5. cheap substrates employed for mass production

Microbial pigments are already in market as a coloring agent for textile and food industries. On the other hand, these chemical compounds have been employed as antioxidants, antimicrobials, antiparasitic, and anticancer.

Advances in metabolic genetic engineering coupled with organic biochemistry have empowered mass pigment production using microbes of interest. Investigating the microbial systems biology to understand the pigment metabolic pathways, recombinant DNA technology like CRISPR-CAS can be employed to reconstruct the genes to increase the production of microbial pigments (He et al., 2017; Lin et al., 2017). Furthermore, suitable fermentation approaches, developing low cost with structured downstream scale-up process, and extraction process could effectively play a crucial role in pigment production.

8.2 MICROBIAL PIGMENTS CRITERIA AND ITS APPLICATIONS

Microorganisms that include bacteria, fungi, actinomycetes, archaea, yeasts, molds, and algae are ubiquitously present in every environmental niche and have multiple roles in nature. Among microbes, bacteria have massive potential to harvest various bioproducts. Generally, all microbes could possibly involve in pigment production; however, a few series of criteria must be satisfied, which are as follows:

i. Microorganisms should be non-pathogenic and non-toxic
ii. Microbes should be able to utilize a wide range of carbon and nitrogen sources from agro-industrial waste
iii. Microbes should be able to produce reasonable yield of pigments
iv. High salt, variable pH, and temperature tolerant microbes
v. Simple methodology should be followed for microbial pigment production and extraction

Natural pigments majorly are produced by the microorganisms such as bacteria, yeast, and molds (Table 8.1) depending on their sources of origin. Pigments extracted from microbial sources have multiple commercial applications listed in Table 8.1. Pigments particularly employed as a food colorant such as riboflavin, beta-carotene, melanin, lycopene, violacein, canthaxanthin, astaxanthin, prodigiosin, and phycocyanin and are more extensively given in Table 8.1. These are not limited to the coloring agent in the food industrial application but also helps to serve as an important additive in food preparations as they are enriched with antioxidant. These microbes are vastly employed in the production of pigments through agro-industrial waste and are best substitutes to synthetic pigments (Lopes and Ligabue-Braun, 2021). Furthermore, in recent years various industries including pharmaceutical, cosmetics, and textile dyeing processes have augmented in exploiting the microbial pigments due to satisfying their series of criteria.

8.3 TYPES OF AGRO/FOOD WASTE

8.3.1 Dairy Industry Waste

Whey is produced during the manufacture of cheese, yogurt, and casein as a by-product. This waste product of dairy industry can cause ecological damage when it is disposed directly into water bodies. But it has the potential to be used as a substrate for microbial fermentations involving lactose, which will make it a high value by-product. It is also a source of bioactive compounds enriched in proteins and peptides. Red pigment has been produced using *Monascus purpureus* using submerged fermentation (Mehri et al., 2021). *Rhodotorula rubra* MTCC 1446 which is a carotenoid biosynthetic yeast has been used to produce a yellowish pink pigment using submerged fermentation using whey supplemented with yeast extract and peptone (Chakraborty, 2019). Cheese whey has been used as a substrate for producing yellow pigments using *Monascus* (Costa et al., 2020). *P. aculeatum* ATCC 10409 has been used to produce yellow pigments using whey media (Afshari et al., 2015).

TABLE 8.1
List of Microorganisms Producing Various Pigment Molecules, Colors, and Its Applications

Microorganisms	Pigment Molecules	Pigments Colors	Application
Bacteria			
Agrobacterium aurantiacum	Astaxanthin, adonixanthin	Pink-red	Food additive, antioxidant
Arthrobacter crystallopoietes	Indigoidine	Dark green	Colorant
Arthrobacter oxidans	Nicotine	Blue	Colorant
Bacillus subtilis	*Riboflavin*	Yellow	Food colorant
Bradyrhizobium sp.	*Canthaxanthin*	Dark-red	Impart color in farmed salmons
Paracoccus carotinifaciens	*Astaxanthin*	Pink-red	Fish feed supplement in the USA
Protomonas extorquens	Rhodoxanthin	Red	Feed additive
Pseudomonas aeruginosa	*Phenazine*	Yellow-orange	Colorant in beverages, cakes, confectionaries, pudding, decoration of food items
Pseudomonas aeruginosa	Fluorescein	Yellow-green	Coloring agent
Actinomycetes			
Gordonia jacobaea	Canaxanthin	Red	Food colorant and cosmetic application
Streptomyces echinoruber	Rubrolone	Red	Antibiotic activity and food colorant
Archaea			
Haloferax mediterranei	Carotenoid	Red	Antitumor, antioxidant, food colorants, and cosmetic application
Fungi			
Ashbya gossypii	Riboflavin (Vitamin B2)	Yellow	Food colorant
Aspergillus cristatus	Catenarin, emodin, physcion, erythroglaucin, rubrocristin, questin	Yellow-red	Food colorant and antibiotic properties
Aspergillus repens	Erythroglaucin, physcion	Yellow-red	Food colorant
Cortinarius	Emodin, dermocybin, dermorubin, flavomannin	Yellow-red	Food colorant and antibiotic properties
Curvularia lunata	Catenarin, chrysophanol cynodontin, erythroglaucin, helminthosporin, tritisporin	Yellow-red	Food colorant and antibiotic properties

(*Continued*)

TABLE 8.1 (*Continued*)
List of Microorganisms Producing Various Pigment Molecules, Colors, and Its Applications

Microorganisms	Pigment Molecules	Pigments Colors	Application
Dermocybe sanguinea	Dermocybin-1-b-D-glycopyranoside, dermorubin, ermolutein, dermoglaucin, 5-chlorodermorubin, emodin, and physcion	Yellow-red	Food colorant and antibiotic properties
Drechslera dictyoides	Catenarin	Red	Food colorant and antibiotic properties
Drechslera graminea	Catenarin	Red	Food colorant and antibiotic properties
Drechslera phlei	Catenarin	Red	Food colorant and antibiotic properties
Drechslera teres	Catenarin	Red	Food colorant and antibiotic properties
Drechslera triticirepenti	Catenarin	Red	Food colorant and antibiotic properties
Fusarium sp	Catenarin, cynodontin, erythroglaucin, helminthosporin, physcion, tritisporin	Yellow-red	Food colorants
Herpotrichia rhodosticta	Averythrin, averythrin-6-monomethyl ether	Orange	Food colorants
Pachybasium candidum	Pachybasin, chrysophanol	Yellow-red	Food colorants
Pencillium islandicum	Skyrin, emodin	Yellow-red	Food colorant and antibiotic properties
Pencillium marneffei	Monascorubrin	Red	Food colorants
Pencillium purpurogenum	Azaphilones	Red	Food colorants
Phoma exigua var. *foveata*	Pachybasin, emodin, chrysophanol, phomarin	Yellow-red	Food colorant and bioactive properties
Talaromyces albobiverticillius	Monascus-like	Red	Antibacterial, food colorant
Talaromyces marneffei	Monascus-like	Red	Antibacterial, food colorant
Talaromyces minioluteus	Monascus-like	Red	Antibacterial, food colorant
Talaromyces purpurogenus	Monascus-like	Red	Antibacterial, food colorant
Talaromyces atroroseus	Mitorubrins, galuconic acid, purpuride	Red	Food colorants
Trichoderma aureoviride	Pachybasin, chrysophanol	Yellow-red	Food colorants
Trichoderma harzianum	Pachybasin, chrysophanol	Yellow-red	Food colorants

(*Continued*)

TABLE 8.1 (*Continued*)
List of Microorganisms Producing Various Pigment Molecules, Colors, and Its Applications

Microorganisms	Pigment Molecules	Pigments Colors	Application
Trichoderma viride	Pachybasin, chrysophanol, emodin 1, 3, 6, 8-tetraHAQN, 2,4,5,7-tetraHAQN	Yellow-red	Food colorant and bioactive properties
Yeast			
Candida famata	Riboflavin (Vitamin B2)	Yellow	Food colorants
Phaffia rhodozyma	Astaxanthin	Pink-red	Feed supplement for salmons, crabs, shrimps, chickens, and egg production
Pichia (*Candida*) *guilliermondii*	Riboflavin (Vitamin B2)	Yellow	Food colorants
Microalgae			
Chlorella fusca	Lutein	Yellow	Food colorant, anticancer
Chlorella zofingiensis	Lutein	Yellow	Food colorant, anticancer
Chlorella protothecoides	Lutein	Yellow	Food colorant, anticancer
Chlorella vulgaris	Lutein	Yellow	Food colorant, anticancer
Chlorococcum citroforme	Lutein	Yellow	Food colorant, anticancer
Coelastrum proboscideum	Lutein	Yellow	Food colorant, anticancer
Muriella aurantiaca	Lutein	Yellow	Food colorant, anticancer
Muriella decolor	Lutein	Yellow	Food colorant, anticancer
Neospondiococcum gelatinosum	Lutein	Yellow	Food colorant, anticancer
Tetracystis aplanosporum	Lutein	Yellow	Food colorant, anticancer
Tetracystis intermedium	Lutein	Yellow	Food colorant, anticancer
Tetracystis tetrasporum	Lutein	Yellow	Food colorant, anticancer

8.3.2 Fruit and Vegetable Waste

When the fruits and vegetables are processed, peel, pulp, and wastewater are generated as wastes and these products contain numerous nutrients which can be used for microbial growth and fermentation. Onion peels, potato skin, mung bean husk, and pea pods were used as substrates for producing pigments, torularhodin, β-carotene, and torulene, using *Rhodotorula mucilaginosa* (Sharma and Ghoshal, 2020). Apple, pomegranate, black carrot, and red beet pulps have been used for pigment production using *Aspergillus carbonarius* (Arikan et al., 2020). Sweet potato-based medium has been used for red pigment production with *Monascus purpureus* using submerged fermentation (Srivastav et al., 2015). Wine industry produces large amounts of grape waste. *Monascus purpureus* has been used for pigment production using grape waste (Mohamed et al., 2012). Jack fruit seeds (Silbir and Goksungur, 2019) and Durian seeds (Srianta et al., 2012) have been used as substrates to produce red pigments using *Monascus.* Carotenoids have been produced using apple pomace as substrate with *Sarcina* sp. (Attri and Joshi, 2005).

8.3.3 Agro Industrial Residue

Husk, bran, cobs, molasses, bagasse, etc. are produced during the harvesting and processing of agricultural products along with the major product. Straw hydrolysate has been used for cost-effective pigment production by *Monascus purpureus* in submerged fermentation (Liu et al., 2020). *Monascus* has been used in the co-solid state fermentation of corn cob powder for the production of orange and red pigments (Embaby et al., 2018). During the process of corn wet milling, corn steep liquor is produced as a by-product and is rich in nutrients. Red pigments have been produced using corn steep liquor with *Monascus ruber* (Hamano and Kilikian, 2006).

A list of agro-industrial wastes which have been employed to produce microbial pigments is summarized in Table 8.2.

8.4 PRE-TREATMENT

Agrowaste is a rich source of lignocellulose, consisting of lignin, cellulose, and hemicellulose in the plant cell wall. To make the glucose present in cellulose and hemicellulose accessible to the microorganisms, the agrowaste must be pre-treated. There are several pre-treatment methods: (1) physical pre-treatment, e.g.: milling, steam explosion, hydrothermal treatment, and irradiation, (2) chemical pre-treatment, e.g.: using NaOH, NH_3, H_2O_2, peroxy formic acid, peroxymonosulftate, (3) biological pre-treatment, using White rot fungi, e.g.: *Bjerkendra adusta*, *Phanerochaete chysoporium*, and *Ceriporiopsis subvermispora*, (4) enzymatic pre-treatment using lignin peroxidases, and (5) combined pre-treatment methods. An effective and economical pre-treatment method should be chosen to make this process cost-effective.

8.5 FERMENTATION PROCESS IN THE DEVELOPMENT OF MICROBIAL PIGMENTS

Microbial metabolism involves in the conversion of agrowaste residues which cause serious problems to value-added products such as alcohol, acids, and gases by the fermentation process, thus decreasing biological oxygen demand (BOD). Recently, many industries and researchers have focused on the processing of agro-industrial wastes for the production of pigments using fermentation and biotechnological processes. To accomplish the anticipated yields of a target pigment, researchers have

Table 8.2
List of Agro-Industrial Residues Used as a Substrate for Microbial Pigment Production

Agro-industrial residues	Microorganisms	Pigment	Type of Fermentation
Bacteria			
Peanut seed oil	*Serratia marcescens* 11E	Prodigiosin	SmF
Sugarcane bagasse	*Planococcus* sp. TRC1	β-carotene	SSF
Liquid pineapple waste	*Chryseobacterium artocarpi* CECT 8497	Yellowish-orange pigment	SmF
Glycerol and soy peptone bagasses	*Serratia marcescens* Xd-1	Prodigiosin	SSF
Liquid pineapple waste	*Chromobacterium violaceum* UTM5	Violacein and deoxyviolacein	SmF
Sugarcane bagasse hydrolysate	*Dietzia maris* NIT-D	Transcanthaxanthin (carotenoid)	SmF
Vegetable cabbage waste	*Pseudomonas* sp.	Melanin	SmF
Sugarcane bagasse	*Chromobacterium violaceum*	Violacein	SmF
Fungi			
Petiole oil palm fronds	*Monascus purpureus* FTC 5357	Red pigments	SSF
Maltose syrup	*Monascus ruber* CCT 3802	Orange, yellow, and red pigments	SmF and SSF
Fruits and vegetable waste	*Blakeslea trispora* MTCC884	Carotenoids	SSF
Corn cob	*Monascus purpureus* ATCC 16436	Orange and red pigments	SSF
Sugarcane bagasse hydrolysate	*Monascus ruber Tieghem* IOC 2225	Red pigment	SmF
Waste orange peels	*Penicillium purpurogenum* CBS 113139	Yellow, orange, and red pigments	SSF, Semi-SSF and SmF
Bakery waste	*Monascus purpureus* ATCC 16365	Orange, yellow, and red pigments	SSF and SmF
Raw glycerol	*Monascus ruber* CCT 3802	Yellow, orange, and red pigments	SmF
Grape waste/cheese whey/soybean meal/rice husk	*Penicillium chrysogenum* IFL1 and IFL2, *Fusarium graminearum* IFL3, *Monascus purpureus* NRRL 1992, *P. vasconiae* IFL4	Yellow, orange, and red pigments	SmF
Corn meal	*Monascus purpureus* CMU001	Red pigments	SSF
Corn cob powder	*Monascus purpureus* KACC 42430	Yellow and red pigments	SSF
Bengal gram husk	*Talaromyces purpureogenus* CFRM02	Red pigments	SmF
Oil palm frond	*Monascus purpureus* FTC 5356	Red pigments	SSF

(Continued)

Table 8.2 (*Continued*)
List of Agro-Industrial Residues Used as a Substrate for Microbial Pigment Production

Agro-industrial residues	Microorganisms	Pigment	Type of Fermentation
Wastes of potato chips manufacturing	*Monascus purpureus* Went NRRL 1992	Red, orange, and yellow pigments	SmF
Yeast			
Onion peels/mung bean husk	*Rhodotorula mucilaginosa* MTCC-1403	β-carotene, phytoene, torulene, and Torularhodin	SmF
Cassava wastewater	*Rhodotorula glutinis* CTT 2182	Carotenoids	SmF
Mesquite pods/corn steep liquor	*Xanthophyllomyces dendrorhous* ATCC 24202	Carotenoids	SmF
Sugarcane juice	*Rhodotorula rubra* 102	Carotenoids	SmF
Coffee husk/pulp extract	*Rhodotorula mucilaginosa* CCMA 0156	Carotenoids	SmF
Crude glycerol/Corn maceration water/ rice parboiling water	*Sporidiobolus salmonicolor* CBS 2636	Carotenoids	SmF
Cassava bagasse	*Rhodotorula mucilaginosa*	Carotenoids	SmF
Olive pomace	*Xanthophyllomyces dendrorhous* ATCC24202 and *Sporidiobolus salmonicolor* ATCC24259	Astaxanthin	SSF
Raw glycerol/corn steep liquor/ sugarcane molasse	*Sporodiobolus pararoseus* CCT 7689	Carotenoids	SmF
Carob pulp syrup/ sugarcane molasses	*Rhodosporidium toruloides* NCYC 921	Carotenoids	SmF
Raw glycerol/corn steep liquor/ parboiled rice water	*Rhodotorula glutinis* ATCC 15125	Carotenoids	SmF
Brewery wastewater	*Rhodotorula glutinis* MT-5	Carotenoids	SmF
Rice bran	Rhodotorula glutinis	β-carotene	SSF

SmF, submerged fermentation; SSF, solid state fermentation; Semi-SSF, semi-solid state fermentation.

been involved in designing and development of a biotechnological fermentation-based pigment process. Further, many critical factors needed to be taken into consideration are selection of bioreactor, raw materials from waste residue and additional chemicals used, microbes, and type of fermentation (batch, fed-batch, or continuous). A fully functional automated bioreactor equipped with multiple devices to maintain certain parameters that influence pigment production including temperature, pH, dissolved oxygen, aeration, and agitation. Ensuring those parameters will help industries to scale up the pigment productivity from research lab (Figure 8.1).

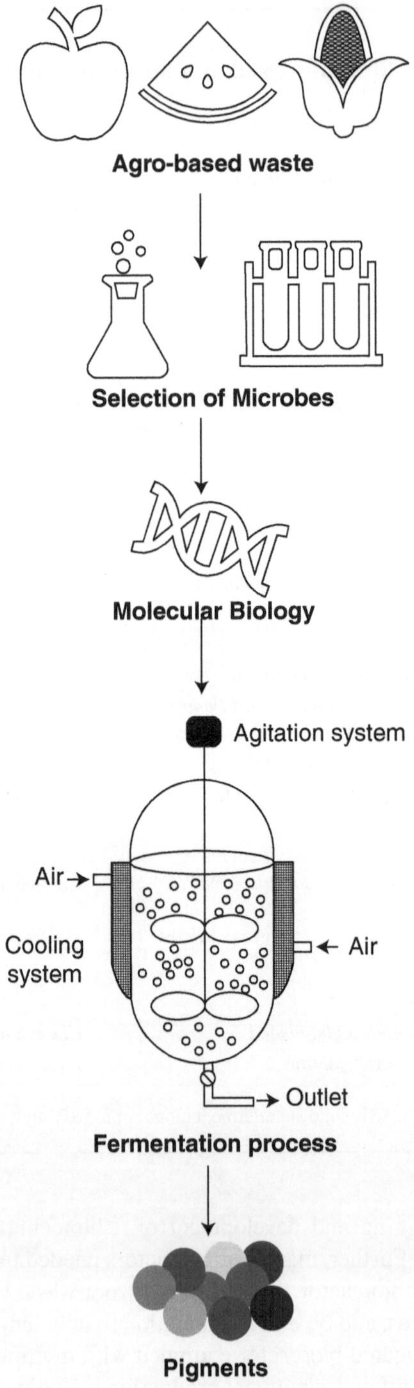

FIGURE 8.1 Schematic representation of microbial pigment production using agricultural biomass residues.

8.6 GENETIC ENGINEERING-BASED STRAIN IMPROVEMENTS FOR ENHANCING PIGMENT PRODUCTION

Microbial carotenoids have been produced using a multivariate modular metabolic engineering-based approach to modify the secondary metabolism (Ajikumar et al., 2010). The metabolic engineering-based approach has been used to manipulate tricarboxylic pathway, lycopene biosynthesis pathway to enhance β-Carotene production and lycopene production, respectively, in *E.coli* (Zhao et al., 2013; Coussement et al., 2017; Usmani et al., 2020). Similar pathway engineering-based approach has been used to improve lycopene biosynthesis in *Rhodobacter sphaeroides* (Su et al., 2018) and β-Carotene production in *Yarrowia lipolytica* (Gao et al., 2017). Genome shuffling-based approach is another way to enhance phenotype which is predominantly used by industries. Genome shuffling has been used successfully to enhance pigment production in *Monascus purpureus* (Ghosh and Dam, 2020). More recently the CRISPR technology for genome editing is being used to manipulate genome for metabolic engineering. *Dunaliella salina* β-carotene hydroxylase has been edited using CRISPR Cas9-based approach, which resulted in significantly higher expression of β-Carotene and Zeaxanthin (Hu et al., 2021).

8.7 CONCLUSION

The agro-industrial waste for producing microbial waste has a huge potential, as we utilize the by-product which can cause environmental pollution, as a substrate for producing microbial pigments, which can be used in a variety of applications. Microbial contamination of the agrowaste substrate, which is the raw material can have deleterious effects as it increases the levels of impurities, which can significantly compromise the product quality. Hence the purity of the strain and purity of the raw materials should be ensured. Another area of concern that limits the usage of natural pigments is their poor stability. Several strategies including encapsulation and nanoemulsion are being tested to improve the stability and shelf life of the pigments. Genome engineering and synthetic biology-based approaches can help in strain improvement and enhancing productivity. Apart from achieving high pigment yield, some concerns regarding the safety of the pigments produced should be ensured as some of the pigment-producing microbes are also associated with toxins. Genetically manipulated strains that lack the production of toxins can be developed and employed to overcome the issue of toxins. Cost-effective strategies to produce the pigments at a large scale will play a pivotal role in bringing up the microbial pigments from lab to market. Nevertheless, the prospect of producing microbial pigments has a promising future.

REFERENCES

Abdulkadir, N. Bacterial pigments and its significance. *MOJ Bioequiv. Bioavailab.* 4, 00073, (2017).

Afshari, M., Shahidi, F., Mortazavi, S. A., Tabatabai, F. & Es'haghi, Z. Investigating the influence of pH, temperature and agitation speed on yellow pigment production by *Penicillium aculeatum* ATCC 10409. *Nat. Prod. Res.* 29, 1300–1306 (2015).

Ajikumar, P. K. et al. Isoprenoid pathway optimization for Taxol precursor overproduction in *Escherichia coli*. *Science* 330, 70–74 (2010).

Arikan, E., Canli, O., Caro, Y., Dufossé, L. & Dizge, N. Production of bio-based pigments from food processing industry by-products (apple, pomegranate, black carrot, red beet pulps) using *Aspergillus carbonarius*. *J. Fungi — Open Access Mycol. J.* 6, 240 (2020).

Attri, D. & Joshi, V. Optimization of apple pomace based medium and fermentation conditions for pigment production by Micrococcus species. *J. Sci. Ind. Res.* 64, 598–601 (2005).

Babitha, S. Microbial pigments. In *Biotechnology for Agro-Industrial Residues Utilisation: Utilisation of Agro-Residues* (eds. Singh nee' Nigam, P. & Pandey, A.) pp. 147–162, Springer, Netherlands (2009). doi:10.1007/978-1-4020-9942-7_8

Carrillo-Nieves, D. et al. Biotransformation of agro-industrial waste to produce lignocellulolytic enzymes and bioethanol with a zero waste. *Biomass Convers. Biorefin.* (2020). doi:10.1007/s13399-020-00738-6

Chakraborty, D. Production and stability analysis of yellowish pink pigments from Rhodotorula rubra MTCC 1446. *Internet J. Microbiol.* (2019). doi:10.5580/245b

Coussement, P., Bauwens, D., Maertens, J. & De Mey, M. Direct combinatorial pathway optimization. *ACS Synth. Biol.* 6, 224–232 (2017).

da Costa, J. P. V., de Oliveira, C. F. D., & Vendruscolo, F. Cheese whey as a potential substrate for *Monascus* pigments production. *AIMS Agric. Food* 5, 785–798 (2020).

Embaby, A. M., Hussein, M. N. & Hussein, A. Monascus orange and red pigments production by Monascus purpureus ATCC16436 through co-solid state fermentation of corn cob and glycerol: An eco-friendly environmental low cost approach. *PLoS One* 13, e0207755 (2018).

Gao, S. et al. Iterative integration of multiple-copy pathway genes in Yarrowia lipolytica for heterologous β-carotene production. *Metab. Eng.* 41, 192–201 (2017).

Ghosh, S. & Dam, B. Genome shuffling improves pigment and other bioactive compound production in Monascus purpureus. *Appl. Microbiol. Biotechnol.* 104, 10451–10463 (2020).

Hamano, P. & Kilikian, B. Production of red pigments by Monascus ruber in culture media containing corn steep liquor. *Brazilian J. Chem. Eng.* 23 (2006).

He, X., Li, Y., Lawson, D. & Xie, D.-Y. Metabolic engineering of anthocyanins in dark tobacco varieties. *Physiol. Plant.* 159, 2–12 (2017).

Hu, L. et al. CRISPR/Cas9-induced β-carotene hydroxylase mutation in *Dunaliella salina* CCAP19/18. *AMB Express* 11, 1–8 (2021).

Lin, C.-H., Lin, T.-H. & Pan, T.-M. Alleviation of metabolic syndrome by monascin and ankaflavin: The perspective of Monascus functional foods. *Food Funct.* 8, 2102–2109 (2017).

Liu, J. et al. Cost-effective pigment production by *Monascus purpureus* using rice straw hydrolysate as substrate in submerged fermentation. *J. Biosci. Bioeng.* 129, 229–236 (2020).

Lopes, F. C. & Ligabue-Braun, R. Agro-industrial residues: Eco-friendly and inexpensive substrates for microbial pigments production. *Front. Sustain. Food Syst.* 5, 65 (2021).

Mehri, D., Perendeci, N. A. & Goksungur, Y. Utilization of whey for red pigment production by *Monascus purpureus* in submerged fermentation. *Fermentation* 7, 75 (2021).

Mohamed, M., Mohamad, R., Manan, M. & Ariff, A. Enhancement of red pigment production by *Monascus purpureus* FTC 5391 through retrofitting of helical ribbon impeller in stirred-tank fermenter. *Food Bioprocess Technol.* 5, 80–91 (2012).

Panesar, R., Kaur, S. & Panesar, P. S. Production of microbial pigments utilizing agro-industrial waste: A review. *Curr. Opin. Food Sci.* 1, 70–76 (2015).

Ravindran, R., Hassan, S. S., Williams, G. A. & Jaiswal, A. K. A review on bioconversion of agro-industrial wastes to industrially important enzymes. *Bioengineering* 5, 93 (2018).

Sadh, P. K., Duhan, S. & Duhan, J. S. Agro-industrial wastes and their utilization using solid state fermentation: A review. *Bioresour. Bioprocess.* 5, 1 (2018).

Sen, T., Barrow, C. J. & Deshmukh, S. K. Microbial pigments in the food industry—challenges and the way forward. *Front. Nutr.* 6, 7 (2019).

Sharma, R. & Ghoshal, G. Optimization of carotenoids production by *Rhodotorula mucilaginosa* (MTCC-1403) using agro-industrial waste in bioreactor: A statistical approach. *Biotechnol. Rep.* 25, e00407 (2020).

Silbir, S. & Goksungur, Y. Natural red pigment production by *Monascus purpureus* in submerged fermentation systems using a food industry waste: Brewer's spent grain. *Foods* 8, (2019).

Srianta, I., Novita, Y. & Kusumawati, N. Production of monascus pigments on durian seed: Effect of supplementation of carbon source. *J. Pure Appl. Microbiol.* 6, 59–63 (2012).

Srivastav, P., Yadav, V. K., Govindasamy, S. & Chandrasekaran, M. Red pigment production by *Monascus purpureus* using sweet potato-based medium in submerged fermentation. *Nutrafoods* 14, 159–167 (2015).

Su, A. et al. Metabolic redesign of *Rhodobacter sphaeroides* for lycopene production. *J. Agric. Food Chem.* 66, 5879–5885 (2018).

Usmani, Z., Sharma, M., Sudheer, S., Gupta, V. K. & Bhat, R. Engineered microbes for pigment production using waste biomass. *Curr. Genomics* 21, 80–95 (2020).

Zhao, J. et al. Engineering central metabolic modules of *Escherichia coli* for improving β-carotene production. *Metab. Eng.* 17, 42–50 (2013).

9 Nanotechnology-Associated Bioremediation for the Elimination of Emerging Contaminants

Alok Tripathi
Indrashil University

Sheeba Narayanan
National Institute of Technology

P. Suresh Kumar
Indian Council of Agricultural Research-National Research Centre for Banana

CONTENTS

DOI: 10.1201/9781003188292-9

9.1 INTRODUCTION

The accelerated population and industrial growth have ignited the intense load of multiple pollutants to the waterbodies. Conventional wastewater treatment techniques and their components are attaining their breaking point to deliver satisfactory results to meet standard needs (Jain et al., 2021). In this regard, advances in nanotechnology provide many possibilities to create cutting-edge wastewater treatment systems. It is being investigated as a promising innovation and has shown astounding achievements in different fields including wastewater treatment (Qu et al., 2013). Nanotechnology-validated technologies not only conquer significant difficulties encountered by current technologies but also build new treatment possibilities that could permit minimum usage of water (Theron et al., 2008). The profoundly productive, adaptive, and multifunctional approaches empowered by nanotechnology are conceived to give elite and reasonable methodologies to treat water and wastewater that are less dependent on enormous infrastructure. By virtue of their small size and immense surface area, nanomaterials exhibit phenomenal possibilities to construct more efficient redox active media and catalysts to treat wastewater (Khan et al., 2019).

Nanobioremediation combines the advantages of bioremediation using nanomaterials. In many treatment processes, the residue generated from the process is a source of major concern for disposal. Nanomaterials when pooled with bioremediation are effective since nanomaterials can immobilize the microorganisms and prevent them from leaching out of the system when they were free cells.

9.2 CONTAMINANTS IN WASTEWATER

Wastewater comprises various hazardous and deleterious contaminants originating from various sectors such as agricultural, sewage, commercial, and industrial as shown in Figure 9.1. Their composition can be distinguished by their actual appearance, substance composition, and microbial stacks (Hakeem, 2016). Wastewater is a complicated grid made out of water, suspended solids, organic and inorganic compounds, heavy metals, dissolved biodegradable contaminants, microorganisms, etc., which contribute to a high chemical oxygen demand and biochemical oxygen demand (Tripathi and Narayanan, 2018).

9.3 BASIC WASTEWATER TREATMENT PROCESS

In recent times, in conjunction with an ascent in industrialization and populace development, the pace of wastewater propagation has been overgrown, which turned into a big threat to the climate and ecosystem. Consequently, a valid wastewater treatment methodology assisted by physical, chemical, and biological methods needs to be implemented for the division and separation of contaminations from wastewater

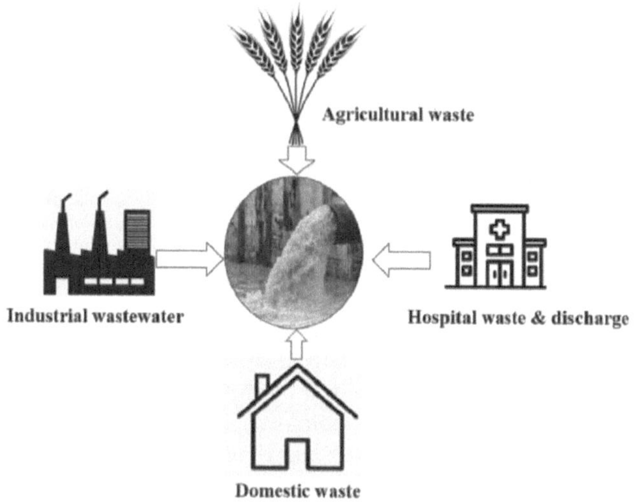

FIGURE 9.1 Sources of wastewater. (Adapted from Jain et al., 2021.)

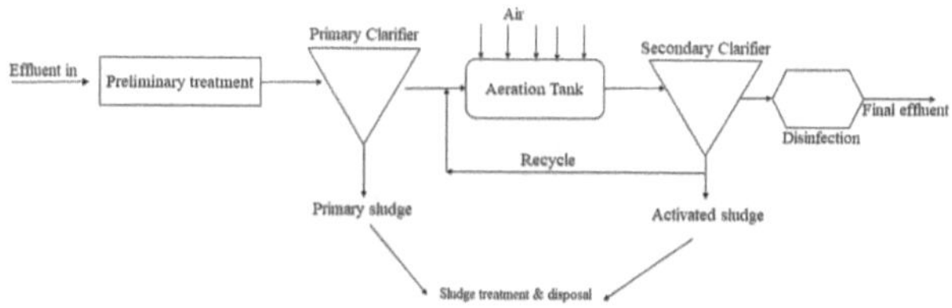

FIGURE 9.2 Overview of wastewater treatment processes. (Adapted from Jain et al., 2021.)

(Tripathi and Narayanan, 2019). The wastewater treatment techniques not only aimed to eliminate the impurities and contaminants underneath the permitted limit but also to retrieve micronutrients and water to evade from ecological and environmental threats (Runguphan and Kitpichai, 2020). The stages required to treat wastewater incredibly rely upon the degree of contamination to be treated (Figure 9.2).

Preliminary treatment is the initial step measure to treat wastewater, which eliminates huge and additionally weighty trash. It involves two-step screening followed by grit removal; the screening system eliminates enormous drifting debris like plastics, papers, clothes, etc. (Jain et al., 2021). Grit removal is followed by screening which essentially eliminates inorganic particles like rock, sand, and other substantial particulate matters. Later, the wastewater moves to primary treatment which prevalently isolates the suspended solids through a sedimentation process. It is a process to hold large volumes of wastewater in tanks to settle the suspended solids at the bottom of the tank. This process removes 80%–90% of suspended solids and 40% of biochemical oxygen demand (Kalfa et al., 2020).

The secondary wastewater treatment process is also known as the biological treatment which is used to remove organic contaminants present in wastewater through microorganisms (Verlicchi et al., 2012). Secondary treatment has been classified into two categories, the first is the aerobic treatment where the microorganisms use oxygen to degrade organic matter present in wastewater, and the second is the anaerobic treatment where the organic contaminants are treated by microorganisms in absence of oxygen. Activated sludge process is an example of a combined aerobic and anaerobic system (Bora and Dutta, 2014). The final stage of wastewater treatment is tertiary treatment, which is used to enhance the quality of water before its discharge. It includes the advanced processes to remove residual organic, inorganic, and microorganisms leftover in primary and secondary processes. It includes filtration, chemical treatment, and ozonation (Qu et al., 2013).

9.4 APPLICATION OF NANOTECHNOLOGY IN WASTEWATER

The materials possessing sizes smaller than 100 nm are termed nanomaterials, so far multifarious nanomaterials were utilized in the wastewater treatment as, for example, self-assembled monolayer on mesoporous supports, carbon-based nanomaterials, polymeric nanoparticles, biopolymers, metal nanoparticles, and many more. The trails through which nanotechnology utilized nanomaterials in wastewater treatment are nano-filtration, adsorption, photocatalysis, bio-sorption, sensing materials, and so on (Qu et al., 2013).

9.5 ADSORPTION

Adsorption is a surface phenomenon used to transfer the pollutant from either a liquid or gas phase to a solid phase under certain experimental conditions. Similar to that bio-sorption involves the use of biomaterials for the same purpose. The application of a few nanomaterials used in the adsorption process is discussed in this section.

9.5.1 Carbon-Based Nanoadsorbents for Adsorption

For adsorption of organic contaminants present in wastewater, carbon nanotubes have demonstrated higher effectiveness as compared to activated carbon (Pan et al., 2008). The external surfaces of carbon nanotubes are the regions for adsorption, and its high adsorption limit predominantly originates from the enormous explicit surface region and the interaction of contaminants with carbon nanotube (Yang and Xing, 2010). In aqueous condition, the carbon nanotubes aggregate due to hydrophobicity, but these aggregates restrain intersectional vacancies and sections, with high contaminants adsorption capacity (Pan et al., 2008).

In comparison to activated carbon, carbon nanotubes have a substantially large amount of micropores accountable for organic impurities (Ji et al., 2009). Significant adsorption for metal ions with persistent kinetics had been observed through oxidized carbon nanotubes. As a consequence of electrostatic attractiveness and chemical bonding, the surface functional groups of carbon nanotubes are proved to be significant adsorption sites (Rao et al., 2007). As compared to activated carbon, numerous studies reported the superior performance of carbon nanotubes to adsorb heavy metals such as Zn^{2+}, Cu^{2+}, and Pb^{2+}, in addition to the extremely attainable sites for adsorption and intragroup distance of diffusion which result in rapid adsorption kinetics (Li et al., 2003; Lu et al., 2006).

Furthermore, the viability of adsorbents can be determined through their regeneration capacity; by virtue of reducing pH of a solution the metal ion adsorption on carbon nanotubes can easily be transposed. At $pH < 2$, 90% and in many cases near to 100% recovery of metal have been observed (Lu et al., 2006; Li et al., 2005), and after regeneration, the adsorption potential remained stable. In a study performed by Lu et al. on the adsorption of Zn^{2+}, it was found that after 10 regeneration and reuse cycles the adsorption capability of single-walled nanotubes and multi-walled nanotubes was reduced to 25%, which for the activated carbon was reduced to 50% (Lu et al., 2006).

9.5.2 Metal-Supported Nanoadsorbent

Aluminium oxides, titanium oxide, and iron oxides are some cost-effective metal oxides used as adsorbents in various applications. The combination of individual metal groups and oxygen restraints the adsorption, which is a binary level process, lateral surface adsorption of metal ions, succeeded by rate-constraining internal diffusion through micropore walls (Trivedi and Axe, 2000). In view of the greater explicit surface region, their nanoscale analogies have high adsorption and accelerated kinetics. An expanded adsorption capacity of magnetite beyond 100 times, as its particle size was reduced against 300–11 nm, was reported by Yean et al., and this was attributed to their structural modification at nanoscale which leads to the formation of new active surface sites (Yean et al., 2005).

In the same way, iron oxide nanoparticles can be superparamagnetic, since the magnetic property is extremely volume reliant as it comes from the aggregate reciprocation of nuclear attractive dipoles. A high magnetic tendency was observed as the size of ferromagnet was reduced to the critical level ~40 nm, along with their reduced size, during countering an extrinsic magnetic field it dissipates permanent magnetic moments and turns into a superparamagnetic particle (Yavuz et al., 2006). These nanomaterials can be either utilized straightforwardly as adsorbents or as core-shell frameworks, where the shell stipulates essential action, whereas the magnetic core acknowledges attractive detachment.

In the past few years, diverse heavy metals (arsenic, chromium, nickel, mercury, cadmium, and lead) have been treated through metal-based nanomaterials such as TiO_2, and nano-sized magnetite has demonstrated excellent performance in comparison to activated carbon to treat arsenic (Deliyanni et al., 2003; Mayo et al., 2007). In conjunction with this metal oxide nanoparticles can be inoculated in the framework of activated carbon to boost its performance to treat arsenic along with organic pollutants (Hristovski et al., 2009a, b). By varying the pH of a solution these metal oxide-based adsorbents can be readily recovered and reused in multiple cycles (Hu et al., 2006), and later their adsorption potential will be declined (Deliyanni et al., 2003).

9.6 MEMBRANE METHODS

The fundamental objective of wastewater treatment is to eliminate undesired pollutants, and depending upon their size membranes enable physical obstruction to such constituents. As a vital part of reuse and treatment, they give a significant degree of automation, in conjunction with less chemical and land requirement. Their commutable arrangements permit an adaptive design (Qu et al., 2013). Apart from this their selectivity and permeability, high energy demand in the case of pressure-driven process, and fouling during operations are significant challenges. The efficient working of the membrane system totally depends on the nature of the material selected, and the amalgamation of various nanomaterials into the membrane frameworks exhibits an improved performance in terms of their thermal and mechanical stability, as well as for pollutant degradation.

9.6.1 Nanocomposite Membranes

There are a number of studies that are dedicated to making concurrence or multi-functional membranes by inclusion of nanomaterials within polymeric or inorganic membrane structures. Metal oxide particles, photocatalytic materials, and antimicrobial nanomaterials are used in such applications. The main purpose of consolidation of these particles in the membrane is to improve their anti-fouling capacity. Powerful fouling resistance, water permeability, and expanded surface hydrophilicity was found in polymeric ultrafiltration membranes by the incorporation of metal oxides nanoparticles such as TiO_2 (Bae and Tak, 2005), alumina (Maximous et al., 2010), silica (Bottino et al., 2001), and zeolite (Pendergast et al., 2010). These materials also assisted to achieve enriched thermal and mechanical stability. Carbon nanotubes and sliver nanoparticles have been used as antimicrobial materials to inhibit biofouling and biofilm development on membrane surfaces (Mauter et al., 2011; Zodrow et al., 2009). Similarly, much research inputs have been dedicated to create photocatalyst-integrated membranes where the combination of physical separation along with reactivity to treat the pollutant was achieved (Choi et al., 2006).

9.6.2 Nanofiber Membrane

These membranes are prepared by the electrospinning technique, which possesses strong porosity and an expanded surface area (Li and Xia, 2004). These membranes are successfully used for air purification systems, and their implementation in the field of water treatment is still undeveloped. Without substantial fouling and high repulse proportion, it can eliminate micro-sized contaminants from water (Ramakrishna et al., 2006). Hence, prior to the reverse osmosis and ultrafiltration they can be opted as a pre-treatment step. In their structural geometry, various nanomaterials can be effectively incorporated during the spinning process (Li and Xia, 2004). For example, ceramic nanoparticles can be reinforced in these membranes to eliminate heavy metals and pollutants in the course of filtration.

9.6.3 Bio-inspired Membranes

These membranes are extremely permeable and selective in nature, in order to improve the performance of a polymeric membrane aquaporin, and a type of protein groove that controls water flow throughout cell membrane has been incorporated (Kumar et al., 2007). Kumar et al. integrated aquaporin-Z derived from *Escherichia coli* to triblock-polymer blisters, which illustrated water penetrability as a minimum over the original blisters, with total dismissal of urea, glucose, salt, and glycerol. It can be prepared by coating aquaporin merged lipid layers on nanofiltration membranes (Kumar et al., 2007).

Similar to that well-coordinated carbon nanotubes were proved a better choice to permeate water, and as per Pendergast and Hoek (2011) membranes with aligned carbon nanotubes have shown higher flux capacity compared to commercial reverse osmosis membrane for seawater (Pendergast and Hoek, 2011). Due to un-uniform diameter at nanoscale, the dismissal of small molecules and salt is a difficult task for these membranes. Hence, to overcome such difficulties carboxyl functional groups were introduced in carbon nanotube-based membranes to achieve 98% exclusion of ferricyanide (Fornasiero et al., 2008). The main issue to use aquaporin and carbon nanotube-based membranes is their commercialized production and fabrication which is a complicated task (Hinds, 2012).

9.7 DECONTAMINATION AND MICROBIAL CONTROL

The implementation of oxidative disinfectants such as chlorine could lead to the formation of disinfectant by products which are difficult to treat, hence in recent trends, ultraviolet-based disinfectant technologies have emerged as an alternative. Apart from this nanomaterial (Ag, TiO_2, ZnO, Carbon nanotubes, Ce_2O_4) based technology has been widely implemented for decontamination and microbial control in wastewater (Li et al., 2008).

Among above-mentioned nanomaterials, silver nanoparticles are well known for their antimicrobial property, and have low toxicity (Xiu et al., 2011; Xiu et al., 2012). Graphite and graphene-based materials have similar antimicrobial properties like carbon nanotubes which kill the bacteria through oxidizing process (Liu et al., 2011). These nanomaterials are projected into bio-film control, bio-fouling control of membranes, and decontamination of wastewater (Brady-Estévez et al., 2010). Silver-based nanoparticles have inherent capability to treat water endured pathogens; the conductive nature and fibrous structure of carbon nanotubes facilitate to development of carbon nanotube filters which efficiently eliminate bacteria and viruses based on their size. The withheld bacteria and viruses can be oxidized directly by applying periodic voltage supply (Rahaman et al., 2012; Vecitis et al., 2011).

9.8 PHOTOCATALYSIS

It is an advanced oxidation process which is a combination of catalysis with photochemistry. In recent years it is extensively implemented in wastewater treatment (Tripathi and Narayanan, 2020a). Photocatalysis follows the use of nanomaterial-based photocatalyst to treat various pollutants, pathogens, and hazardous materials. The mechanism of photocatalysis has been explained in the following equations (Tripathi and Narayanan, 2020b):

$$\text{Photocatalyst} + h\vartheta \rightarrow \text{Photocatalyst}\left(e^- + h^+\right) \tag{9.1}$$

$$H_2O + h^+ \rightarrow OH^\circ + H^+ \tag{9.2}$$

$$O_2 + e^- \rightarrow O_2^- \tag{9.3}$$

$$O_2^- + H^+ \rightleftarrows HOO \quad (9.4)$$

$$2HOO \rightarrow H_2O_2 + O_2 \quad (9.5)$$

$$H_2O_2 \rightarrow 2OH^{\circ} \quad (9.6)$$

Photocatalysis process initiates with the photo-excitation of electron from valence band to conduction band, and the created vacancies in valence band react with water to form oxidizing radicals. These radicals react with oxygen to produce anionic superoxide radical, which is also involved in the oxidation process (Tripathi and Narayanan, 2018).

9.8.1 Types of Catalysts Used in Photocatalysis Process

Based on current and past research, photocatalytic materials can be classified into different categories, namely: binary and ternary semiconductors photocatalysts, type-II heterojunction nanocomposites, and Z-scheme photocatalysts.

Figures 9.3 and 9.4 show the classification of various binary and ternary semiconductor photocatalysts, and Tables 9.1 and 9.2 illustrate their photocatalytic applications.

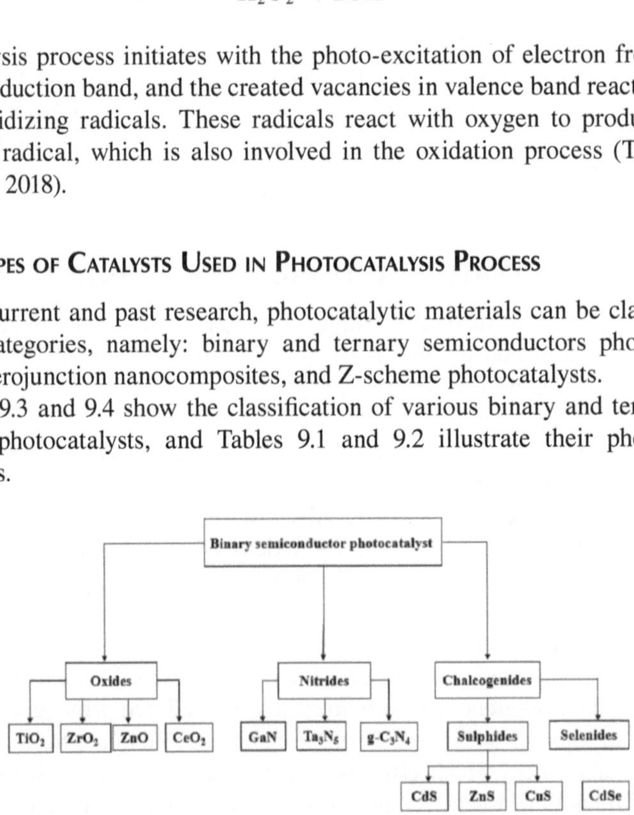

FIGURE 9.3 Classification of binary semiconductor-based photocatalysts. (Adapted from Djurišić et al., 2020.)

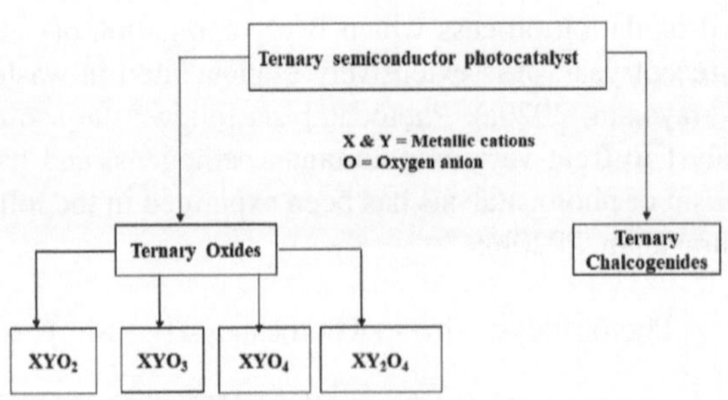

FIGURE 9.4 Classification of ternary semiconductor-based photocatalysts. (Adapted from Djurišić et al., 2020.)

TABLE 9.1
Applications of Binary and Ternary Semiconductor Photocatalysts

Photocatalyst	Source of Illumination	Application	References
TiO_2	15W blue lamp	Mineralization of sucrose	Teoh et al. (2005)
ZnO	UV-lamp	Degradation of methyl orange	Hong et al. (2009)
ZrO_2	300W high-pressure mercury lamp	Degradation of rhodamine B	Shu et al. (2012)
CeO_2	250W high-pressure mercury lamp	Degradation of amido black and acridine orange	Khan et al. (2011)
ZnS	125W high-pressure mercury lamp	Photodegradation of eosin B	Hu et al. (2005)
CdS	350W xenon lamp	Water splitting	Jing and Guo (2006)
CdSe	300W xenon lamp	Water splitting	Holmes et al. (2012)
GaN	200W mercury lamp	Decolouration of orange II	Jung et al. (2008)
Ta_3N_5	300W xenon lamp	Oxygen evolution from water oxidation	Hisatomi et al. (2012)
CuS	500W xenon lamp	Degeneration of methylene blue and methyl orange	Xu et al. (2015)
α-$AgGaO_2$	Xenon lamp with glass filter	Decomposition of isopropanol	Ouyang et al. (2009)
$SrTiO_3$	450 W high-pressure mercury lamp	Nitric oxide degradation	Kobayashi et al. (2018)
$BiVO_4$	300W xenon lamp	O_2 evolution from an aqueous $AgNO_3$ solution	Yu and Kudo (2006)
$AgInS_2$	300W xenon arc lamp	Degradation of 4-nitrophenol under visible irradiation.	Hossein et al. (2017)

9.9 NANOTECHNOLOGY-ASSISTED BIOREMEDIATION

This method combines the advantages of nanoparticles to improve the microbial degradation of contaminants and pollutants. It is considered to be an integrated approach for the treatment and recovery of contaminants. It is expected to give more efficiency, less time, and less harm to nature. This integrated approach is developed to overcome the disadvantages associated with nanotechnology and bioremediation-only processes. Besides the positive impact of the combined process, the effect of nanomaterials on the flora and fauna of the ecosystem is a matter of concern. Strategies to combine the processes are underway to mitigate or balance the effect of nanomaterials on the ecosystem.

There are different types of nanomaterials and they are prepared by different processes such as solvothermal, hydrothermal, solgel, CVD, electrochemical, photochemical, and biological. Biological nanoparticles are viruses, proteins, and plasmids.

Literature reports many advantages of combining nanoparticles with the process of bioremediation. Since the size of nanoparticles is in the nano range, the available surface area per gram of the material is more, thereby enhancing the reactivity in

TABLE 9.2
Type-II Nanocomposite Systems with Their Synthesis Approach and Photocatalytic Applications

Photocatalyst	Source of Illumination	Application	References
TiO_2 nanorods	320W xenon lamp	H_2 generation from an aqueous ethanol	Vu et al. (2014)
TiO_2/ZnO composite	300W xenon lamp	H_2 evolution from an aqueous methanol solution	Hussein et al. (2013)
TiO_2/ZnS	Fluorescent lamp	Degradation of aqueous solution of Orange II dye	Štengl et al. (2008)
ZnO/In_2S_3 core/shell nanorods	500W xenon lamp	Degradation of Rhodamine B	Khanchandani et al. (2013)
SnO_2/Fe_2O_3	1000W xenon lamp	Degradation of acid blue 62 dye	Xia et al. (2008)
SnO_2/SnS_2	1000W xenon lamp	Degradation of methyl orange	Zhang et al. (2011)
CdS/ZnS core/shell nanowires	300W xenon lamp	degradation of 4-chlorophenol and methylene blue	Wang et al. (2009)
In_2O_3/Ta_2O_5	300W xenon lamp	H_2 production from aqueous methanol solution	Xu et al. (2011)

bioremediation. Since the nanoparticles display a quantum effect, the requirement of activation energy is less for a specific reaction to be feasible. Many materials exhibit the surface plasmon resonance effect which is beneficial in recognition of toxic material.

There are many applications of nanoparticle-assisted bioremediation such as water remediation (both groundwater and wastewater), remediation of solid waste, remediation of heavy metals (water as well as soil), hydrocarbon remediation, and remediation of uranium.

Several nanomaterials have been tested in combination with living organisms. Further, the selection of nanomaterial is dependent upon the nature of contaminant to be removed. If the contaminants are organic, then carbon-based nanomaterials are preferred, and iron-based nanomaterials are desirable for contaminants with magnetic properties. The category of biological systems also plays a major role in the efficacy of the combined process such as the nature of plants and species-specific to contaminants. A combination of plants and microorganisms is beneficial since the plants possess major advantages in the removal of contaminants.

9.9.1 Nanobioremediation for Treatment of Polluted Soil

The nature of a soil is a vital parameter and requires careful monitoring as it is used for a variety of purposes such as construction, plantation, and agriculture. Soil is regarded as life-sustaining medium as it supports the growth of plants and vegetation. It is composed of both organic and inorganic constituents. It has many layers from the top such as humus or organic layer, top sand, leached organic matter layer, subsoil, parent material, and finally bedrock.

Soil can be polluted in many ways and are mostly man-made. Soil pollution is defined as reducing the quality of soil through toxic compounds, chemicals, radioactive substances, and pathogens which will also restrict the growth of plants and vegetation. Some of the most active sources of soil pollution are discharge of industrial effluents, unwarranted use of fertilizers and chemicals, leachate from various waste streams, etc. The majority of the pollutants are absorbed into soil while some are adsorbed on the top surface of soil.

Conventional soil remediation techniques involve bioremediation which involves the use of fungi and microorganisms which can break down the complex organic compounds into small easily biodegradable components (Prasad, 2021). It is classified as in-situ and ex-situ bioremediation. In the former, it is the treatment of soil in its original place whereas in the latter the soil is treated in a place other than its natural location. Bioremediation is well suited for organically degrading pollutants in the soil as the process is completely dependent on the nature of soil. However, this process cannot be applied to certain chemicals.

Thermal desorption method involves the use of thermal energy or heat to release the volatile components from the polluted soil. These volatile components are collected for further treatments. The disadvantage of this process is that some harmful chemicals when vapourized and not contained or treated will be released into the environment causing air pollution.

Surfactant enhanced remediation utilizes the injection of solutions into the soil with or without additives. This method exploits the solubility of contaminants in water and is defined by the ability of soil to enhance solubility. Various types of surfactants are used in this process. Recovery of these surfactants without further contaminating the soil is a difficult task.

Pump and treat method is widely used in the treatment of polluted groundwater, since the soil is polluted with wastewater from many chemical and metallurgical industries. Wells are constructed to drain the water from the soil and it is then directed to conventional treatment methods.

In-situ oxidation is another conventional technology which utilizes the oxidants such as ozone, hydrogen peroxides, and potassium permanganate. When these are applied to soil, the pollutants are oxidized. But few microbes and naturally occurring elements are also affected in this process.

The use of nanoparticles synthesized from poly(ethylene) glycol modified urethaneacrylate (PMUA) to increase the absorption of phenanthrene (PHEN) had demonstrated that these engineered NPs are capable of capturing and further degradation by bacteria. The recovery of PMUA can be done by recovery bioreactors (Tungittiplakorn et al., 2005). The use of bimetallic nanoparticles (Pd/nFe) for dechlorination of Anchor 1248 had shown promising results with 99% removal for trichlorinated bipheyls which were biodegraded by *Burkholderia xetonovorans* LB400. The toxicity of the residues after degradation was reduced to around one/third of the value before treatment (Le et al., 2015). Murugesan et al. (2011) evaluated the effect of nFe–Pd as a catalytic reductant for degradation of triclosan and the intermediate product 2-phenoxyphenol was successfully degraded by the biocatalyst

Sphingomonas sp. PH-07 strain in contaminated soil using a nano–bio hybrid process (Murugesan et al., 2011). The gamma isomer of 1,2,3,4,5,6-hexachlorocyclohexane (-HCH), Lindane which is used for the control of pests in agriculture had been identified as a potential threat to the environment and had been banned throughout the world. However, in an attempt to remediate the Lindane-contaminated soils, a study was conducted using zerovalent nano iron particles in combination with CMC-Pd/nFe0 and *Sphingomonas* sp. strain for the degradation of the γ isomer. The results indicated that the reducing property of zerovalent nano iron had impacted the integrated process through a synergistic effect (Singh et al., 2013).

Single enzyme nanoparticles are also employed as conjugate enzymes by combining them with magnetic nanoparticles. Synthetic enzymes are found to be more beneficial as they show higher resistance to oxidation and hence a prolonged lifetime (Qiang et al., 2019). Two different enzymes, trypsin and peroxidase, were used in conjugate with core-shell magnetic nanoparticles. The nanoparticles could be readily recovered using magnetic field. Soil polluted by Carbazole is a threat to the environment as they are mutagenic and readily undergo radical transformation into more dangerous derivatives. Wang et al. (2007) used Fe_3O_4 nanoparticles/gellan gum gel beads with microbial cells (*Sphingomonas* sp. strain XLDN2–5 cells) embedded in the nanoparticles. This combined approach was found to be effective in the degradation of Carbazole than the system without immobilization. A biocomposite formed by the combination of Fe_3O_4 nanoparticles onto the surface of *Sphingomonas* sp. XLDN2–5 cells was used in a similar study in the degradation of Carbazole. In addition to its degradation process, the composite was found to exhibit outstanding reusability because of its magnetic properties (Li et al., 2013). The most common deadly chemical 2,3,7,8-TeCDD found in soil and sediments is highly recalcitrant in nature and possesses high resistance towards bioremediation. A laboratory system was developed using palladized iron nanoparticles through a process of reductive dechlorination followed by oxidative transformation of dibenzo-p-dioxin using *Sphingomonas wittichii* RW1 (DSM 6014) (Bokare et al., 2012). The Cr (VI) ions are accumulated in soil and water due to the release of large volumes of wastewater from leather industries, metal industries, and tanning processes. In a similar study of conversion of hexavalent chromium, the performance of the species *S. oneidensis* MR-1 immobilized in Ca-alginate/Carbon nanotubes beads was studied (Yan et al., 2013). The electron transfer ability of the CNT was found to have an enhanced effect on the conversion of Cr (VI) to trivalent chromium. Ravikumar et al. (2016) successfully described a mechanism using nano zerovalent iron-immobilized calcium alginate beads (nZVI–C–A beads) in a continuous film reactor. A biofilm was formed on the immobilized beads using the consortium of bacteria including *Bacillus subtilis* VITSUKMW1, *E. coli* VITSUKMW3, and *Acinetobacter junii* VITSUKMW2. The process demonstrated 92% removal of the contaminant in the laboratory studies and they found that the removal was enhanced in the presence of biofilm. Chlorinated solvents like Tricholoroethylene remain in the subsurface of contaminated soil and treatment of these chemicals is difficult at the source due to low rates of dechlorination, detrimental effect of these chemicals to the bacteria. However, nanoscale zerovalent iron in the presence of *Dehalococcoides* sp. is effectively dechlorinated and converted to ethane after a lag period (Xiu et al., 2010). In a study conducted to detoxify the halogenated organic pollutants in the soil, the bioPd nanoparticles obtained from the bioreduction of Pd (II) by *Shewanella oneidensis* MR-1 could dehalogenate the Polychlorinated Biphenyls in soil and sediment matrices. The bioPd so obtained had higher reactivity in the dehalogenation process (Windt et al., 2005).

9.9.2 Nanobioremediation for Treatment of Waste Water

Nanoadsorbents prepared from the *Cynomorium coccineum* extract were used successfully for the removal of methylene blue dye. The extract was used for the synthesis of CuO nanoparticles using copper sulphate as the substrate. The study is beneficial in exploring new nanoparticles or adsorbents for treating contaminated water (Sebeia et al., 2020). Nano zerovalent iron and bacterium *Sphingomonas* sp. PH-07 were employed for the reductive-oxidative process for the sequential degradation of deca-BDE and the effect of nano zerovalent iron on survival of the aerobic species were carried out. The outcome of the treatment process could be applied for the treatment of higher halogenated species of contaminants in wastewater (Kim et al., 2012). The efficacy of nanocellulose decorated with bacteria was experimentally evaluated for diuron degradation in water. The nanocomposite achieved not only degraded the diuron but also the metabolite 3,4-dichloroaniline. Such a matrix of nanocomposite will lead the way forward for a combined functional biological system with nanomaterials in the treatment of various herbicides in water as well as soil (Liu et al., 2018). A one-pot facile method for the synthesis of enzymatically active carbon nanotube in combating the organophosphates through bioremediation was suggested by Mechrez et al. (2014). A model compound of methyl paraoxon was subjected to filtration of the organophosphate hydrolase carbon nanotube membrane. A significant reduction in the model compound is identified through various cycles of filtration. The enzymatic activity was retained in the CNT matrix over a number of cycles (Mechrez et al., 2014). Another study to elucidate the potential prospects of supported immobilized biosorbents for bioremediation of polluted water using CNT matrix showed improved performance. Multi walled carbon nanotubes because of their size and structure exhibited superior performance over Single-walled carbon nanotubes (Mishra and Scrivener Publishing Llc, 2014).

Few studies have documented the effect of combining the biological process with the nanoparticles in a hybrid system. These studies have shown promising results. They are presented below. Cholorophenol with aromatic ring structure is usually found in wastewater and is termed as carcinogenic. Many attempts for the degradation of chlorophenols through physical and chemical processes were reported, and it was found that they can be effectively decomposed using biological methods. Magnetically k-carrageenan immobilized *Rhodococcus rhodochrous* cells with the optimum Fe_3O_4 nanoparticle could break the barrier of mass transfer resistance with improved recovery of cells in addition to an efficient degradation compared to the free cell embedded nanoparticle (Hou et al., 2016). The association of Gram-negative bacterium *Halomonas* sp. with polyvinylpyrrolidone covered iron oxide nanoparticles in the remediation of metals was studied with reference to lead and cadmium removal. In addition to the removal of metals, it was found that the Fe was used up by the species as nutrients suggesting the support rendered by the nanoparticle in the growth of species which can accelerate the bioremediation mechanism (Cao et al., 2020).

Enzymes immobilized in nanoparticles have been widely used in the treatment of textile wastewater. Enzyme immobilization had been developed predominantly to overcome the difficulties associated with the retrieval of free enzyme from the reaction solution as well as the instability. In a study conducted by Wang et al. (2013) the degradation of phenolic azo dyes laccase immobilized on magnetic Fe_3O_4/SiO_2 indicated remarkable colour degradation to the extent of 80% due to the interruption in the mass transfer limitations caused due to the smaller size of nanoparticles. In another study conducted for the treatment of phenolic wastewater and dye, phospholipid-templated titania particles synthesized from dodecylamine were used for encapsulating horseradish peroxidase, and nanomaterial combined biological process exhibited around 93% removal in the first cycle followed by a minimal reduction in the efficiency for the repeated cycles (Jiang et al., 2014). Enzyme lignin peroxidase isolated from *Pseudomonas aeruginosa* strain OS4 was encapsulated on surface modified Fe_3O_4 magnetic nanoparticles subjected to decolourization of textile industry effluent containing Reactive Blue azo dye. The laboratory experiments showed promising results in decolourization to the extent of 97% for 76 h (Darwesh et al., 2015). Iron oxide nanoparticles because of their magnetic properties are found to exhibit degradation and reusability after separation from the mixture. The immobilization of enzyme glucose oxidase by the iron oxide nanoparticles for the decolourization of Acid yellow 12 from dye wastewater was studied by Aber et al. (2016). The process variables were optimized for colour removal in the bio-fenton process. A nanocomposite prepared by the conjugation of P*p*PD with Iron oxide was used to immobilize Laccase enzyme. This composite is found to exhibit excellent conductivity property, stability, and removal of RB-19 from the solution. The nanocomposite was found to have around 80% removal efficiency and was higher than the free counterparts (Liu et al., 2016). Magnetic graphene oxide nanomaterial was employed in immobilizing the copper-containing enzyme, Laccase and experimented for the colour removal efficiency of crystal violet, malachite green, and brilliant green in an aqueous solution. The investigation revealed colour removal efficiency of 94.7% for Crystal violet, 95.6% of malachite green, and 91.4% of brilliant green respectively suggesting the Laccase immobilize magnetic GO for treatment of industrial wastewater (Chen et al., 2017). Process of biocatalyses for the removal of Indigo Carmine by the Laccase immobilized on EDTA-TMS surface modified magnetic nanoparticle exhibited 97% recovery of enzymatic activity. The conjugate was stable and only 27% of the activity was deteriorated over five cycles of usage of the catalyst (Fernandes et al., 2017).

9.10 CONCLUSION

Nanotechnology has penetrated many walks of human life and the energy and environmental applications are the most promising fields. The unique properties of materials in the nanoscale have revolutionized many industries such as food, cosmetics, energy, IT, and agriculture. These properties show tremendous output in environmental applications, especially in the water treatment sector. Contaminants are pollutants which render the wastewater objectionable and are found to degrade our ecosystem. These contaminants are easily adsorbed, converted, or reduced by the use of nanomaterials, nanocomposites, and nanomatrix. Bioremediation assisted by nanomaterials has been in existence and is equally competitive to other alternate processes with an added advantage of an ecofriendly process. Nanomaterials were once branded as an eco-toxic material but the studies conducted in bioremediation for soil and water treatment prove that nanomaterials bind themselves to the microorganisms, and in fact, the growth of microorganisms is well supported by the nanonutrients thus contributing to sustainability. The immobilization of microorganisms with nanomaterials improves the microbial activity in a reaction. Further aspects of the mechanism of reaction, new nanomaterial-enzyme combinations, reusability of the matrix, and the enzymes are further areas to be explored.

REFERENCES

Aber, Soheil, Ehsan Mahmoudikia, and Afzal Karimi. 2016. "Immobilization of Glucose Oxidase on Fe_3O_4 Magnetic Nanoparticles and Its Application in the Removal of Acid Yellow 12." *Water, Air, & Soil Pollution* 227 (93): 1–11. doi:10.1007/s11270-016-2754-x.

Bae, Tae Hyun, and Tae Moon Tak. 2005. "Effect of TiO_2 Nanoparticles on Fouling Mitigation of Ultrafiltration Membranes for Activated Sludge Filtration." *Journal of Membrane Science* 249 (1–2): 1–8. doi:10.1016/j.memsci.2004.09.008.

Bokare, Varima, Kumarasamy Murugesan, Jae-Hwan Kim, Eun-Ju Kim, and Yoon-Seok Chang. 2012. "Integrated Hybrid Treatment for the Remediation of 2, 3, 7, 8-Tetrachlorodibenzo-p-Dioxin." *Science of the Total Environment* 435–436: 563–566. doi:10.1016/j.scitotenv.2012.07.079.

Bora, Tanujjal, and Joydeep Dutta. 2014. "Applications of Nanotechnology in Wastewater Treatment—A Review." *Journal of Nanoscience and Nanotechnology* 14 (1): 613–626. doi:10.1166/jnn.2014.8898.

Bottino, A., G. Capannelli, V. D'Asti, and P. Piaggio. 2001. "Preparation and Properties of Novel Organic-Inorganic Porous Membranes." *Separation and Purification Technology* 22–23: 269–275. doi:10.1016/S1383-5866(00)00127-1.

Brady-Estévez, Anna S., Mary H. Schnoor, Seoktae Kang, and Menachem Elimelech. 2010. "SWNT-MWNT Hybrid Filter Attains High Viral Removal and Bacterial Inactivation." *Langmuir* 26 (24): 19153–19158. doi:10.1021/la103776y.

Cao, Xiufeng, Amjed Alabresm, Yung Pin, Alan W Decho, and Jamie Lead. 2020. "Science of the Total Environment Improved Metal Remediation Using a Combined Bacterial and Nanoscience Approach." *Science of the Total Environment* 704: 135378. doi:10.1016/j.scitotenv.2019.135378.

Chen, Jing, Juan Leng, Xiai Yang, Liping Liao, Liangliang Liu, and Aiping Xiao. 2017. "Enhanced Performance of Magnetic Graphene Oxide-Immobilized Laccase and Its Application for the Decolorization of Dyes." *Molecules* 22 (221): 1–11. doi:10.3390/molecules22020221.

Choi, Hyeok, Elias Stathatos, and Dionysios D. Dionysiou. 2006. "Sol-Gel Preparation of Mesoporous Photocatalytic TiO_2 Films and TiO2/Al2O3 Composite Membranes for Environmental Applications." *Applied Catalysis B: Environmental* 63 (1–2): 60–67. doi:10.1016/j.apcatb.2005.09.012.

Darwesh, Osama M, Hassan Moawad, Olfat S Barakat, and Wafaa M Abd El-Rahim. 2015. "Bioremediation of Textile Reactive Blue Azo Dye Residues Using Nanobiotechnology Approaches." *Research Journal of Pharmaceutical, Biological and Chemical Sciences*, 6 (1): 1202–1211.

Deliyanni, E. A., D. N. Bakoyannakis, A. I. Zouboulis, and K. A. Matis. 2003. "Sorption of As(V) Ions by Akaganéite-Type Nanocrystals." *Chemosphere* 50 (1): 155–163. doi:10.1016/S0045-6535(02)00351-X.
Djurišić, Aleksandra B., Yanling He, and Alan M.C. Ng. 2020. "Visible-Light Photocatalysts: Prospects and Challenges." *APL Materials* 8 (3). AIP Publishing, LLC. doi:10.1063/1.5140497.
Fernandes, Raquel A, Ana Luísa Daniel-da-silva, Ana P M Tavares, and Ana M R B Xavier. 2017. "EDTA-Cu (II) Chelating Magnetic Nanoparticles as a Support for Laccase Immobilization." *Chemical Engineering Science* 158:599–605. doi:10.1016/j.ces.2016.11.011.
Fornasiero, Francesco, Hyung Gyu Park, Jason K Holt, Michael Stadermann, Costas P Grigoropoulos, Aleksandr Noy, Olgica Bakajin, and Robert H Austin. 2008. "Grigoropoulos-Ion Exclusion by Sub-2-Nm Carbon Nanotube Pores.Pdf." *Proceedings of the National Academy of Sciences* 105 (45): 17250–17255.
Hakeem, Khalid Rehman, Javaid Akhtar, and Muhammad Sabir. 2016. "Soil Science: Agricultural and Environmental Prospectives." In *Soil Science: Agricultural and Environmental Prospectives*, pp. 1–430. doi:10.1007/978-3-319-34451-5.
Hinds, Bruce. 2012. "Dramatic Transport Properties of Carbon Nanotube Membranes for a Robust Protein Channel Mimetic Platform." *Current Opinion in Solid State and Materials Science* 16 (1): 1–9. doi:10.1016/j.cossms.2011.05.003.
Hisatomi, Takashi, Kazuhiko Maeda, Yosuke Moriya, and Kazunari Domen. 2012. "2012-JACS-Enhanced Water Oxidation on Ta_3N_5 Photocatalysts by Modification.Pdf." *Journal of the American Chemical Society* 5: 3–6.
Holmes, Michael A., Troy K. Townsend, and Frank E. Osterloh. 2012. "Quantum Confinement Controlled Photocatalytic Water Splitting by Suspended CdSe Nanocrystals." *Chemical Communications* 48 (3): 371–373. doi:10.1039/c1cc16082f.
Hong, R. Y., J. H. Li, L. L. Chen, D. Q. Liu, H. Z. Li, Y. Zheng, and J. Ding. 2009. "Synthesis, Surface Modification and Photocatalytic Property of ZnO Nanoparticles." *Powder Technology* 189 (3): 426–432. doi:10.1016/j.powtec.2008.07.004.
Hossein, Amir, Cheshme Khavar, and Moslem Jafarisani. 2017. "Photocatalytic Degradation of 4-Nitro Phenol in Aqueous Solution by the $AgInS_2$ Nanoparticles Synthesized via Microwave Heating Technique." *International Journal of Health Studies* 3 (1): 19–25. doi:10.22100/ijhs.v3i1.205.
Hou, Jianfeng, Feixia Liu, Nan Wu, Jiansong Ju, and Bo Yu. 2016. "Efficient Biodegradation of Chlorophenols in Aqueous Phase by Magnetically Immobilized Aniline - Degrading Rhodococcus Rhodochrous Strain." *Journal of Nanobiotechnology*, 1–8. doi:10.1186/s12951-016-0158-0.
Hristovski, Kiril D., Hanhphuc Nguyen, and Paul K. Westerhoff. 2009a. "Removal of Arsenate and 17α-Ethinyl Estradiol (EE2) by Iron (Hydr)Oxide Modified Activated Carbon Fibers." *Journal of Environmental Science and Health - Part A Toxic/Hazardous Substances and Environmental Engineering* 44 (4): 354–361. doi:10.1080/10934520802659695.
Hristovski, Kiril D., Paul K. Westerhoff, Teresia Möller, and Paul Sylvester. 2009b. "Effect of Synthesis Conditions on Nano-Iron (Hydr)Oxide Impregnated Granulated Activated Carbon." *Chemical Engineering Journal* 146 (2): 237–243. doi:10.1016/j.cej.2008.05.040.
Hu, Jin Song, Ling Ling Ren, Yu Guo Guo, Han Pu Liang, An Min Cao, Li Jun Wan, and Chun Li Bai. 2005. "Mass Production and High Photocatalytic Activity of ZnS Nanoporous Nanoparticles." *Angewandte Chemie - International Edition* 44 (8): 1269–1273. doi:10.1002/anie.200462057.
Hu, Jing, Guohua Chen, and Irene M. C. Lo. 2006. "Selective Removal of Heavy Metals from Industrial Wastewater Using Maghemite Nanoparticle: Performance and Mechanisms." *Journal of Environmental Engineering* 132 (7): 709–715. doi:10.1061/(asce)0733-9372(2006)132:7(709) .

Hussein, Abdulmenan M., Luther Mahoney, Rui Peng, Harrison Kibombo, Chia Ming Wu, Ranjit T. Koodali, and Rajesh Shende. 2013. "Mesoporous Coupled ZnO/TiO_2 Photocatalyst Nanocomposites for Hydrogen Generation." *Journal of Renewable and Sustainable Energy* 5 (3). doi:10.1063/1.4808263.

Jain, Keerti, Anand S. Patel, Vishwas P. Pardhi, and Swaran Jeet Singh Flora. 2021. "Nanotechnology in Wastewater Management: A New Paradigm towards Wastewater Treatment." *Molecules* 26 (6). doi:10.3390/molecules26061797.

Ji, Liangliang, Wei Chen, Lin Duan, and Dongqiang Zhu. 2009. "Mechanisms for Strong Adsorption of Tetracycline to Carbon Nanotubes: A Comparative Study Using Activated Carbon and Graphite as Adsorbents." *Environmental Science and Technology* 43 (7): 2322–2327. doi:10.1021/es803268b.

Jiang, Yanjun, Wei Tang, Jing Gao, Liya Zhou, and Ying He. 2014. "Enzyme and Microbial Technology Immobilization of Horseradish Peroxidase in Phospholipid-Templated Titania and Its Applications in Phenolic Compounds and Dye Removal." *Enzyme and Microbial Technology* 55: 1–6. doi:10.1016/j.enzmictec.2013.11.005.

Jing, Dengwei, and Liejin Guo. 2006. "A Novel Method for the Preparation of a Highly Stable and Active CdS Photocatalyst with a Special Surface Nanostructure." *Journal of Physical Chemistry B* 110 (23): 11139–11145. doi:10.1021/jp060905k.

Jung, Hye Seong, Young Joon Hong, Yirui Li, Jeonghui Cho, Yong Jin Kim, and Gyu Chul Yi. 2008. "Photocatalysis Using GaN Nanowires." *ACS Nano* 2 (4): 637–642. doi:10.1021/nn700320y.

Kalfa, Ayelet, Barak Shapira, Alexey Shopin, Izaak Cohen, Eran Avraham, and Doron Aurbach. 2020. "Capacitive Deionization for Wastewater Treatment: Opportunities and Challenges." *Chemosphere* 241: 125003. doi:10.1016/j.chemosphere.2019.125003.

Khan, Ibrahim, Khalid Saeed, and Idrees Khan. 2019. "Nanoparticles: Properties, Applications and Toxicities." *Arabian Journal of Chemistry* 12 (7): 908–931. doi:10.1016/j.arabjc.2017.05.011.

Khan, Sher Bahadar, M. Faisal, Mohammed M. Rahman, and Aslam Jamal. 2011. "Exploration of CeO_2 Nanoparticles as a Chemi-Sensor and Photo-Catalyst for Environmental Applications." *Science of the Total Environment* 409 (15): 2987–2992. doi:10.1016/j.scitotenv.2011.04.019.

Khanchandani, Sunita, Simanta Kundu, Amitava Patra, and Ashok K. Ganguli. 2013. "Band Gap Tuning of ZnO/In_2S_3 Core/Shell Nanorod Arrays for Enhanced Visible-Light-Driven Photocatalysis." *Journal of Physical Chemistry C* 117 (11): 5558–5567. doi:10.1021/jp310495j.

Kim, Young-mo, Kumarasamy Murugesan, Yoon-young Chang, Eun-ju Kim, and Yoon-seok Chang. 2012. "Degradation of Polybrominated Diphenyl Ethers by a Sequential Treatment with Nanoscale Zero Valent Iron and Aerobic Biodegradation," *Journal of Chemical Technology & Biotechnology* 87: 216–224. doi:10.1002/jctb.2699.

Kobayashi, Mariko, Yoshikazu Suzuki, Tomoyo Goto, Sung Hun Cho, Tohru Sekino, Yusuke Asakura, and Shu Yin. 2018. "Low-Temperature Hydrothermal Synthesis and Characterization of $SrTiO_3$ Photocatalysts for NOx Degradation." *Journal of the Ceramic Society of Japan* 126 (2): 135–138. doi:10.2109/jcersj2.17195.

Kumar, Manish, Mariusz Grzelakowski, Julie Zilles, Mark Clark, and Wolfgang Meier. 2007. "Highly Permeable Polymeric Membranes Based on the Incorporation of the Functional Water Channel Protein Aquaporin Z." *Proceedings of the National Academy of Sciences of the United States of America* 104 (52): 20719–20724. doi:10.1073/pnas.0708762104.

Le, Thao Thanh, Khanh Hoang Nguyen, Jong Rok Jeon, Arokiasamy J. Francis, and Yoon Seok Chang. 2015. "Nano/Bio Treatment of Polychlorinated Biphenyls with Evaluation of Comparative Toxicity." *Journal of Hazardous Materials* 287: 335–341. doi:10.1016/j.jhazmat.2015.02.001.

Li, Dan, and Younan Xia. 2004. "Electrospinning of Nanofibers: Reinventing the Wheel?" *Advanced Materials* 16 (14): 1151–1170. doi:10.1002/adma.200400719.

Li, Qilin, Shaily Mahendra, Delina Y. Lyon, Lena Brunet, Michael V. Liga, Dong Li, and Pedro J.J. Alvarez. 2008. "Antimicrobial Nanomaterials for Water Disinfection and Microbial Control: Potential Applications and Implications." *Water Research* 42 (18): 4591–4602. doi:10.1016/j.watres.2008.08.015.

Li, Yan Hui, Zechao Di, Jun Ding, Dehai Wu, Zhaokun Luan, and Yanqiu Zhu. 2005. "Adsorption Thermodynamic, Kinetic and Desorption Studies of Pb^{2+} on Carbon Nanotubes." *Water Research* 39 (4): 605–609. doi:10.1016/j.watres.2004.11.004.

Li, Yan Hui, Jun Ding, Zhaokun Luan, Zechao Di, Yuefeng Zhu, Cailu Xu, Dehai Wu, and Bingqing Wei. 2003. "Competitive Adsorption of Pb^{2+}, Cu^{2+} and Cd^{2+} Ions from Aqueous Solutions by Multiwalled Carbon Nanotubes." *Carbon* 41 (14): 2787–2792. doi:10.1016/S0008-6223(03)00392-0.

Li, Yufei, Xiaoyu Du, Chao Wu, Xueying Liu, Xia Wang, and Ping Xu. 2013. "An Efficient Magnetically Modified Microbial Cell Biocomposite for Carbazole Biodegradation," *Nanoscale Research Letters*, 8 (1): 1–5.

Liu, Jie, Eden Morales-narváez, Teresa Vicent, and Arben Merkoçi. 2018. "Microorganism-Decorated Nanocellulose for e Ffi Cient Diuron Removal." *Chemical Engineering Journal* 354 (August): 1083–1091. doi:10.1016/j.cej.2018.08.035.

Lu, Chungsying, Huantsung Chiu, and Chunti Liu. 2006. "Removal of Zinc(II) from Aqueous Solution by Purified Carbon Nanotubes: Kinetics and Equilibrium Studies." *Industrial and Engineering Chemistry Research* 45 (8): 2850–2855. doi:10.1021/ie051206h.

Liu, Shaobin, Tingying Helen Zeng, Mario Hofmann, Ehdi Burcombe, Jun Wei, Rongrong Jiang, Jing Kong, and Yuan Chen. 2011. "Antibacterial Activity of Graphite, Graphite Oxide, Graphene Oxide, and Reduced Graphene Oxide: Membrane and Oxidative Stress." *ACS Nano* 5 (9): 6971–6980. doi:10.1021/nn202451x.

Liu, Youxun, Mingyang Yan, Yuanyuan Geng, and Juan Huang. 2016. "Laccase Immobilization on Poly (p -Phenylenediamine)/ Fe_3O_4 Nanocomposite for Reactive Blue 19 Dye Removal." *Applied Sciences* doi:10.3390/app6080232.

Mauter, Meagan S., Yue Wang, Kaetochi C. Okemgbo, Chinedum O. Osuji, Emmanuel P. Giannelis, and Menachem Elimelech. 2011. "Antifouling Ultrafiltration Membranes via Post-Fabrication Grafting of Biocidal Nanomaterials." *ACS Applied Materials and Interfaces* 3 (8): 2861–2868. doi:10.1021/am200522v.

Maximous, Nermen, G. Nakhla, K. Wong, and W. Wan. 2010. "Optimization of Al_2O_3/PES Membranes for Wastewater Filtration." *Separation and Purification Technology* 73 (2): 294–301. doi:10.1016/j.seppur.2010.04.016.

Mayo, J. T., C. Yavuz, S. Yean, L. Cong, H. Shipley, W. Yu, J. Falkner, A. Kan, M. Tomson, and V. L. Colvin. 2007. "The Effect of Nanocrystalline Magnetite Size on Arsenic Removal." *Science and Technology of Advanced Materials* 8 (1–2): 71–75. doi:10.1016/j.stam.2006.10.005.

Mechrez, Guy, Maksym A Krepker, Yifat Harel, and Jean-Paul Lellouche. 2014. "Biocatalytic Carbon Nanotube Paper: A 'One-Pot' Route for Fabrication of Enzyme-Immobilized Membranes for Organophosphate Bioremediation." *Journal of Materials Chemistry B* 38: 915–922. doi:10.1039/c3tb21439g.

Mishra, Ajay Kumar, Scrivener Publishing Wiley Salem, Massachusetts. 2014. "Prospects for Immobilization of Microbial Sorbents on Carbon Nanotubes for Biosorption : Bioremediation of Heavy." In *Application of Nanotechnology in Water Research*, pp. 39–59.

Murugesan, Kumarasamy, Varima Bokare, Jong Rok Jeon, Eun Ju Kim, Jae Hwan Kim, and Yoon Seok Chang. 2011. "Effect of Fe-Pd Bimetallic Nanoparticles on Sphingomonas Sp. PH-07 and a Nano-Bio Hybrid Process for Triclosan Degradation." *Bioresource Technology* 102 (10): 6019–6025. doi:10.1016/j.biortech.2011.02.099.

Ouyang, Shuxin, Naoki Kikugawa, Di Chen, Zou Zhigang, and Ye Jinhua. 2009. "A Systematical Study on Photocatalytic Properties of Agmo2 (m) Al, Ga, in): Effects of Chemical Compositions, Crystal Structures, and Electronic Structures." *Journal of Physical Chemistry C* 113 (4): 1560–1566. doi:10.1021/jp806513t.

Pan, Bo, Daohui Lin, Hamid Mashayekhi, and Baoshan Xing. 2008. "Adsorption and Hysteresis of Bisphenol A and 17α-Ethinyl Estradiol on Carbon Nanomaterials." *Environmental Science and Technology* 42 (15): 5480–5485. doi:10.1021/es8001184.

Pendergast, Marytheresa M., and Eric M.V. Hoek. 2011. "A Review of Water Treatment Membrane Nanotechnologies." *Energy and Environmental Science* 4 (6): 1946–1971. doi:10.1039/c0ee00541j.

Pendergast, Mary Theresa M., Jodie M. Nygaard, Asim K. Ghosh, and Eric M.V. Hoek. 2010. "Using Nanocomposite Materials Technology to Understand and Control Reverse Osmosis Membrane Compaction." *Desalination* 261 (3): 255–263. doi:10.1016/j.desal.2010.06.008.

Prasad, Majeti Narasimha Vara. 2021. *Handbook of Assisted and Amendment: Enhanced Sustainable Remediation Technology*. doi:10.1002/9781119670391.

Qiang, You, Sharma Amit, Andrzej Paszczynski, and Daniel Meyer. 2019. "Conjugates of Magnetic Nanoparticle-Enzyme for Bioremediation." In *2007 Cleantech Conference and Trade Show Cleantech 2007*, 95–97.

Qu, Xiaolei, Pedro J J Alvarez, and Qilin Li. 2013. "Applications of Nanotechnology in Water and Wastewater Treatment." *Water Research* 47 (12): 3931–3946. doi:10.1016/j.watres.2012.09.058.

Rahaman, Md Saifur, Chad D. Vecitis, and Menachem Elimelech. 2012. "Electrochemical Carbon-Nanotube Filter Performance toward Virus Removal and Inactivation in the Presence of Natural Organic Matter." *Environmental Science and Technology* 46 (3): 1556–1564. doi:10.1021/es203607d.

Ramakrishna, Seeram, Kazutoshi Fujihara, Wee Eong Teo, Thomas Yong, Zuwei Ma, and Ramakrishna Ramaseshan. 2006. "Electrospun Nanofibers: Solving Global Issues." *Materials Today* 9 (3): 40–50. doi:10.1016/S1369-7021(06)71389-X.

Rao, Gadupudi Purnachadra, Chungsying Lu, and Fengsheng Su. 2007. "Sorption of Divalent Metal Ions from Aqueous Solution by Carbon Nanotubes: A Review." *Separation and Purification Technology* 58 (1): 224–231. doi:10.1016/j.seppur.2006.12.006.

Ravikumar, K V G, Deepak Kumar, Gaurav Kumar, P Mrudula, Chandrasekaran Natarajan, and Amitava Mukherjee. 2016. "Enhanced Cr(VI) Removal by Nanozerovalent Iron-Immobilized Alginate Beads in the Presence of a Bio Fi Lm in a Continuous-Flow Reactor," doi:10.1021/acs.iecr.6b01006.

Runguphan, T., and J. Kitpichai. 2020. "Coaction of Bio-Sorption and Bio-Filtration for the Remediation of Domestic and Agricultural Wastewater Contaminated with Heavy Metal." *IOP Conference Series: Materials Science and Engineering* 965 (1). doi:10.1088/1757-899X/965/1/012010.

Sebeia, Nouha, Mahjoub Jabli, Adel Ghith, and Tawfik A Saleh. 2020. "Eco-Friendly Synthesis of Cynomorium Coccineum Extract for Controlled Production of Copper Nanoparticles for Sorption of Methylene Blue Dye." *Arabian Journal of Chemistry* 13 (2): 4263–4274. doi:10.1016/j.arabjc.2019.07.007.

Shu, Zhanxia, Xiuling Jiao, and Dairong Chen. 2012. "Synthesis and Photocatalytic Properties of Flower-like Zirconia Nanostructures." *CrystEngComm* 14 (3): 1122–1127. doi:10.1039/c1ce06155k.

Singh, Ritu, Natesan Manickam, Mohana Krishna Reddy Mudiam, Ramesh Chandra Murthy, and Virendra Misra. 2013. "An Integrated (Nano-Bio) Technique for Degradation of γ-HCH Contaminated Soil." *Journal of Hazardous Materials* 258–259: 35–41. doi:10.1016/j.jhazmat.2013.04.016.

Štengl, Václav, Snejana Bakardjieva, Nataliya Murafa, Vendula Houšková, and Kamil Lang. 2008. "Visible-Light Photocatalytic Activity of TiO_2/ZnS Nanocomposites Prepared by Homogeneous Hydrolysis." *Microporous and Mesoporous Materials* 110 (2–3): 370–378. doi:10.1016/j.micromeso.2007.06.052.

Teoh, Wey Yang, Lutz Mädler, Donia Beydoun, Sotiris E. Pratsinis, and Rose Amal. 2005. "Direct (One-Step) Synthesis of TiO_2 and Pt/TiO_2 Nanoparticles for Photocatalytic Mineralisation of Sucrose." *Chemical Engineering Science* 60 (21): 5852–5861. doi:10.1016/j.ces.2005.05.037.

Theron, J., J. A. Walker, and T. E. Cloete. 2008. "Nanotechnology and Water Treatment: Applications and Emerging Opportunities." *Critical Reviews in Microbiology* 34 (1): 43–69. doi:10.1080/10408410701710442.

Tripathi, Alok, and Sheeba Narayanan. 2018. "Impact of TiO_2 and TiO_2/g-C_3N_4 Nanocomposite to Treat Industrial Wastewater." *Environmental Nanotechnology, Monitoring & Management* 10 (January): 280–291. doi:10.1016/j.enmm.2018.07.010.

Tripathi, Alok, and Sheeba Narayanan. 2019. "Skeletal Tailoring of Two-Dimensional π-Conjugated Polymer (g-C_3N_4) through Sodium Salt for Solar-Light Driven Photocatalysis." *Journal of Photochemistry and Photobiology A: Chemistry* 373 (September): 1–11. doi:10.1016/j.jphotochem.2018.12.031.

Tripathi, Alok, and Sheeba. Narayanan. 2020a. "Stimulation of n–π*Transition of g-C_3N_4 through ZnAl-Layered Double Hydroxide for Solar Light Assisted Phenol Degradation." *Materials Science in Semiconductor Processing* 108. doi:10.1016/j.mssp.2019.104892.

Tripathi, Alok, and Sheeba Narayanan. 2020b. "Structural Modification of a 2D π-Conjugated Polymeric Material (g-C_3N_4) through Boron Doping for Extended Visible Light Absorption." *Synthetic Metals* 260. doi:10.1016/j.synthmet.2019.116284.

Trivedi, P., and L. Axe. 2000. "Modeling Cd and Zn Sorption to Hydrous Metal Oxides." *Environmental Science and Technology* 34 (11): 2215–2223. doi:10.1021/es991110c.

Tungittiplakorn, Warapong, Claude Cohen, and Leonard W. Lion. 2005. "Engineered Polymeric Nanoparticles for Bioremediation of Hydrophobic Contaminants." *Environmental Science and Technology* 39 (5): 1354–1358. doi:10.1021/es049031a.

Vecitis, Chad D., Mary H. Schnoor, Md Saifur Rahaman, Jessica D. Schiffman, and Menachem Elimelech. 2011. "Electrochemical Multiwalled Carbon Nanotube Filter for Viral and Bacterial Removal and Inactivation." *Environmental Science and Technology* 45 (8): 3672–3679. doi:10.1021/es2000062.

Verlicchi, Paola, M. Al Aukidy, and Elena Zambello. 2012. "Occurrence of Pharmaceutical Compounds in Urban Wastewater: Removal, Mass Load and Environmental Risk after a Secondary Treatment-A Review." *Science of the Total Environment* 429: 123–155. doi:10.1016/j.scitotenv.2012.04.028.

Vu, Thi Thuy Duong, Frej Mighri, Abdellah Ajji, and Trong On Do. 2014. "Synthesis of Titanium Dioxide/Cadmium Sulfide Nanosphere Particles for Photocatalyst Applications." *Industrial and Engineering Chemistry Research* 53 (10): 3888–3897. doi:10.1021/ie403718n.

Wang, Hongxia, Wei Zhang, Jingxiang Zhao, Lulu Xu, Chunyan Zhou, Lin Chang, and Liyan Wang. 2013. "Rapid Decolorization of Phenolic Azo Dyes by Immobilized Laccase with Fe_3O_4/SiO_2 Nanoparticles as Support." *Industrial & Engineering Chemistry Research* 52: 4401–4407.

Wang, Le, Hongwei Wei, Yingju Fan, Xinzheng Liu, and Jinhua Zhan. 2009. "Synthesis, Optical Properties, and Photocatalytic Activity of One-Dimensional CdS@ZnS Core-Shell Nanocomposites." *Nanoscale Research Letters* 4 (6): 558–564. doi:10.1007/s11671-009-9280-3.

Wang, Xia, Zhonghui Gai, Bo Yu, Jinhui Feng, Changyong Xu, Yong Yuan, Zhixin Lin, and Ping Xu. 2007. "Degradation of Carbazole by Microbial Cells Immobilized in Magnetic Gellan Gum Gel Beads." *Applied and Environmental Microbiology* 73 (20): 6421–6428. doi:10.1128/AEM.01051-07.

Windt, Wim De, Peter Aelterman, and Willy Verstraete. 2005. "Bioreductive Deposition of Palladium (0) Nanoparticles on Shewanella Oneidensis with Catalytic Activity towards Reductive Dechlorination of Polychlorinated Biphenyls" 7: 314–325. doi:10.1111/j.1462-2920.2004.00696.x.

Xia, Huili, Huisheng Zhuang, Tao Zhang, and Dongchang Xiao. 2008. "Visible-Light-Activated Nanocomposite Photocatalyst of Fe_2O_3/SnO_2." *Materials Letters* 62 (6–7): 1126–1128. doi:10.1016/j.matlet.2007.07.062.

Xiu, Zong-ming, Zhao-Hui Jin, Tie-Long Li, Shaily Mahendra, Gregory V Lowry, and Pedro J J Alvarez. 2010. "Bioresource Technology Effects of Nano-Scale Zero-Valent Iron Particles on a Mixed Culture Dechlorinating Trichloroethylene." *Bioresource Technology* 101 (4): 1141–1146. doi:10.1016/j.biortech.2009.09.057.

Xiu, Zong-ming, Jie Ma, and Pedro J J Alvarez. 2011. "Differential Effect of Common Ligands and Molecular Oxygen on.Pdf," 9003–9008.

Xiu, Zong Ming, Qing Bo Zhang, Hema L. Puppala, Vicki L. Colvin, and Pedro J.J. Alvarez. 2012. "Negligible Particle-Specific Antibacterial Activity of Silver Nanoparticles." *Nano Letters* 12 (8): 4271–4275. doi:10.1021/nl301934w.

Xu, Leilei, Jianguo Guan, Liang Gao, and Zhigang Sun. 2011. "Preparation of Heterostructured Mesoporous In_2O_3/Ta_2O_5 Nanocomposites with Enhanced Photocatalytic Activity for Hydrogen Evolution." *Catalysis Communications* 12 (6): 548–552. doi:10.1016/j.catcom.2010.11.027.

Xu, Wence, Shengli Zhu, Yanqin Liang, Zhaoyang Li, Zhenduo Cui, Xianjin Yang, and Akihisa Inoue. 2015. "Nanoporous CuS with Excellent Photocatalytic Property." *Scientific Reports* 5: 1–11. doi:10.1038/srep18125.

Yan, Fang-fang, Chao Wu, Yuan-yuan Cheng, Yan-rong He, Wen-wei Li, and Han-qing Yu. 2013. "Carbon Nanotubes Promote Cr(VI) Reduction by Alginate-Immobilized Shewanella Oneidensis MR-1." *Biochemical Engineering Journal* 77: 183–189. doi:10.1016/j.bej.2013.06.009.

Yang, Kun, and Baoshan Xing. 2010. "Adsorption of Organic Compounds by Carbon Nanomaterials in Aqueous Phase: Polanyi Theory and Its Application." *Chemical Reviews* 110 (10): 5989–6008. doi:10.1021/cr100059s.

Yavuz, Cafer T., J. T. Mayo, William W. Yu, Arjun Prakash, Joshua C. Falkner, Sujin Yean, Lili Cong, et al. 2006. "Low-Field Magnetic Separation of Monodisperse Fe_3O_4 Nanocrystals." *Science* 314 (5801): 964–967. doi:10.1126/science.1131475.

Yean, S., L. Cong, C. T. Yavuz, J. T. Mayo, W. W. Yu, A. T. Kan, V. L. Colvin, and M. B. Tomson. 2005. "Effect of Magnetite Particle Size on Adsorption and Desorption of Arsenite and Arsenate." *Journal of Materials Research* 20 (12): 3255–3264. doi:10.1557/jmr.2005.0403.

Yu, Jianqiang, and Akihiko Kudo. 2006. "Effects of Structural Variation on the Photocatalytic Performance of Hydrothermally Synthesized $BiVO_4$." *Advanced Functional Materials* 16 (16): 2163–2169. doi:10.1002/adfm.200500799.

Zhang, Yong Cai, Zhen Ni Du, Kun Wei Li, Ming Zhang, and Dionysios D. Dionysiou. 2011. "High-Performance Visible-Light-Driven SnS_2/SnO_2 Nanocomposite Photocatalyst Prepared via in Situ Hydrothermal Oxidation of SnS_2 Nanoparticles." *ACS Applied Materials and Interfaces* 3 (5): 1528–1537. doi:10.1021/am200102y.

Zodrow, Katherine, Léna Brunet, Shaily Mahendra, Dong Li, Anna Zhang, Qilin Li, and Pedro J.J. Alvarez. 2009. "Polysulfone Ultrafiltration Membranes Impregnated with Silver Nanoparticles Show Improved Biofouling Resistance and Virus Removal." *Water Research* 43 (3): 715–723. doi:10.1016/j.watres.2008.11.014.

10 Phytoremediation Potential of Some Bioenergy Crops
A Review

V. Anbuganesan, R. Vishnupradeep, A. S. Archana, S. Soundarya, L. Benedict Bruno, and M. Rajkumar
Bharathiar University

CONTENTS

DOI: 10.1201/9781003188292-10

10.1 INTRODUCTION

Soil pollution as a result of increased deposition of contaminants is a vital environmental and agricultural issue that the world faces today. The contaminants such as heavy metals (HM), polyaromatic hydrocarbons, pesticides and herbicides originated from different sources including natural sources, agricultural practices, industrial and domestic effluent, and atmospheric sources, which increased the contaminant concentration and availability in the soil, resulting in various negative effects on ecosystem (Ibrahim and Afandi, 2020; Zhang et al., 2022). Among the various soil contaminants, HM/metalloid is one of the major toxic substances with the highest negative impacts on soil's physical, chemical and biological properties (Cachada et al., 2018; Mishra et al., 2015). HM (As, Cd, Cr, Cu, Hg, Ni, Pb and Zn) contamination in soil may come as a consequence of natural sources (weathering of ore bodies, volcanic activity and forest fires) and anthropogenic sources such as disposal of urban and industrial wastes, pesticides usages, mining activities, smelting processes, mineral fertilizer application, fossil fuel combustion, use of agrochemicals, sewage and atmospheric deposition from traffic emissions such as motor vehicles and combustion fuel (Cachada et al., 2018; Sharma et al., 2018; Weissmannová and Pavlovský, 2017).

In recent decades, the concentration of these metals is increasing in soil and poses serious environmental issues at local, regional and global levels. For example, due to industrial expansion in China, the HM contaminations have increased in agricultural soil and deteriorated agricultural production. Whereas in India, the maximum contamination of HM is found in regions such as Odisha, Karnataka, Uttar Pradesh, Telangana, Maharashtra, and Jharkhand due to rapid industrialization and population increase. In particular, the prevalent type of soil contaminants in southern (Karnataka), northern (Uttar Pradesh) and eastern (Odisha) India is Cr and Ni; in central (Telangana) India is As and Pb; in western (Maharashtra) and eastern (Jharkhand) India is Zn and Cu, respectively (Adimalla, 2020). In general, HM have a direct impact on human health through consumption, inhalation, skin contact and dermal absorption (Ahmad et al., 2021). In addition, HM entry into the food chain causes severe problems to animal and human health causing skin lesions, skin cancer, cardiovascular diseases, brain cancer and other carcinogenic effects (Khan et al., 2017; Sardar et al., 2013). Apart from the human health effect, high concentrations of HM in soils cause serious problems to agriculture. Although plants require some metals as essential nutrient for their growth, metabolism and other vital processes, excessive concentration is lethal and toxic to the plants which cause reduced seed germination, stunted growth, decreased yield and damages to other vital biochemical processes (Basir-Cyio et al., 2020; Zulfiqar et al., 2019). The prominent effects of soil metal pollution on human health and agriculture are represented in Table 10.1.

Clean-up of excess soil metal contamination is tedious and also the existing remediation technologies such as physical and chemical methods are expensive and have several technical difficulties. Phytoremediation, the use of plants for decontamination of soil, has received distinct attention in the past three decades due to the technical feasibility, low investments in technology and eco-friendly nature. Additionally,

TABLE 10.1
The Impacts of the Different HM Soil Pollutants on Human Health and Agriculture

	Impact on Human Health				
Contaminants	**Health Effects**	**Exposure**	**Reference**	**Impacts on Agriculture**	**Reference**
Nickel	• Affects important cellular processes such as oxidative phosphorylation and ATP synthesis • Lung cancer • Fibrosis • Cardiovascular diseases • Epigenetic effects	• Inhalation • Skin contact	Carre et al. (2017); Zambelli et al. (2016)	• Reduced chlorophyll content • Stomatal conductivity affects the Calvin cycle and CO_2 uptake • Reduce plant nutrient uptake • Reduce shoot and root growth, and wilt of leaves of tree	Ahmad and Ashraf (2012)
Mercury	• Affects central nervous system (CNS) and gastrointestinal toxicity • Affects brain development • Causes protein damage in cellular function • Congenital malformations • Perinatal mortality	• Exposure via eating contaminated seafood	Espana et al. (2018)	• Stunted growth, reduced tiller and panicle formation • Reduced yield • In vivo accumulation in seedling shoots and roots • Reduced germination rate • Reduced flower and fruit weight • Plant bleaching	Basir-Cyio et al. (2020)
Copper	• Anaemia • Arthritis • Diabetes • Heart attack • Liver dysfunction • Autism • Cancer • Hyper tension • Hair loss	• Inhalation • Ingestion	Lokeshappa et al. (2012)	• Stunted growth • Decreased biomass yield	Bruno et al. (2021)

(*Continued*)

TABLE 10.1 (*Continued*)
The Impacts of the Different HM Soil Pollutants on Human Health and Agriculture

Contaminants	Impact on Human Health			Impacts on Agriculture	Reference
	Health Effects	Exposure	Reference		
Arsenic	• Brain damage • Cardiovascular and respiratory disorder • Conjunctivitis • Dermatitis • Skin cancer	• Dermal contact • Inhalation • Ingestion of contaminated food and water	Ayangbenro and Babalola (2017); Li et al. (2019); Rasheed et al., (2016)	• Reduced seed germination • Reduced fruit yield, stunting, and wilting	Alloway (2013)
Cadmium	• Liver and urinary organ injury • Low bone density • Itai-itai illness • Erectile dysfunction • Nephron toxicity	• Ingestion of contaminated food and water • Bioaccumulation	Khan et al. (2017)	• Stunted growth of roots and shoots • Reduced nutrient content • Poor plant seed germination	McLaughlin and Singh (1999)
Zinc	• Cardiovascular diseases • Chest pain • Dermatitis • Dizziness • Dry cough • Shortness of breath • Headache • Kidney diseases • Lung and nasal cancer • Nausea	• Ingestion • Inhalation • Skin contact	Qu et al. (2012)	• Decreased germination and biomass yield • Reduced plant chlorophyll, carotenoid, starch and amino acid content	Moffett et al. (2003)

(*Continued*)

TABLE 10.1 (*Continued*)
The Impacts of the Different HM Soil Pollutants on Human Health and Agriculture

	Impact on Human Health				
Contaminants	**Health Effects**	**Exposure**	**Reference**	**Impacts on Agriculture**	**Reference**
Chromium	• Damages kidney • Carcinogenic effect • Haemolysis • Renal and liver failure • Asthma • Hair loss in humans	• Ingestion • Thermal contact	ATSDR, (2012); Rahman and Singh (2019); Sheehan et al. (1991)	• Reduction in seed germination • Causes plant vigour, and iron intake in plants	Rahman and Singh (2019)
Lead	• Harms nervous, urinary and reproductive system • Anaemia • Bone deterioration • Cardiovascular disease • Nephrosis	• Ingestion of contaminated soil or dust.	Havugimana et al. (2015); Mishra et al. (2019)	• Inhibits seed germination and growth • Poor CO_2 fixation • Reduces the growth of plant proteins	Zulfiqar et al. (2019)

the utilization of bioenergy crops in phytoremediation process has an added advantage over conventional phytoremediation technique such as conversion of biomass into biofuel. It is well known that the utilization of fossil fuel for energy production is increasing since the last century due to increasing population and global needs. Therefore, considering the energy necessity and remediation feasibility exploiting non-edible bioenergy crops is regarded as a worthy alternate and discussed in this chapter.

10.2 HEAVY METAL REMEDIATION PROCESSES

HM can stay in the environment for a long time after they are introduced. The extent of pollution depends upon the type of HM and soil. In-situ or ex-situ, on-site or off-site, biological, physical and chemical remediation procedures are all employed to clean up heavy metal(loid)s contaminated soils (Ali et al., 2013). The combination of these strategies is frequently used to provide a more cost-effective and efficient clean-up of a contaminated site. The overall view of existing remediation processes is represented in Figure 10.1

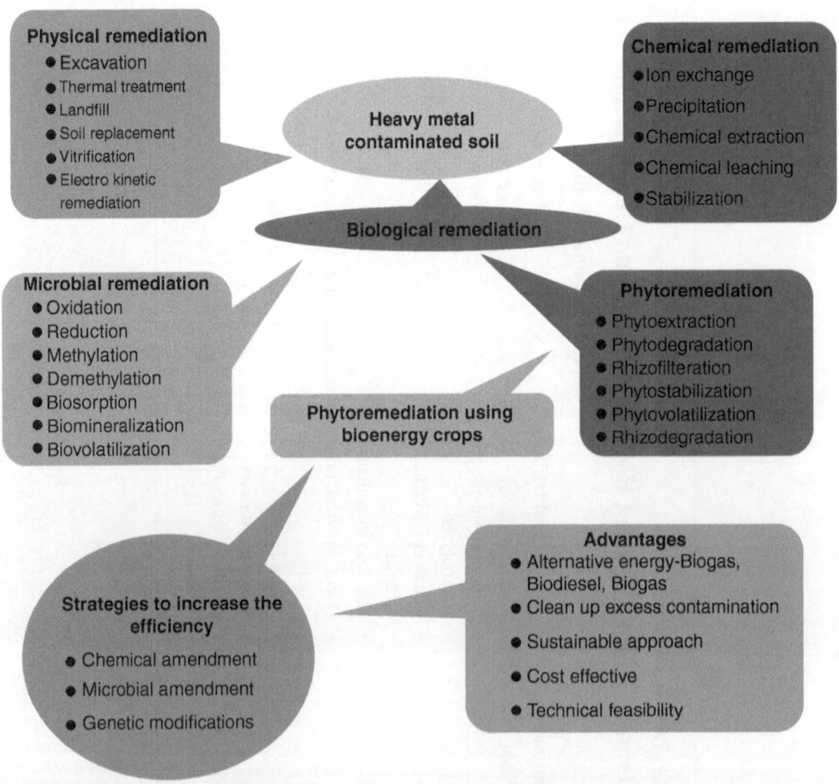

FIGURE 10.1 Overall methods in decontamination of soil heavy metal.

10.2.1 Physical and Chemical Method

HM have been claimed to be removed using a wide range of physical processes, involving detoxifying the polluted system by using metals' physicochemical properties. The physical method of remediation includes soil replacement (Yao et al., 2012), soil washing (Abumaizar and Smith, 1999), soil isolation (Zheng and Wang, 2002), soil adsorption (Muharrem and Olcay, 2017), electrokinetic method (Sivapullaiah et al., 2015), membrane filtration (Khulbe and Matsuura, 2018), granular activated carbon (Sani et al., 2017), vitrification (Mallampati et al., 2015) and photocatalysis (Tahir et al., 2019). Earlier soil replacement, washing and isolation approaches successfully isolate polluted soil and ecosystem, reducing environmental impact. These processes dilute the concentration of HM in the soil and render increased potential in soil functionality. Despite its advantages, because of the significant labour requirements, these techniques are only suitable for extremely contaminated soils with a limited space as well in case agricultural fields there exist a high risk of losing soil fertility. The process of soil vitrification includes the involvement of high temperature in the HM-contaminated soil site in order to encourage the formation of materials for preventing the movement of HM across the contaminated soil site. The tons of Zn- and Pb-rich ceramic wastes were cleaned up by using in-field Joule heating vitrification at about 1850 °C (Dellisanti et al. 2016). Solar technology was used by Navarro et al. (2013) to vitrify waste from Ag–Pb mines in Spain. They discovered that vitrification rendered Zn, Mn, Fe and Cu immobile in the contaminated soil itself. The thermal treatment at high temperature (1350°C) immobilized the HM (Zn, Ni, Mn and Cu) and restricted the leaching out from the soil, thereby reducing the environmental risk. Soil electrokinetic remediation works on the basis of establishing an appropriate electric field gradient on two sides of an electrolytic tank holding saturated contaminated soil. The usage of ideal nanomaterials such as nano-photocatalyst could improve the remediation of HM in the soil. These photocatalysts have many specific properties with high adsorption ability for HM, and the ability to convert high toxic elements into low toxic effluents at lower costs (Tahir et al., 2019).

The remediation of hazardous HM from the contaminated soil could be done using chemical processes. The chemical methods in the HM-contaminated soil brought changes to the chemical characteristics of HM and thereby diminish its hazardous nature. Various chemical processes include chemical precipitation (Djedidi et al., 2009), ion exchange (Lee et al., 2007) and coagulation and flocculation (Renault et al., 2009). Chemical treatments are highly successful at the field scale, but they have the disadvantage of forming by-products, which adds to the number of downstream processing stages (Rajendran et al., 2022). Immobilization of heavy metal(loid)s in soil is usually accomplished by adding organic and inorganic amendments to the soil. Both the physical and chemical methods of HM remediation have several disadvantages including:

- Limited to small areas and specific geographic locations
- Techniques are expensive
- Loss of land cropping function

- Require more land for trash storage
- Limited to certain compounds
- Disposal cost is high
- Induce groundwater and air pollution

10.2.2 Biological Methods

Nevertheless, biological approaches have certain advantages over the existing chemical and physical methods. Biological methods employ microbes and plants to remediate the HM-contaminated soils. Microbes including bacteria, algae, fungi and yeast are utilized for processes such as bioleaching, immobilization, bioaugmentation, biosorption, biological stabilization, composting and volatilization (Alidou-Arzika et al., 2021). Most of the microbes produce several metal-chelating compounds such as siderophores which can sequester the metals and stabilize the cell walls. Several microbes secrete exo- and endo-enzymes which can mineralize the metals and reduce the toxicity of the HM in the soils. In addition, the extracellular polysaccharides producing ability of the microbes play a critical role in mitigating HM toxicity. The microbial exopolysaccharide possess negatively charged functional groups that induce adsorption through ionic interaction which is energy independent and with no metabolic reaction involved (Alidou-Arzika et al., 2021; Bruno et al., 2021; Karthik et al., 2017). These microbial-mediated bioremediations may be considered an effective safer remediation technology, but the bottleneck in microbial remediation is it cannot be employed in highly contaminated areas. In this scenario, phytoremediation is a widely accepted and efficient method for cleaning up large contaminated areas due to their cost-effectiveness and eco-friendly nature. The efficiency of this process is determined by the features of the plants, the area to be remediated and the contaminant to be remediated (Elicker et al., 2014).

10.2.2.1 Phytoremediation

The utilization of plants to remove, transport, stabilize and/or decompose pollutants in soil, sediment and water is known as phytoremediation. Plants are used as filters in phytoremediation technology, a bioremediation approach, to collect, immobilize and change pollutants into a less hazardous form (Parmar and Singh, 2015). Phytoremediation has the following advantages: can be utilized for a larger area, for various contaminants, does not create secondary pollution and does not excavate the soil from the sites. Phytoremediation aspect involves phytoaccumulation, phytoextraction, phytostabilization, phytovolatilization, rhizofiltration and rhizodegradation. Phytoaccumulation is the process by which plants absorb pollutants from contaminated locations, as well as the other nutrients and water they need to grow. In phytoaccumulation, the contaminants absorbed by the plant are not eliminated, but rather accumulate in the shoots, leaves and other components of the plant (Muthusaravanan et al., 2018). Whereas in phytostabilization the mobility and bioavailability of pollutants are reduced in the environment, thus preventing their migration to groundwater or their entry into the food chain by root absorption and accumulation, adsorption onto roots or precipitation within the root zone (rhizosphere) (Etim, 2012; Padmavathiamma and Li, 2007). While phytovolatilization is a process of using plants to absorb contaminants from the soil, convert them to a volatile state and transpire them into the atmosphere (Awa and Hadibarata, 2020). In rhizodegradation, the plant exudates and organic compounds degraded the pollutants in the rhizosphere and converted them into minerals or comparatively less toxic substances (Awa and Hadibarata, 2020; Ali et al., 2013).

10.3 PHYTOREMEDIATION OF HEAVY METAL-POLLUTED SOILS BY BIOENERGY CROPS

Currently, most HM phytoremediation approaches are prone to uncertainty of causing secondary pollution. While disposal and burning of biomass, by which the accumulated pollutants can be liberated into the environment such as SO_2, CO_2 and suspended particles, have substantial consequences on human health and endanger human survival and the ecosystem (Moosavi et al., 2018). Therefore, environmental challenges and risks that accompany phytoremediation have to be addressed along with economic feasibility in order to implement this technology for a wider application. In recent years, the utilization of non-edible bioenergy crops is getting popular in the scientific community due to their reusability and environmental friendliness. The use of non-edible energy crops in phytoremediation to remediate contaminated lands is considered as a sustainable process and can be an alternative approach to overcome the raising concern of secondary pollution caused by conventional phytoremediation technique (Yadav et al., 2019). In addition, bioenergy crops can be utilized for ecological restoration, soil conservation, contaminated land repair and as an attractive and clean-up plant along roadsides (Wang et al., 2019). Further, with the ability to generate huge amounts of biomass under a variety of growing situations, the utilized non-edible plants can exploit as a feedstock for the conversion of biofuel including ethanol, biodiesel and biogas.

10.3.1 Potential of Bioenergy Crops

The bioenergy crops are fast growing, water and nutrient efficient, have low invasive potential and feature excessive tolerance for stress (Moosavi et al., 2018). Furthermore, bioenergy crop cultivars are more resistant to biotic and abiotic stressors, allowing them to develop more quickly than conventional crops. Bioenergy crops also require less biological, chemical or physical pre-treatments, lowering the cost of biomass processing (Yadav et al., 2019). They reduce the risk of energy poverty and contribute to economic development in developing countries (Carere et al., 2008; Schroder et al., 2018).

10.3.2 Types of Bioenergy Crops

Generally, the bioenergy crops can be divided into three types: first-generation bioenergy crops, second-generation crops, and third-generation crops. The first-generation bioenergy crops consist of food crops such as sugarcane, corn and rapeseed which were utilized for the phytoremediation processes. The utilization of these crops creates an issue of food security and increases the cost of the food products generated from these crops. To overcome these issues in phytoremediation, the high lignocellulose-based second-generation crops such as switchgrass, miscanthus, alfalfa, and reed canary grass were utilized. These crops can be grown in marginal and other contaminated lands and the bioenergy can be extracted from the lignocellulosic biomass. However, the biomass produced from these second-generation crops is considerably less. Therefore, the third-generation bioenergy crops were employed to produce high biomass content to reduce the production cost of the bioenergy. The third-generation crops include boreal plants, eucalyptus and crassulacean acid metabolism (CAM) plants, where these plants can able to produce high biomass which has the advantages of cost-effectiveness and environmental friendly (Chen et al., 2021; Han et al., 2011; Hussain et al., 2019).

10.3.3 Biomass Producing Efficiency of Bioenergy Crops during Metal Remediation

The efficiency and cost-effectiveness of the phytoremediation process using bioenergy crops lie in the high biomass production, stress tolerance and metal uptake ability (Jiang et al., 2015). In general, plants have the innate capacity to uptake metals and metalloids from soil through chelation and translocation as micronutrients. However, based on the HM severity, the biomass production ability may get affected and decline (Meers et al., 2008; Saleh et al., 2004; Tsao, 2003; Zhao et al., 2009). Therefore, it is important to select the plants with adequate growth rate, high biomass production along with metal tolerance. Several bioenergy crops exhibit higher biomass production and metal uptake ability coined as hyperaccumulators which can be utilized to remediate the metal-contaminated soil (Vamerali et al., 2010). These hyperaccumulators are belonging to the natural vegetation of metal-enriched soils (Pollard et al., 2000). The bioenergy crops such as *Miscanthus* sp., *Miscanthus sinensis, M. sacchariflorus, M. floridulus, M. xgiganteu, Jatropacurcas* and *Ricinus* sp. are widely utilized for phytoremediation with high biomass production. For example, Han et al. (2011) utilized the bioenergy crop *Miscanthus* to remediate the soil HM contamination, and reported an increase in the above-ground biomass that can be exploited for the production of bioethanol. Similarly, Aggangan et al. (2017) utilized metal-tolerant *Jatropha curcus* L. for the reclamation of HM-contaminated soil which is a source of biodiesel production. In another study, the high biomass producing bioenergy crop *Ricinus cummunis* was employed for remediating copper-contaminated soil (Andreazza et al., 2013). Further, the bioenergy crops such as *Arundo donax L.* (Miao et al., 2012), *Glycin max* L. (Hussain et al., 2019), *Pennisetum purpureum* (Liu et al., 2009) and *Pongamia pinnata* (Kanwal et al., 2018) were reported for high biomass production during remediation of HM-contaminated soil.

10.3.4 Metal Removal/Stabilization/Accumulation Efficiency of Bioenergy Crops

Several bioenergy crops have a high potential to remediate the HM-polluted soils through phytostabilization, phytoaccumulation and phytoextraction processes. The process depends on the factors such as plant species, cultivars, metal speciation and translocation ability from root to shoot. For example, it is reported that the phytostabilization ability of *Ricinus communis* is comparatively higher than other bioenergy crops (Huang et al., 2011). Similarly, the phytoextraction ability of the *Helianthus annuus* was reportedly high due to the increased translocation of HM from root to shoot (Chauhan et al., 2020). Besides, several reports suggested that a single bioenergy crop can be exploited for remediating multi-metal-contaminated sites (Gonzalez and Gonzalez-Chavez, 2006; Kumar et al., 2008; Yadav et al., 2010). For instance, *Jatropha curcas* was reported for remediating multiple metals such as Al, Ar, Fe, Cr, Cd, Mn, Pd, Ni and Zn (Ahmadpour et al., 2010; Gonzalez and Gonzalez-Chavez, 2006; Jamil et al., 2009; Kumar et al., 2008; Pandey et al., 2012; Yadav et al., 2009). The metal remediation ability of the bioenergy crops is summarized in Table 10.2.

TABLE 10.2
Heavy Metal Accumulation/Removal Efficiency of Bioenergy Crops

Plant Species	Heavy Metal	Reported Accumulation Concentration/Percentage Removal	Metal Remediation Mechanism	Reference
Ricinus communis L.	Cd	1086.36 mg/kg in roots, 200.13 mg/kg in shoots	Phytostabilization and highest metal removal	Bauddh and Singh (2012)
Helianthus annuus L. DRSF-108	Pb	Accumulation of Pb in shoot, root, leaves and flower by 201.94, 319.25, 53.95, 1.109 mg/kg, respectively	Phytoextraction (increased metal accumulation in tissues of the plant)	Chauhan et al. (2020)
Helianthus annuus L. DRSF-113	Pb	Accumulation of Pb in shoot, root, leaves and flower by 120.16, 241.95, 40.76, 0.779 mg/kg, respectively	Phytoextraction (increased metal accumulation in tissues of the plant)	Chauhan et al. (2020)
Helianthus annuus L. LSFH-171	Pb	Accumulation of Pb in shoot, root, leaves and flower by 106.71, 229.7, 38.519, 0.455 mg/kg, respectively	Phytoextraction (increased metal accumulation in tissues of the plant)	Chauhan et al. (2020)
Helianthus annuus L. PBH	Pb	Accumulation of Pb in shoot, root, leaves and flower by 224.30, 394.32, 72.37, 1.319 mg/kg, respectively	Phytoextraction (increased metal accumulation in tissues of the plant)	Chauhan et al. (2020)
Helianthus annuus L. KBSH-44	Pb	Accumulation of Pb in shoot, root, leaves and flower by 98.40, 208.1, 26.09, 0,663 mg/kg, respectively	Phytoextraction (increased metal accumulation in tissues of the plant)	Chauhan et al. (2020)
Miscanthus lutarioriparius Xiangnadi NO4,	Cd	Cd accumulation in root, shoot, leaves by 132.47, 6.73, 5.26 mg/kg, respectively	Phytostabilization (reduced translocation from root to shoot)	Chen et al. (2021)

(*Continued*)

TABLE 10.2 (*Continued*)
Heavy Metal Accumulation/Removal Efficiency of Bioenergy Crops

Plant Species	Heavy Metal	Reported Accumulation Concentration/Percentage Removal	Metal Remediation Mechanism	Reference
Miscanthus sinensis Xiangmang NO1,	Cd	Cd accumulation in root, shoot and leaves by 66.14, 1.98, 5.66 mg/kg, respectively	Phytostabilization (reduced translocation from root to shoot)	Chen et al. (2021)
M. lutarioriparius×M. sinensis hybrid Xiangzamang NO1	Cd	Cd accumulation in root, shoot and leaves by 153.07, 3.49, 6.43 mg/kg, respectively	Phytostabilization (reduced translocation from root to shoot)	Chen et al. (2021)
M. floridulus Wujiemang NO1	Cd	Cd accumulation in root, shoot and leaves by 160.74, 4.22, 5.56 mg/kg, respectively	Phytostabilization (reduced translocation from root to shoot)	Chen et al. (2021)
Azadirecta indica	Pb Zn Ni	119. 1 mg/kg in roots 1.5 mg/kg in roots 17.2 mg/kg in roots	Phytoextraction and increased metal accumulation	Collina et al. (2017)
Pennisetum purpureum	Cu	485.63 mg/kg in roots and 194.07 mg/kg in shoots	Phytoextraction (increased metal accumulation in tissues of the plant)	Liu et al. (2009)
Phragmites australis	Cu	179.40 mg/kg in roots and 30.8% mg/kg in shoots	Phytoextraction (increased metal accumulation in tissues of the plant)	Liu et al. (2009)
Glycin max L	Pb Zn	46 % of total Pb uptake by roots 91% of total Zn uptake by roots	Phytoextraction (increased root metal uptake)	Murakami and Ae (2009)
Arundo donax L	As, Cu, Cd, Cr, Ni, Fe, Pb, Zn	47% removal 58% removal 56% removal 56% removal 54% removal 62% removal 60% removal 62% removal	Rhizofiltration	Rai (2021)
Pongamia glabra	Cr	68.2 mg/kg in root 27.9 mg/kg in shoot	Phytodegradation, and increased root nodule	Unnikannan et al. (2013)
Jatropha curcas L	Cr	16.46 mg/kg in roots, 2.74 mg/kg in shoots	Phytostabilization (maximum root accumulation due to conversion of Cr(IV) into Cr(III))	Yadav et al. (2010)

10.3.5 Strategies to Increase Phytoremediation Potential of Bioenergy Crops – Enhanced Phytoremediation

Although phytoremediation of HM through bioenergy crops could be an effective method, certain constraints reduce its efficiency by decreasing the germination rate and growth of the plants in high metal-contaminated areas. Several approaches have been employed to increase stress tolerance, germination rate, growth and metal uptake by utilizing some soil amendments such as chemical amendments (acetic acid, biochar, citric acid, compost, ethylene diamine tetra acetic acid (EDTA) and oxalic acid), plant growth-promoting microbes (bacteria and fungi) and using of genetically engineered crops. The strategies for improving the phytoremediation of efficiency of the bioenergy crops are represented in Figure 10.2.

10.3.5.1 Chemical-Assisted Phytoremediation with Bioenergy Crops: Organic or Inorganic Amendments

In order to increase the phytoremediation potential of the bioenergy crops, several chemicals were used as an amendment to chelate, changing metal speciation and reducing the mobilization. In general, organic and inorganic chemicals such as humic substances, dissolved organic matter, citric acid, oxalic acid, EDTA, Ethylene

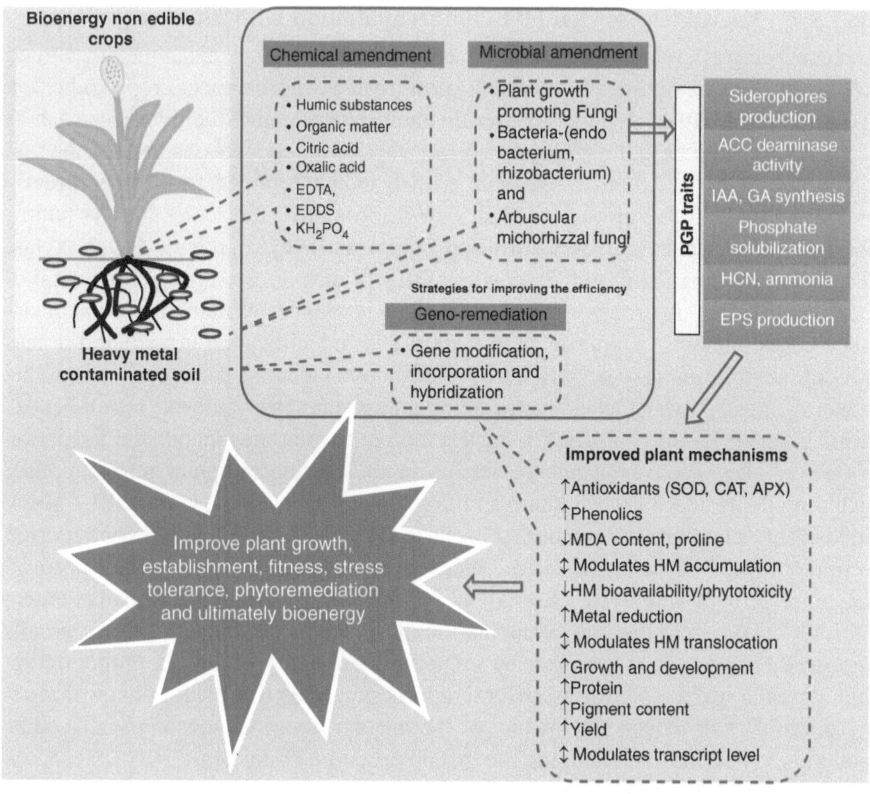

FIGURE 10.2 Strategies to improve the phytoremediation efficiency of bioenergy crops.

diamine-N, N'-disuccinic acid (EDDS), KH_2PO_4 and tetrasodium pyrophosphate were utilized to increase the efficiency of the phytoremediation (Turgut et al., 2004; Zhang et al., 2016). For instance, Miao et al. (2012) reported that the organic amendments such as citric acid and acetic acid have the ability to decrease the toxicity of the HM by forming metal-ligand complexes, thereby improving the plant growth and remediation efficiency. Other amendments such as EDTA and sepiolite reduced the mobilization of the metal by chelation mechanism and also it has been reported that these amendments reduced the oxidative damages in plants and thus increased the phytoremediation efficiency and growth of the bioenergy crops (Miao et al., 2012; Qureshi et al., 2020; Turgut et al., 2005). In another study it has been reported that the organic amendments such as dissolved organic matter, compost and citric acid involved the change in the metal speciation from toxic form to less toxic form, thereby improving the tolerance level of the plant and enhancing the growth and metal remediation of the bioenergy crops (Aggangan et al., 2017; Chen et al., 2020). Recently, biochar-based amendments were also utilized to reduce the bioavailability of metal in contaminated areas. These biochar amendments assist plant growth by decreasing the phytotoxicity by immobilizing the metals and thus decreasing the plant oxidative damage (Bashir et al., 2021). Table 10.3 summarizes the chemical-assisted phytoremediation of bioenergy crops and their mechanisms.

10.3.5.2 Microbial-Assisted HM Phytoremediation with Bioenergy Crops

In recent years microbial assistance and its interactions with plants in metal-polluted soil have received significant attention to improve plant tolerance, crop production and phytoremediation efficiency. Several studies reported that the microbes such as bacteria and fungi have the ability to tolerate various abiotic stresses, reduce the toxicity of the metals and promote the plant growth and phytoremediation either directly or indirectly by producing various plant growth-promoting molecules such as siderophores, indole acetic acid, gibberlic acid, and 1-aminocyclopropane-1-carboxylate deaminase (Wiangkham and Prapagdee, 2018; Zhang et al., 2018). The metabolites produced by microbes increase the plant tolerance by inducing metal resistance genes, forming complexes with metals, and inducing plant growth and fitness through stimulating root growth and proliferation, inducing plant nutrient uptake, reducing stress ethylene level, synthesizing antioxidant enzymes, etc. (Bruno et al., 2021, Vishnupradeep et al., 2022). Furthermore, the microbes reduce the formation of free radicles, reactive oxygen species formation and improve plant nutrient uptake including Fe, K and P (Wiangkham and Prapagdee, 2018; Zhang et al., 2018). Many rhizospheric plant growth-promoting bacteria (PGPB) and fungi have been reported to immobilize the HM on its surface and reduced the bioavailability and improved the plant growth indirectly (Kumar et al., 2021). For instance, Rojjanateeranaj et al. (2017) reported that the augmentation of *Arthrobacter* sp. with *Glycin max* L. improved the growth of the plant by reducing the toxicity of Cd via immobilizing the Cd on the surface. Similarly, several reports suggested that plant growth-promoting microbes can reduce the toxicity of the metal via various mechanisms such as reduction, oxidation and changing the metal speciation (Bilal et al., 2020). Recently, Vishnupradeep et al. (2022) reported that the Cr-reducing plant growth-promoting bacteria increased the growth of the *Zea mays* plant by reducing the Cr toxicity by

TABLE 10.3
Chemical-Assisted Phytoremediation Using Bioenergy Crops

Chemical Amendments	Plants Species	Heavy Metal	Improved Plant Mechanism	References
Compost (500 g/plant)	*Jatropha curcas* L.	Cu, Cd, Zn, Pb contaminated soil	Increased plant height (28%), stem diameter (78%), root length (46%), root dry weight (307%), shoot dry weight (241%) and leaf area (207%)	Aggangan et al. (2017)
Rice straw biochar (20 g/kg)	*Helianthus annuus* L.	Cd	Decreased SOD (49%), POD (41%), CAT (47%), Chl (46%) and fresh biomass (78%)	Bashir et al. (2021)
Wheat straw biochar (20 g/kg)	*Helianthus annuus* L.	Cd	Decreased SOD (43%), POD (34%), CAT (40%), Chl (36%) and fresh biomass (52%)	Bashir et al. (2021)
Acacia biochar (20 g/kg)	*Helianthus annuus* L.	Cd	Decreased SOD (37%), POD (33%), CAT (32%), Chl (9%) and fresh biomass (51%)	Bashir et al. (2021)
Sugarcane bagasse biochar (20 g/kg)	*Helianthus annuus* L.	Cd	Decreased SOD (20%), POD (12%), CAT (25%), Chl (19%) and fresh biomass (24%)	Bashir et al. (2021)
EDDS (7.5 mmol/kg)	*Helianthus annuus* L.	Cd	Increased MDA Hydrogen peroxide, shoot biomass (3.28%–30.31%), root biomass (0.73%–23.81%) and reduce total chlorophyll	Chen et al. (2020)
Citric acid (5 mmol/kg	*Glycin max* L.	Cd, Cr, Cu, Ni (industrial contaminated soil)	Increased plant biomass up to 25%, Chl a (48%), Chl b (15%), carotenoid (23%) and decreased proline up to 10%	Hussain et al. (2019)
Citric acid (5 mmol/kg	*Glycin max* L.	Cd (100 mg/kg)	Increased biomass (24 %), dry biomass (20%), Chl a (28%), Chl b (28%), carotenoid (25%) and decreased proline (10%)	Hussain et al. (2019)
Citric acid (5 mmol/kg	*Glycin max* L.	Cd (200 mg/kg)	Increased Chl a (27%), Chl b (30%), carotenoid (25%) and decreased proline up to 28%	Hussain et al. (2019)
Prosopis juliflora biochar (50 g/kg)	*Ricinus communis* L.	Pb (800 mg/kg)	Increased chl a (38%), chl b (52%), total chl (42%), protein (72%) and reduced anthocyanin (41%), proline (19%), MDA (29%), hydrogen peroxidase (14%) compared to Pb treatment	Kiran and Prasad (2019)

(*Continued*)

TABLE 10.3 (*Continued*)
Chemical-Assisted Phytoremediation Using Bioenergy Crops

Chemical Amendments	Plants Species	Heavy Metal	Improved Plant Mechanism	References
Rice husk ash (50 g/kg)	*Ricinus communis* L.	Pb (800 mg/kg)	Increased chl a (31%), chl b (10%), total chl (22%), protein (77%) and reduced anthocyanin (24%), proline (45%), MDA (26%), hydrogen peroxidase (27%) compared to Pb treatment	Kiran and Prasad (2019)
KH_2PO_4	*Pennisetum purpureum*	Cu	Reduce phytotoxicity (41 %) and improve photosynthesis under Cu stress.	Liu et al. (2009)
Citric acid (5 mmol/kg	*Arundo donax* L.	As (13.7 mg/kg), Cd (1.07 mg/kg), Pb (52.4 mg/kg) Contaminated soil	Increased shoot biomass (25%), Chl (72%), SOD (3.9%), CAT (10%)	Miao et al. (2012)
Acetic acid (5 mmol/kg	*Arundo donax* L.	As (13.7 mg/kg), Cd (1.07 mg/kg), Pb (52.4 mg/kg) Contaminated soil	Increased SOD (21%), CAT (80%) decreased shoot biomass (34%), Chl (68%)	Miao et al. (2012)
EDTA (5 mmol/kg	*Arundo donax* L.	As (13.7 mg/kg), Cd (1.07 mg/kg), Pb (52.4 mg/kg) Contaminated soil	Increased SOD (39%), CAT (49%) decreased Chl (25%)	Miao et al. (2012)
Sepiolite (40 g/kg)	*Arundo donax* L.	As (13.7 mg/kg), Cd (1.07 mg/kg), Pb (52.4 mg/kg) Contaminated soil	Improved Chl (87%), CAT (10%) and reduced biomass, SOD (38%)	Miao et al. (2012)
Citric acid EDTA	*Ricinus communis* L.	Cr	Increased SOD (EDTA – 17%; citric acid – 8%), POD (EDTA -3.5%; citric acid – 2%), CAT (EDTA -3%; citric acid – 18%), Reduce oxidative stress, MDA and hydrogen peroxide	Qureshi et al. (2020)
EDTA	*Helianthus annuus* L.	Cr	Improves translocation (42%) of HM from soil	Turgut et al. (2005)
Biosludge	*Jatropha curcas* L.	Cr (250 mg/kg)	Increased APX, CAT, GSH, GST	Yadav et al. (2010)

converting Cr (VI) in to Cr (III). Further, it has been reported that several metal-mobilizing bacteria enhanced the phytoremediation efficiency by increasing the plant metal uptake and also the metabolites produced by these bacteria improved the plant tolerance to these metals by altering the metabolites related to stress tolerance (Govarthanan et al., 2018). For example, Bruno et al. (2021) reported the utilization of metal-mobilizing plant growth-promoting bacteria increased the Cd, Pb, Ni and Zn uptake of *Zea mays* and improved the plant growth by altering the proline, malondialdehyde content, enzymatic and non-enzymatic antioxidant level. The interactive effects of microbe and bioenergy crops and their important impact on phytoremediation are summarized in Table 10.4.

10.3.5.3 Genetic Engineering of Bioenergy Crops to Enhance HM Phytoremediation

Recently, genetic modification approaches have been investigated to increase the plant tolerance and phytoremediation ability of bioenergy crops. Several approaches such as gene modification, incorporation and hybridization were utilized to improve the plant metal tolerance, accumulation and degradation (Pasricha et al., 2021). Many transgenic plants can be genetically modified at callus level to tolerate HM. For instance, the expression of modified genes such as *merA*, *merB* and *AtMRP7* increased the metal resistance and metal accumulation in the transgenic plants (Lyyra et al., 2007; Wojas et al., 2009). Similarly, Watanabe et al. (2005) incorporated metalothinein gene (CUP1) in bioenergy crop *Helianthus annuus*, and found that overexpression of this gene improved the plant Cd tolerance, detoxification, growth and phytoremediation ability. In another study, it has been reported that the incorporation of *hpt* and *gut* genes improved the plant tolerance to HM stress and protected the plants from the toxic effect of the contaminant (Trivedi et al., 2009). The overall approaches of genetic engineering for improving phytoremediation efficiency of bioenergy crops are represented in Figure 10.3. The use of such strategies will bring us closer to the goal of improved phytoremediation using bioenergy crops; however, still knowledge gap remains in using genetically modified bioenergy crops, and therefore more research is required to fulfil the gap. Recent examples of genetically engineered bioenergy crops to enhance phytoremediation potential are summarized in Table 10.5.

10.3.6 Energy Production from Utilized Bioenergy Crops

Plant-based biofuels are environmentally sustainable alternatives to fossil fuels that have the potential to reduce global warming, climate change, environmental foot print and improve soil quality (Sharma et al., 2018). The bioenergy crops employed for phytoremediation can be converted into the generation of liquid and gaseous biofuels such as bioethanol, biodiesel and biohydrogen. The three most common commercially available first-generation biofuels are biodiesel, ethanol and biogas (Sagar and Kartha, 2007). Using conventional methods, the first-generation biofuels can be produced from high sugar- and starch-containing edible crops, grains and vegetables (Naik et al., 2010). Second-generation biofuels are derived from lingocellulosic biomass (crop straw, husks, forest residue or perennial grasses) or non-food oil

TABLE 10.4
Microbial-Assisted Phytoremediation Using Bioenergy Crops

Microbial Amendments	Plants Species	Heavy Metal	Improved Plant Mechanism	References
Funneliformis mosseae (AMF)	*Glycin max* L.	Cu, Pb, Zn (100, 100, 300 mg/kg)	Increased root colonization (60-70%), plant height, leaf area, shoot P nutrient (2.5%–3%), root P nutrient (1.5%–2%)	Adeyemi et al. (2021)
Pseudomonas koreensis AGB-1	*Miscanthus sinensis*	Metal contaminates mining soils	Increased plant biomass (54%), protein content (28%), SOD (33%), CAT (31%) and chl (27%). Reduced MDA (31%)	Babu et al. (2015)
Sphingomonas sp. (4×10^8 CFU)	*Glycin max* L.	Cr (5 mM)	Increased MDA, GSH, CAT (45%), SOD, POD (72%) compared to non-inoculated plant, increased Chl (78%) compared to metal control plant	Bilal et al. (2018)
Rhizophagusir regularis (AMF)	*Phragmites australis*	Cd	Increase the root Cd concentration 1252.82–1546.22 mg/kg and prohibit translocation	Huang et al. (2017)
Pseudomonas lurida	*Helianthus annuus* L.	Cu	Increased shoot length, leaf mass area, leaf density, microbial population in leaf	Kumar et al. (2020)
Pseudomonas sp. PjM15	*Ricinus communis* L.	Ni, Cu, Zn	Increased shoot dry weight (20%) and root dry weight (25%)	Rajkumar and Freitas (2008)
Pseudomonas Jessenii PsM6	*Ricinus communis* L.	Ni, Cu, Zn	Increased shoot dry weight (15%) and root dry weight (18%)	Rajkumar and Freitas (2008)
Glomus geosporum (AMF)	*Azadirecta indica*	Tannery effluent (Cd, Cr, Cu, Pb and Zn)	Restricts HM translocation from soil to plant parts. (Cu, Pb and Zn, respectively, in 49.83, 96.85, 149.21 ppm in root tissues and 37.43, 25.71, 21.89 ppm in shoot tissues)	Thangaswamy et al. (2015)
Vasicular arbuscular myccorhiza	*Pongamia pinnata*	Cu	Limits high levels of Cu translocation (0.0407%) within the roots and delimits copper toxicity	Tulod et al. (2012)
Arbuscular mycorrhizal fungi	*Phragmites australis*	Zn, Cd	Alleviate toxic effects to the plants (Zn reduction 10%–57%)	You et al. (2021)

seed crops (pongamia, jatropha). The mostly used crops for bioenergy production are castor, canola, jatropha, wild artichoke, jojoba, miscanthus, poplar, eucalyptus, cotton, sunflower, sugarcane, sugar beet, soybean, branched millet, kenaf and millet. To

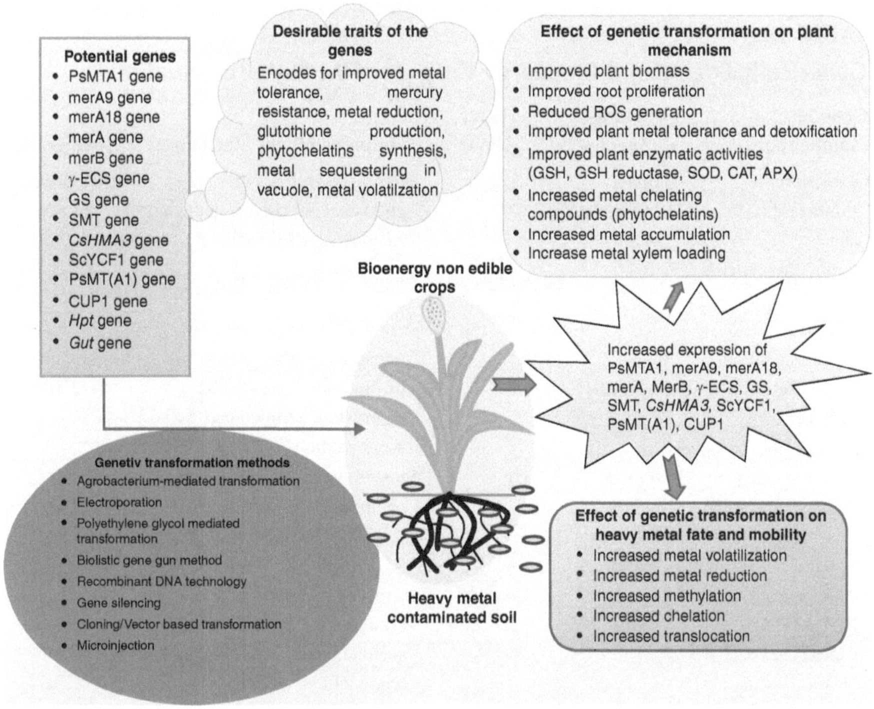

FIGURE 10.3 Overview of genetic engineering approaches to improve the phytoremediation efficiency of bioenergy crops.

TABLE 10.5
Genetically Engineered Bioenergy Crops for HM Phytoremediation

Genetic Modifications	Plants Species	Heavy Metal	Improved Plant Mechanism	References
PsMTA1 Gene	*Populus alba*	Cu	Increased Cu tolerance, reduced ROS accumulation	Balestrazzi et al. (2009)
merA9 and merA18 genes	*Populus deltoids*	Hg	Increased expression of mercuric ion reductase and biomass Increased Hg accumulation	Che et al. (2003)
γ-glutamylcysteine synthetase (γ-ECS)	*Populus tremula×P. alba*	Cd	Increased total thiols, glutathiones (GSH), oxidized GSH and GSH reductase activity Decreased ROS generation including singlet oxygen and hydrogen peroxide concentration	He et al. (2015)

(*Continued*)

TABLE 10.5
Genetically Engineered Bioenergy Crops for HM Phytoremediation

Genetic Modifications	Plants Species	Heavy Metal	Improved Plant Mechanism	References
Glutathione synthetase (GS) and γ-glutamylcysteine synthetase (γ-ECS)	*Populus tremula x P. alba*	Cd	Increased synthesis of phytochelatin (PC) content and cd concentration in tissues	Koprivova et al. (2002)
Selenocysteine methyltransferase, SMT	Indian mustard	Se	Increased selenocysteine methyltransferase (SMT) expression, Se tolerance, Se accumulation	LeDuc et al. (2006)
merA and merB	*Populus deltoides* Bartr. ex Marsh	Hg	Increased detoxification of Hg compounds by volatilization, resistance to Hg	Lyyra et al. (2007)
HMA (heavy metal P1B-ATPase) genes (*CsHMA3*)	*Camelina sativa*	Cd, Pb and Zn	Increased root growth, leaf width, Pb tolerance, Pb and Zn accumulation, translocation, and seed yield	Park et al. (2014)
ScYCF1 (yeast cadmium factor 1)	*Populus alba X P. tremula* var. *glandulosa*	Multiple metals (Cd, Zn, and Pb)	Increased metal resistance, root growth and metal accumulation Reduced toxicity	Shim et al. (2013)
Metallothioneins type 2 gene [PsMT(A1)]	*Poplar*	Zn and Cu	Increased translocation and accumulation of Zn and Cu Increased metal tolerance Modulates SOD CAT and APX activity Decreased ROS generation	Turchi et al. (2012)
Metallothionein gene (CUP1)	*Helianthus annuus* L.	Cd	Increase Cd tolerance and plant fresh weight	Watanabe et al. (2005)

convert the biomass into bioenergy several processes are employed such as anaerobic fermentation, pyrolysis, distillation, gasification, thermo-conversion, esterification, transesterification and hydrolysis (Bauddh et al., 2017; He et al., 2019; Li et al., 2010). For instance, Dhiman et al. (2017) employed enzymatic saccharification process to convert the *Helianthus annuus* biomass after phytoremediation, where they reported the hyperaccumulator bioenergy plant could increase the phytoremediation process and yielded 11.4 g/L of bioethanol. Similarly, Hunce et al. (2019) studied the biogas potential of bioenergy crops through transesterification and reported that the biomass from *Helianthus annuus* and *Silybummarianum* after phytoremediation process was

TABLE 10.6
Biomass Conversion Techniques to Produce Biofuels from Energy Plants

Conversion Technologies	Products	Usages	References
Pyrolysis	Biochar	Solid fuel in boilers or as pre-material for activated carbon production	Bastabak et al. (2021)
	Bio-oil and Syn gas	Biofuel and biomaterial	Khiari et al. (2020)
Anaerobic fermentation	Biogas	Heat and electricity generation	Arici and Koçar (2015); Wu et al. (2019)
Microbial fermentation	Bioethanol	Suitable to blend with conventional fuel	Derman et al. (2018)
Jatropha curcus L. Crude extract	Biodiesel	Used for alternation of Petro-diesel	Lu et al. (2009)

able to yield 130 to 223 ml g^{-1} of biogas. Table 10.6 highlights the overall energy conversion process from the bioenergy plants.

10.4 CONCLUSION AND FUTURE PERSPECTIVE

It is well known that increasing population and industrialization increase soil pollution and energy scarcity all around the globe. Over the past years, various technologies have been employed to clean up metal-contaminated soil. Phytoremediation holds great promise to remediate metal-contaminated soil, in addition utilizing bioenergy crops to metal remediation has simultaneous advantages such as conversion of biogas, bioethanol and bio hydrogen. Phytoremediation through bioenergy crops that do not compete with food crops could be the best approach for sustainable soil reclamation and to reduce the increasing energy demand. These non-edible bioenergy crops such as *Populus, Jatropha, Helianthus, Ricinus,* and *Miscanthus* exhibited a high potential to remediated metal-contaminated soil as well as they are the best candidate for producing bioenergy. Furthermore, genetic modification in bioenergy crops is a powerful approach that increases the efficiency of the crop metal tolerance, growth and remediation under HM-contaminated soil. This genetic approach improves the plant metabolites and antioxidant defence mechanism which plays a major role in improving the growth and tolerance of the bioenergy crops in high metal-contaminated soil. In recent years, the approach of inserting single gene (mer a, mer b, GSH, or γ-ECS) responsible for metal tolerance or metal reduction has been successfully generated in genetically modified bioenergy crops that respond to one particular mechanism. These modified bioenergy crops with one desirable gene were successfully tested for a single mechanism such as metal accumulation, increased growth, stress tolerance and metal speciation. However, more experiments should be carried out to incorporate multiple genes that possess desirable traits (combination of genes) in one genotype to express different responses in bioenergy crops to tolerate, detoxify and accumulate metal under various environmental conditions. In addition, several countries have strict regulations for utilizing and experimenting genetically modified crops that limit the application of the genetically engineered bioenergy crops in metal phytoremediation. Therefore we should consider producing a safer and non-dispersing transgene technology to overcome these limitations. Moreover, it is important to implement a long-term field trail testing for assessing the efficiency of the transgenic bioenergy crops in multiple stress conditions. These long-term field trials may provide a clear scenario of the efficiency and transgene dispersion that may lead to acceptance and change in regulations in many countries.

REFERENCES

Abumaizar RJ, Smith EH. 1999. Heavy metal contaminants removal by soil washing. *Journal of Hazardous Materials B*. 70(1–2); 71–86.

Adeyemi NO, Atayese MO, Sakariyawo OS, Azeez JO, Sobowale SPA, Olubode A, Mudathir R, Adebayo R, Adeoye S. 2021. Alleviation of heavy metal stress by arbuscular mycorrhizal symbiosis in *Glycine max* (L.) grown in copper, lead and zinc contaminated soils. *Rhizosphere*. 18: 100325.

Adimalla N. 2020. Heavy metals pollution assessment and its associated human health risk evaluation of urban soils from Indian cities: a review. *Environmental Geochemistry and Health*. 42(1): 173–190.

Aggangan N, Cadiz N, Llamado A, Raymundo A. 2017. *Jatropha Curcas* for bioenergy and bioremediation in mine tailing area in Mogpog, Marinduque, Philippines. *Energy Procedia*. 110: 471–478.

Ahmad MSA, Ashraf M. 2012. Essential roles and hazardous effects of nickel in plants. In *Reviews of Environmental Contamination and Toxicology*, 214: 125–167.

Ahmad W, Alharthy RD, Zubair M, Ahmed M, Hameed A, Rafique S. 2021. Toxic and heavy metals contamination assessment in soil and water to evaluate human health risk. *Scientific Reports*. 11(1): 1–12.

Ahmadpour P, Nawi AM, Abdu A, Abdul-Hamid H, Daljit SK, Hassan A, Majid NMN, Shamshuddin J. 2010. Uptake of heavy metals by *Jatropha curcas* L. planted in soils containing sewage sludge. *American Journal of Applied Science*. 7(10): 1291–1299.

Ali H, Khan E, Sajad MA. 2013. Phytoremediation of heavy metals—concepts and applications. *Chemosphere*. 91(7): 869–881.

Alidou-Arzika I, Lebrun M, Miard F, Nandillon R, Bayçu G, Bourgerie S, Morabito D. 2021. Assessment of compost and three biochars associated with *Ailanthus altissima* (Miller) Swingle for lead and arsenic stabilization in a post-mining technosol. *Pedosphere*. 31(6): 944–953.

Alloway BJ. 2013. Sources of heavy metals and metalloids in soils. In: Alloway B (Ed.), *Heavy Metals in Soils*. Environmental Pollution, Springer, Dordrecht, 22: pp. 11–50.

Andreazza R, Bortolon L, Pieniz S, Camargo FAO. 2013. Use of high-yielding bioenergy plant castor bean (*Ricinus communis* L.) as a potential phytoremediaton for copper-contaminated soils. *Pedosphere*. 23(5): 651–66.

Arici S, Koçar G. 2015. The effect of adding maize silage as a co-substrate for anaerobic animal manure digestion. *International Journal of Green Energy*. 12: 453–460.

ATSDR S. 2012. Toxicological profile for chromium.agency for toxic substances and disease registry. Public Health Service, US Department of Health and Human Services. http://www.atsdr.cdc.gov/toxprofiles/tp.asp.

Awa SH, Hadibarata T. 2020. Removal of heavy metals in contaminated soil by phytoremediation mechanism: a review. *Water, Air, & Soil Pollution*. 231(2): 1–15.

Ayangbenro AS, Babalola OO. 2017. A new strategy for heavy metal polluted environments: a review of microbial biosorbents. *International Journal of Environmental Research and Public Health* 14(1): 94.

Babu AG, Shea PJ, Sudhakar D, Jung I, Oh B. 2015. Potential use of *Pseudomonas koreensis* AGB-1 in association with *Miscanthus sinensis* to remediate heavy metal(loid)-contaminated mining site soil. *Journal of Environmental Management.* 151: 160–166.

Balestrazzi A, Botti S, Zelasco S, Biondi S, Franchin C, Calligari P, Racchi M, Turchi A, Lingua G, Berta G, Carbonera D. 2009. Expression of the PsMTA1 gene in white poplar engineered with the MAT system is associated with heavy metal tolerance and protection against 8-hydroxy-2'-deoxyguanosine mediated-DNA damage. *Plant Cell Reports.* 28(8): 1179–1192.

Bashir S, Qayyum MA, Husain A, Bakhsh A, Ahmed N, Hussain MB, Elshikh MS, Alwahibi MS, Hussain BMAAR, Wang Y, Zhou Y, Diao Z. 2021. Efficiency of different types of biochars to mitigate Cd stress and growth of sunflower (*Helianthus*; L.) in wastewater irrigated agricultural soil. *Saudi Journal of Biological Sciences.* 28: 2453–2459.

Basir-Cyio M, Isrun-Baso M, Nakazawa K, Mahfudz-Muchtar T, Napitupulu M, Anshary A, Laude S. 2020. The effect of traditional gold mining to land degradation, mercury contamination and decreasing of agricultural productivity. *Bulgarian Journal of Agricultural Science.* 26(3): 612–621.

Bastabak B, G€odekmerdan E, Koçar GA. 2021. Holistic approach to soil contamination and sustainable phytoremediation with energy crops in the Aegean Region of Turkey. *Chemosphere.* 276: 130192.

Bauddh K, Singh RP. 2012. Growth, tolerance efficiency and phytoremediation potential of *Ricinus communis (L.) and Brassica juncea (L.)* in salinity and drought affected cadmium contaminated soil. Ecotoxicology and Environmental Safety. 85: 13–22.

Bauddh K, Singh B, Korstad, J. 2017. *Phytoremediation Potential of Bioenergy Plants.* Springer, Singapore.

Bilal S, Khan AL, Shahzad R, Kim Y, Imran M, Khan MJ, Al-Harrasi A, Kim TH, Lee I. 2018. Mechanisms of Cr (VI) resistance by endophytic *Sphingomonas* sp. LK11 and its Cr(VI) phytotoxic mitigating effects in soybean (*Glycine max* L.). *Ecotoxicology and Environmental Safety.* 164: 648–658.

Bilal S, Shahzad R, Imran M, Jan R, Kim KM, Lee I. 2020. Synergistic association of endophytic fungi enhances *Glycine max* L. resilience to combined abiotic stresses: heavy metals, high temperature and drought stress. *Industrial Crops & Products.* 143: 111931.

Bruno LB, Anbuganesan V, Karthik C, Kumar A, Banu RJ, Freitas H, Rajkumar M. 2021. Enhanced phytoextraction of multi-metal contaminated soils under increased atmospheric temperature by bioaugmentation with plant growth promoting *Bacillus cereus. Journal of Environmental Management.* 289(24): 112553.

Cachada A, Rocha-Santos T, Duarte AC. 2018. Soil Pollution .In: Duarte AC,Cachada A, and Rocha-Santos T (Eds.), *Soil and pollution: an introduction to the main issues*, , Elsevier, pp. 1–28..

Carere CR, Sparling R, Cicek N, Levin DB. 2008. Third generation biofuels via direct cellulose fermentation. *International Journal of Molecular Sciences.* 9(7): 1342–1360.

Carre F, Caudeville J, Bonnard R, Bert V, Boucard P, Ramel M. 2017. Global Soil Security In: Field DJ, Morgan CLS, McBratney AB (Eds.), *Soil contamination and human health: a major challenge for global soil security.* , Springer, Cham, pp. 275–295.

Chauhan P, Rajguru AB, Dudhe MY, Mathur J. 2020. Efficacy of lead (Pb) phytoextraction of five varieties of *Helianthus annuus* L. from contaminated soil. *Environmental Technology & Innovation.* 18: 100718.

Che D, Meagher RB, Heaton AC, Lima A, Rugh CL, Merkle SA. 2003. Expression of mercuric ion reductase in Eastern cottonwood (*Populus deltoides*) confers mercuric ion reduction and resistance. *Plant Biotechnology Journal*. 1: 311–319

Chen L, Yang J, Wang D. 2020. Phytoremediation of uranium and cadmium contaminated soils by sunflower (*Helianthus annuus* L.) enhanced with biodegradable chelating agents. *Journal of Cleaner Production*. 263: 121491.

Chen ZJ, Tian W, Li Y, Sun L, Chen Y, Zhang H, Li Y, Han H. 2021. Responses of rhizosphere bacterial communities, their functions and their network interactions to Cd stress under phytostabilization by *Miscanthus* spp. *Environmental Pollution*. 287: 117663.

Collina K, Junior FM, Nnamdi N, Janfa N. 2017. Comparative studies on the efficacy of *Azadirachta indica* and *Moringa oleifera* in phytoremediation of some selected heavy metals from contaminated soil. *Asian Journal of Environment & Ecology*. 5(3): 1–11.

Dellisanti, F, Rossi PL, Valdra G. 2016. In-field remediation of tons of heavy metal-rich waste by Joule heating vitrification. *International Journal of Mineral Processing*. 93: 239–245.

Derman E, Abdulla R, Marbawi H, Sabullah MK. 2018. Oil palm empty fruit bunches as a promising feedstock for bioethanol production in Malaysia. *Renewable Energy*. 129: 285–298.

Dhiman SS, Zhao X, Li J, Kim D, Kalia VC, Kim IW, Kim JY, Lee JK. 2017. Metal accumulation by sunflower (*Helianthus annuus* L.) and the efficacy of its biomass in enzymatic saccharification. *PLoS One*. 12: e0175845

Djedidi Z, Bouda M, Souissi MA, Cheikh R, Mercier G, Tyagi RD, Blais JF. 2009. Metals removal from soil, fly ash and sewage sludge leachates by precipitation and dewatering properties of the generated sludge. *Journal of Hazardous Materials*. 172(2): 1372–1382.

Elicker C, Sanches-Filho PJ, Castagno KRL. 2014. Electroremediation of heavy metals in sewage sludge. *Brazilian Journal of Chemical Engineering*. 31: 365–371.

Espana VAA, Pinilla ARR, Bardos P, Naidu R. 2018. Contaminated land in Colombia: a critical review of current status and future approach for the management of contaminated sites. *Science of the Total Environment*. 618: 199–209.

Etim EE. 2012. Phytoremediation and its mechanisms: a review. *International Journal of Environment and Bioenergy*. 2(3): 120–136.

Gonzalez RC, Gonzalez-Chavez MCA. 2006. Metal accumulation in wild plants surrounding mining wastes. *Environmental Pollution*. 144: 84–92.

Govarthanan M, Mythili R, Selvankumar T, Kannan SK, Kim H. 2018. Myco-phytoremediation of arsenic- and lead-contaminated soils by *Helianthus annuus* and wood rot fungi, *Trichoderma* sp. isolated from decayed wood. *Ecotoxicology and Environmental Safety*. 151: 279–284.

Han M, Kim Y, Koo BC, Choi GW. 2011. Bioethanol production by Miscanthus as a lingo cellulosis biomass: focus on high efficient conversion to glucose and ethanol. *BioResources*. 6: 1939–1953.

Havugimana H, Bhople BS, Kumar A, Byiringiro E, Mugabo JP, Kumar A. 2015. Soil pollution–major sources and types of soil pollutants. *Environmental Science and Engineering*. 11: 53–86.

He J, Li H, Ma C, Zhang Y, Polle A, Rennenberg H, Luo ZB. 2015. Overexpression of bacterial γ-glutamylcysteine synthetase mediates changes in cadmium influx, allocation and detoxification in poplar. *New Phytologist*. 205: 240–254.

He J, Strezov V, Kumar R, Weldekidan H, Jahan S, Dastjerdi BH, Zhou X, Kan T. 2019. Pyrolysis of heavy metal contaminated *Avicennia marina* biomass from phytoremediation: characterisation of biomass and pyrolysis products. *Journal of Cleaner Production*. 234: 1235–1245.

Huang H, Yu N, Wang L, Gupta DK, He Z, Wang K, Zhu Z, Yan X, Li T, Yang X. 2011. The phytoremediation potential of bioenergy crop *Ricinus communis* for DDTs and cadmium co-contaminated soil. *Bioresource Technology*. 102(23): 11034–11038.

Huang X, Ho SH, Zhu S, Ma F, Wu J, Yang J, Wang L. 2017. Adaptive response of arbuscular mycorrhizal symbiosis to accumulation of elements and translocation in *Phragmites australis* affected by cadmium stress. *Journal of Environmental Management*. 197: 448–455.

Hunce SY, Clemente R, Bernal MP. 2019. Energy production potential of phytoremediation plant biomass: *Helianthus annuus* and *Silybum marianum*. *Industrial Crops and Products*. 135: 206–216

Hussain A, Kamrand MA, Javed MT, Hayat K, Farooq MA, Alij N, Ali M, Manghwar H, Jani F, Chaudhary HJ. 2019. Individual and combinatorial application of *Kocuria rhizophila* and citric acid on phytoextraction of multi-metal contaminated soils by *Glycine max* L. *Environmental and Experimental Botany*. 159: 23–33.

Ibrahim N, Afandi GE. 2020. Phytoremediation uptake model of heavy metals (Pb, Cd and Zn) in soil using Nerium oleander. *Heliyon*. 6: 04445.

Jamil S, Abhilash PC, Singh N, Sharma PN. 2009. *Jatropha curcas*: a potential crop for phytoremediation of coal fly ash. *Journal of Hazardous Material*. 172: 269–275.

Jiang Y, Lei M, Duan L, Longhurst P. 2015. Integrating phytoremediation with biomass valorisation and critical element recovery: a UK contaminated land perspective. *Biomass and Bioenergy*. 83: 328–339.

Kanwal A, Ali S, Farhan M. 2018. Heavy metal phytoextraction potential of indigenous tree species of the family fabaceae. *International Journal of Phytoremediation*. 21(3): 251–258.

Karthik C, Barathi S, Pugazhendhi A, Ramkumar VS, Thi NBD, Arulselvi PI. 2017. Evaluation of Cr(VI) reduction mechanism and removal by *Cellulosimicrobium funkei* strain AR8, a novel haloalkaliphilic bacterium. *Journal of Hazardous Material*. 333: 42–53.

Khan MA, Khan S, Khan A, Alam M. 2017. Soil contamination with cadmium, consequences and remediation using organic amendments. *Science of the Total Environment*. 601: 1591–1605.

Khiari B, Ghouma I, Ferjani AI, Azzaz AA, Jellali S, Limousy L, Jeguirim M. 2020. Kenaf stems: thermal characterization and conversion for biofuel and biochar production. *Fuel*. 262: 116654.

Khulbe KC, Matsuura T. 2018. Removal of heavy metals and pollutants by membrane adsorption Techniques. *Applied Water Science*. 8(1):19–49.

Kiran BR, Prasad MNV. 2019. Biochar and rice husk ash assisted phytoremediation potentials of *Ricinus communis* L. for lead-spiked soils. *Ecotoxicology and Environmental Safety*. 183: 109574.

Koprivova A, Kopriva S, Jäger D, Will B, Jouanin L, Rennenberg H. 2002. Evaluation of transgenic poplars over-expressing enzymes of glutathione synthesis for phytoremediation of cadmium. *Plant Biology*. 4: 664–670

Kumar A, Tripti, Maleva M, Bruno LB, Rajkumar M. 2021. Synergistic effect of ACC deaminase producing *Pseudomonas* sp. TR15a and siderophore producing *Bacillus aerophilus* TR15c for enhanced growth and copper accumulation in *Helianthus annuus* L. *Chemosphere*. 276: 130038.

Kumar A, Tripti, Voropaeva O, Maleva M, Panikovskaya K, Borisova G, Rajkumar M, Bruno LB. 2020. Bioaugmentation with copper tolerant endophyte *Pseudomonas lurida* strain EOO26 for improved plant growth and copper phytoremediation by *Helianthus annuus*. *Chemosphere*. 266: 128983.

Kumar GP, Yadav SK, Thawale PR, Singh SK, Juwarkar AA. 2008. Growth of *Jatropha curcas* on heavy metal contaminated soil amended with industrial wastes and azotobacter—a greenhouse study. *Bioresource Technology*. 99: 2078–2082.

LeDuc DL, AbdelSamie M, Móntes-Bayon M, Wu CP, Reisinger SJ, Terry N. 2006. Overexpressing both ATP sulfurylase and selenocysteine methyltransferase enhances selenium phytoremediation traits in Indian mustard. *Environmental Pollution*. 144: 70–76

Lee IH, Kuan YC, Chern JM. 2007. Equilibrium and kinetics of heavy metal ion exchange. *Journal of the Chinese Institute of Chemical Engineers*. 38(1); 71–84.

Li C, Zhou K, Qin W, Tian C, Qi M, Yan X, Han W. 2019. A review on heavy metals contamination in soil: effects, sources, and remediation techniques. *Soil and Sediment Contamination: An International Journal*. 28(4): 380–394.

Li X, Hou S, Su M, Yang M, Shen S, Jiang G, Liu, G. 2010. Major energy plants and their potential for bioenergy development in China. *Environmental Management*. 46(4): 579–589.

Liu X, Shen Y, Lou L, Ding C, Cai Q. 2009. Copper tolerance of the biomass crops Elephant grass (*Pennisetum purpureum* Schumach), Vetiver grass (*Vetiveria zizanioides*) and the upland reed (*Phragmites australis*) in soil culture. *Biotechnology Advances*. 27: 633–640.

Lokeshappa B, Shivpuri K, Tripathi V, Dikshit AK. 2012. Assessment of toxic metals in agricultural produce. *Food and Public Health*. 2(1): 24–29.

Lu H, Liu Y, Zhou H, Yang Y, Chen M, Liang B. 2009, Production of biodiesel from *Jatropha curcus* L. oil. *Computers and Chemical Engineering*. 33: 1091–1096.

Lyyra S, Meagher RB, Kim T, Heaton A, Montello P, Balish RS, Merkle SA. 2007. Coupling two mercury resistance genes in Eastern cottonwood enhances the processing of organomercury. *Plant Biotechnology Journal*. 5: 254–262.

Mallampati SR, Mitoma Y, Okuda T, Simion C, Lee BK. 2015. Dynamic immobilization of simulated radionuclide 133 Cs in soil by thermal treatment/vitrification with nanometallic Ca/CaO composites. *Journal of Environmental Radioactivity*. 139: 118–124

McLaughlin MJ, Singh BR. 1999. Cadmium in soils and plants. In: McLaughlin MJ, Singh BR (Eds.),. *Developments in Plant and Soil Sciences*. Springer, Dordrecht 85: pp. 1–9.

Meers E, Tack FMG, Slycken SV, Ruttens A, Laing GD, Vangronsveld J, Ver-loo MG. 2008. Chemically assisted phytoextraction: a review of potential soil amendments for increasing plant uptake of heavy metals. *International Journal of Phytoremediation*. 10: 390–414.

Miao Y, Xi-yuan X, Xu-feng M, Zhao-hui G, Feng-yong W. 2012. Effect of amendments on growth and metal uptake of giant reed (*Arundo donax* L.) grown on soil contaminated by arsenic, cadmium and lead. *The Transactions of Nonferrous Metals Society of China*. 22: 1462–1469.

Mishra RK, Mohammad N, Roychoudhury N. 2015. Soil pollution: causes, effects and control. *Tropical Forest Research Institute*. 3(1): 20–30.

Mishra S, Bharagava RN, More N, Yadav A, Zainith S, Mani S, Chowdhary P. 2019. Heavy metal contamination: an alarming threat to environment and human health. In *Environmental Biotechnology: For Sustainable Future*, pp. 103–125. Springer, Singapore.

Moffett BF, Nicholson FA, Uwakwe NC, Chambers BJ, Harris JA, Hill TC. 2003. Zinc contamination decreases the bacterial diversity of agricultural soil. *FEMS Microbiology Ecology*. 43(1): 13–19.

Moosavi SA, Aghaalikhani M, Ghobadian B, Fayyazi E. 2018. Okra: a potential future bioenergy crop in Iran. *Renewable and Sustainable Energy Reviews*. 93: 517–524.

Muharrem I, Olcay KI. 2017. An overview of adsorption technique for heavy metal removal from water/wastewater: a critical review. *International Journal of Pure Applied Science*. 3(2); 10–19.

Murakami M, Ae N. 2009. Potential for phytoextraction of copper, lead, and zinc by rice (*Oryza sativa* L.) soybean (*Glycine max* [L.] Merr.), and maize (*Zea mays* L.). *Journal of Hazardous Materials*. 162: 1185–1192.

Muthusaravanan S, Sivarajasekar N, Vivek JS, Paramasivan T, Naushad M, Prakashmaran J, Al-Duaij OK. 2018. Phytoremediation of heavy metals: mechanisms, methods and enhancements. *Environmental Chemistry Letters*. 16(4): 1339–1359.

Naik SN, Goud VV, Rout PK, Dalai AK. 2010. Production of first and second generation biofuels: a comprehensive review. *Renewable and Sustainable Energy Reviews*. 14(2): 578–597.

Navarro A, Cardellach E, Cañadas I, Rodríguez J. 2013. Solar thermal vitrification of mining contaminated soils. *International Journal of Mineral Processing*. 119; 65–74.

Padmavathiamma, PK, Li LY. 2007. Phytoremediation technology: hyper-accumulation metals in plants. *Water, Air, and Soil Pollution*. 184(1): 105–126.

Pandey VC, Singh K, Singh JS, Kumar A, Singh B, Singh RP. 2012. *Jatropha curcas*: a potential biofuel plant for sustainable environmental development. *Renewable & Sustainable Energy Reviews*. 16(5): 2870–2883.

Park W, Feng Y, Ahn SJ. 2014. Alteration of leaf shape, improved metal tolerance, and productivity of seed by overexpression of CsHMA3 in *Camelina sativa*. *Biotechnology for Biofuels*. 7: 96.

Parmar S, Singh V. 2015. Phytoremediation approaches for heavy metal pollution: a review. *Journal of Plant Science and Research*. 2(2): 135.

Pasricha S, Mathur V, Garg A, Lenka S, Verma K, Agarwal S. 2021. Molecular mechanisms underlying heavy metal uptake, translocation and tolerance in hyperaccumulators-an analysis heavy metal tolerance in hyperaccumulators. *Environmental Challenges*. 4: 100197.

Pollard AJ, Dandridge KL, Shee EM. 2000. Phytoremediation of Contaminated Soils and Waters. In: Terry N, Bañuelos G (Eds.), *Ecological genetics and the evolution of trace element hyperaccumulation in plants*. CRC Press, Boca Raton, pp. 251–264.

Qu CS, Ma ZW, Yang J, Liu Y, Bi J, Huang L. 2012. Human exposure pathways of heavy metals in a lead-zinc mining area, Jiangsu Province, China. *PloS One*. 7(11): 46793.

Qureshi FF, Ashraf MA, Rasheed R, Ali S, Hussain I, Ahmed A, Iqbal M. 2020. Organic chelates decrease phytotoxic effects and enhance chromium uptake by regulating chromium-speciation in castor bean (*Ricinus communis* L.). *Science of the Total Environment*. 716: 137061.

Rahman Z, Singh VP. 2019. The relative impact of toxic heavy metals (THMs) (arsenic (As), cadmium (Cd), chromium (Cr)(VI), mercury (Hg), and lead (Pb)) on the total environment: an overview. *Environmental Monitoring and Assessment*. 191(7): 1–21.

Rai PK. 2021. Heavy metals and arsenic phytoremediation potential of invasive alien wetland plants *Phragmites karka* and *Arundo donax*: Water-Energy-Food (W-E-F) Nexus linked sustainability implications. *Bioresource Technology*. 15: 100741.

Rajendran S, Priya TAK, Khoo KS, Hoang TKA, Ng H-S, Munawaroh HSH, Karaman C, Orooji Y, Show PL. 2022. A critical review on various remediation approaches for heavy metal contaminants removal from contaminated soils. *Chemosphere*. 287: 132369.

Rajkumar M, Freitas H. 2008. Influence of metal resistant-plant growth-promoting bacteria on the growth of *Ricinus communis* in soil contaminated with heavy metals. *Chemosphere*. 71: 834–842.

Rasheed H, Slack R, Kay P. 2016. Human health risk assessment for arsenic: a critical review. *Critical Reviews in Environmental Science and Technology*. 46(19–20): 1529–1583.

Renault F, Sancey B, Badot PM, Crini G. 2009. Chitosan for coagulation/flocculation processes—an eco-friendly approach. *European Polymer Journal*. 45(5): 1337–1348.

Rojjanateeranaj P, Sangthong C, Prapagdee B. 2017. Enhanced cadmium phytoremediation of *Glycine max* L. through bioaugmentation of cadmium-resistant bacteria assisted by biostimulation. *Chemosphere*. 185: 764–771.

Sagar AD, Kartha S. 2007. Bioenergy and sustainable development? Annual Review of Environment and Resources. *Journal of Sustainable Bioenergy Systems*. 32: 131–167.

Saleh S, Huang X, Greenberg BM, Glick BR. 2004. Phytoremediation of persistent organic contaminants in the environment. In: Singh A, Ward OP (Eds,). *Applied Bioremediation and Phytoremediation*. Soil Biology, Springer, Berlin, Heidelberg 1: pp. 115–131.

Sani A, Hussaini K, Sani HM. 2017. Evaluation of removal efficiency of heavy metals by low-cost activated carbon prepared from African palm fruit. *Applied Water Science*. 7(6): 3151–3155.

Sardar K, Ali S, Hameed S, Afzal S, Fatima S, Shakoor MB, Tauqeer HM. 2013. Heavy metals contamination and what are the impacts on living organisms. *Greener Journal of Environmental Management and Public Safety*. 2(4): 172–179.

Schroder P, Beckers B, Daniels S, Gnädinger F, Maestri E, Marmiroli N, Sæbø, A. 2018. Intensify production, transform biomass to energy and novel goods and protect soils in Europe- a vision how to mobilize marginal lands. *Science of the Total Environment*. 616: 1101–1123.

Sharma S, Tiwari S, Hasan A, Saxena V, Pandey LM. 2018. Recent advances in conventional and contemporary methods for remediation of heavy metal-contaminated soils. *Biotechnology*. 8(4): 1–18.

Sheehan PJ, Meyer DM, Sauer MM, Paustenbach DJ. 1991. Assessment of the human health risks posed by exposure to chromium-contaminated soils. *Journal of Toxicology and Environmental Health, Part A Current Issues*. 32(2): 161–201.

Shim D, Kim S, Choi YI, Song WY, Park J, Youk ES, Jeong SC, Martinoia E, Noh EW, Lee Y. (2013) Transgenic poplar trees expressing yeast cadmium factor 1 exhibit the characteristics necessary for the phytoremediation of mine tailing soil. *Chemosphere*. 90(4), 1478–1486.

Sivapullaiah PV, Prakash SN, Suma BN. 2015. Electrokinetic removal of heavy metals from soil. *Journal of Electrochemical Science and Engineering*. 5(1): 47–65.

Tahir MB, Kiran H, Iqbal T. 2019. The detoxification of heavy metals from aqueous environment using nano-photocatalysis approach: a review. *Environmental Science and Pollution Research*. 26: 10515–10528.

Thangaswamy S, Manjunatha B, Suarez JP, Babu M, Ponnuswamy G, Reddy GVS, Mariadoss S. 2015. Phytoremediation of tannery effluent polluted soils of Dindigul, Tamil Nadu, using Arbuscularmycorrhizal fungi inoculated *Azadirachta indica*. *Journal of Chemical and Pharmaceutical Research*. 7(7): 905–914.

Trivedi S, Gaudani H, Gupta M, Gupta N, Patil P, Gupta G, Krishna KV, Reddy MP. 2009. Establishment of *Agrobacterium*-mediated genetic transformation in *Jatropha curcas* L. *International Journal of Agriculture Sciences*. 1(2): 11–20.

Tsao DT. 2003. Overview of phytotechnologies. In: Scheper T, Tsao D (Eds.), *Advances in Biochemical Engineering Biotechnology*. Springer-Verlag, Berlin, pp. 1–50.

Tulod AM, Castillo ASA, Carandang WM, Pampolina NM. 2012. Growth performance and phytoremediation potential of *Pongamia pinnata* (L.) Pierre, *Samanea saman* (Jacq.) Merr. and *Vitex parviflora* Juss. in copper contaminated soil amended with zeolite and VAM. *The Asian International Journal of Life Sciences*. 21(2): 499–522.

Turchi A, Tamantini I, Camussi AM, Racchi ML. 2012. Expression of a metallothionein A1 gene of *Pisum sativum* in white poplar enhances tolerance and accumulation of zinc and copper. *Plant Science*. 183: 50–56.

Turgut C, Pepe MK, Cutright TJ. 2004. The effect of EDTA and citric acid on phytoremediation of Cd, Cr, and Ni from soil using *Helianthus annuus*. *Environmental Pollution*. 131: 147–154.

Turgut C, Pepe MK, Cutright TJ. 2005. The effect of EDTA on *Helianthus annuus* uptake, selectivity, and translocation of heavy metals when grown in Ohio, New Mexico and Colombia soils. *Chemosphere*. 58: 1087–1095.

Unnikannan P, Baskaran L, Chidambaram ALA, Sundaramoorthy P. 2013. Chromium phytotoxicity in tree species and its role on phytoremediation. *Insight Botany*. 3(1): 15–25.

Vamerali T, Bandiera M, Mosca G. 2010. Field crops for phytoremediation of metal contaminated land. A review. *Environmental Chemistry Letter*. 8(1): 1–17.

Vishnupradeep R, Bruno LB, Taj Z, Karthik C, Challabathula D, Tripti, Kumar A, Freitas H, Rajkumar M. 2022. Plant growth promoting bacteria improve growth and phytostabilization potential of *Zea mays* under chromium and drought stress by altering photosynthetic and antioxidant responses. *Environmental Technology & Innovation*. 25: 102154.

Wang W, Li R, Wang H, Qi B, Jiang X, Zhu Q, Zhao Q. 2019. Sweet cane (*Erianthus arundinaceus*) as a native bioenergy crop with environmental remediation potential in southern China: a review. *GCB Bioenergy*. 11(9): 1012–1025.

Watanabe M, Shinmachi F, Noguchi A, Hasegawa I. 2005. Introduction of yeast metallothionein gene *(CUP1)* into plant and evaluation of heavy metal tolerance of mansgenic plant at the callus stage. *Journal of Soil Science and Plant Nutrient.* 51(1): 129–133.

Weissmannová HD, Pavlovský J. 2017. Indices of soil contamination by heavy metals- methodology of calculation for pollution assessment (minireview). *Environmental Monitoring and Assessment.* 189(12): 1–25.

Wiangkham N, Prapagdee B. 2018. Potential of Napier grass with cadmium-resistant bacterial inoculation on cadmium phytoremediation and its possibility to use as biomass fuel. *Chemosphere.* 201: 511–518.

Wojas S, Hennig J, Plaza S, Geisler M, Siemianowski O. 2009. Ectopic expression of Arabidopsis ABC transporter MRP7 modifies cadmium root-to-shoot transport and accumulation. *Environmental Pollution.* 157(10): 2781–2789.

Wu D, Li L, Zhao X, Peng Y, Yang P, Peng X. 2019. Anaerobic digestion: a review on process monitoring. *Renewable and Sustainable Energy Reviews.* 103: 1–12.

Yadav P, Priyanka P, Kumar D, Yadav A, Yadav K. 2019. Bioenergy crops: recent advances and future outlook. In: Rastegari A, Yadav A, Gupta A. (Eds.), *Prospects of Renewable Bioprocessing in Future Energy Systems.* Biofuel and Biorefinery Technologies, Springer, Cham, 10: pp. 315–335.

Yadav SK, Dhote M, Kumar P, Sharma J, Chakrabarti T, Juwarkara AA. 2010. Differential antioxidative enzyme responses of *Jatrophacurcas* L. to chromium stress. *Journal of Hazardous Materials.* 180: 609–615.

Yadav SK, Juwarkar AA, Kumar GP, Thawale PR, Singh SK, Chakrabarti T. 2009. Bioaccumulation andphyto-translocation of arsenic, chromium and zinc by *Jatropha curcas* L.: impact of dairy sludge and biofertilizer. *Bioresource Technology.* 100: 4616–4622.

Yao Z, Li J, Xie H, Yu C. 2012. A review on remediation technologies of soil contaminated by heavy metals. *Procedia Environmental Science.* 16: 722–729.

You Y, Wang L, Ju C, Wang G, Ma F, Wang Y, Yang D. 2021. Effects of arbuscularmycorrhizal fungi on the growth and toxic element uptake of *Phragmitesaustralis*(Cav.) Trin. ex Steud under zinc/cadmium stress. *Ecotoxicology and Environmental Safety.* 213: 112023.

Zambelli B, Uversky VN, Ciurli S. 2016. Nickel impact on human health: an intrinsic disorder perspective. *Biochimica et Biophysica Acta.* 1864(12): 1714–1731.

Zhang H, Guo Q, Yang J, Mab J, Chen G, Chen T, Zhu G, Wang J, Zhang G, Wang X, Shao C. 2016. Comparison of chelates for enhancing *Ricinus communis* L. Phytoremediation of Cd and Pb contaminated soil. *Ecotoxicology and Environmental Safety.* 133: 57–62.

Zhang X, Zeng B, Li H, Huang J, Jiang L, Zhang X, Tan Z, Wu Z, Qin X, Feng C, Huang Z. 2022. Soil heavy metals and phytoremediation by *Populus deltoides* alter the structure and function of bacterial community in mine ecosystems. *Applied Soil Ecology.* 172: 104359.

Zhang Y, Hu J, Bai J, Wang J, Yin R, Wang J, Lin X. 2018. Arbuscular mycorrhizal fungi alleviate the heavy metal toxicity on sunflower *(Helianthus annuus* L.) plants cultivated on a heavily contaminated field soil at a WEEE-recycling site. *Science of the Total Environment.* 628–629: 282–290.

Zhao FJ, Ma JF, Meharg AA, McGrath SP. 2009. Arsenic uptake and metabolism in plants. *New Phytologist.* 181: 777–794.

Zheng C, Wang, PP. 2002. A field demonstration of the simulation optimization approach for remediation system design. *Ground Water.* 40: 258–265.

Zulfiqar U, Farooq M, Hussain S, Maqsood M, Hussain M, Ishfaq M, Anjum MZ. 2019. Lead toxicity in plants: impacts and remediation. *Journal of Environmental Management.* 250: 109557.

11 Sustainable Approach for the Extraction of Precious Metals from Electronic Waste Materials

Alaa El Din Mahmoud
Environmental Sciences Department, Faculty of Science, Alexandria University, Egypt
Green Technology Group, Faculty of Science, Alexandria University, Egypt

CONTENTS

11.1 INTRODUCTION

Nowadays, sustainable development goals are the main driver in most social, economic, political, and environmental decisions to conserve natural resources and ensure prosperous lives for everyone by 2030. Rapid urbanization, industrialization, and population growth have resulted in an exponential surge in the need for smart electronic and electrical equipment (EEEs). For instance, TVs, mobile phones, computers, coffee machines, refrigerators, etc. have become an indispensable part of our society. However, the fast-changing technology and their limited repair options combined with the availability of better alternatives encourage the growing turning of electronics into E-waste (Ahirwar and Tripathi, 2021), which is mostly disposed into landfills informally with other solid wastes (Alam et al., 2021).

E-waste refers to any form of non-functional and discarded electrical or electronic equipment, which may also be referred to as Waste Electrical or Electronic Equipment (WEEE). E-waste is a broad category of items that are divided into categories based on functional similarities, material composition, average weight, and

DOI: 10.1201/9781003188292-11

TABLE 11.1
Different Classes of E-waste According to European Union Classification

Small Equipment	Small Information Technology IT	Large Equipment	Lamps	Screens and Monitors	Heat exchange Equipment
Microwaves	Printers	Dishwashers	Fluorescent	Flat display panels	Air conditioners
Vacuum cleaners	Desktop computers	Heating systems	Light-emitting diode	Cathode ray tubes	Fridges
Video	Mobiles	Kitchen equipment	-	TVs	Freezers
Projectors	Game consoles	Ventilation	-	-	Dispensers
Speakers					
Toys					
Household tools					

their obsolescence attributes. The composition of WEEE composition might vary significantly across electronic device components, functions, capabilities, and models in terms of period of manufacture (Xiao et al., 2020). Chen et al. (2021) concluded that WEEE product categories possess 4–6 toxicity magnitude orders associated with various concentrations of Cr, Pb, Ni, Zn, Hg, Cd, Cu, Al, and Fe.

Even with the direction to low carbon technologies (i.e., wind turbines, photocatalytic cells, electric vehicles), these still require metals for production. For example, wind turbines use 4.7 tonnes Cu and 3 tonnes Al, while electric vehicles require 1.7–11x Cu more than conventional cars (CDA, 2017). Therefore, it is critical to have stable supplies of 17 metals/materials (Al, Cr, Co, Cu, Fe, Pb, Li, Mn, Mo, Ni, Ag, Ti, V, Zn, etc.) in the next ~40 years for the success of clean energy transition (Tabelin et al., 2021).

Nowadays, there are approximately 54 product-centric categories that can be divided into six classes (Forti et al., 2020). Previously, the European Union directive in 2002 divided E-waste into ten categories, including toys, medical equipment, sports gear, and automated dispensers. Table 11.1 lists the different classes of E-waste and their associated products according to the classification of the European Union.

Improper management of WEEE is an alarming global environmental problem due to the presence of a large variety of toxic substances embedded in the devices (Kiddee et al., 2013). Despite the trace metals are physiologically needed, the high concentration of these metals becomes harmful and toxic (El Din Mahmoud and Fawzy, 2016; Mahmoud et al., 2022). That is because enormous metals such as Pb, Cd, Hg, and Cr can reach soil or water bodies/groundwater and increase the toxicity levels of ecosystem (Mahmoud, 2020; Mahmoud et al., 2021a; Mahmoud and Fawzy, 2021; Mahmoud et al., 2020; Mahmoud et al., 2021b).

Dumped electronics in landfills can leach dangerous chemical substances into the groundwater. The large quantity of heavy metals in leached water could result in severe harm to the human blood, kidneys, and apprehensive structures (Badr et al., 2020; Dotaniya et al., 2022). It is predicted that by 2040, the carbon emissions

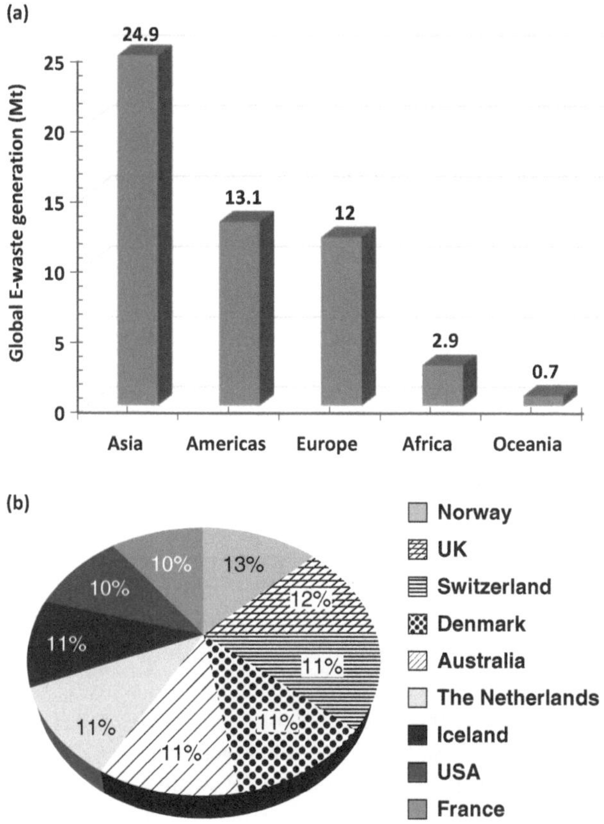

FIGURE 11.1 (a) Global generation of E-waste and (b) countries rank based on their E-waste generation worldwide in 2019.

from the manufacturing and use of electronics will attain 14% of overall emissions (Belkhir and Elmeligi, 2018).

The global EEE consumption increases by around 2.5 million metric tonnes (Mt) annually. Figure 11.1 shows that Asia generates the most global E-waste followed by the Americas, Europe, and then Africa with a world total of 53.6 Mt in 2019 according to Forti et al. (2020). They stated that 17.4% of the collected E-wastes in 2019 was recycled, while the rest ended up either in landfills, dumps, or incinerated.

E-wastes are rich in precious metals like Gold (Au), Silver(Ag), and Platinum (Pt) along with other useful metals such as Aluminium (Al), Copper (Cu), Silica (Si), and Iron (Fe) (Fungaro et al., 2021; Robinson, 2009). Because of their unique physical and chemical properties, precious metals are commonly used as catalysts in a variety of fields, including agriculture and medicine (Ramesh et al., 2008). Precious metals have also traditionally been valuable as currencies and continue to be important as investment commodities. Under ISO 4217, gold (Au), silver (Ag), platinum (Pt), and palladium (Pd) are all known as types of currency. Since precious metals are in short supply, recovering them from aqueous and waste solutions is commercially appealing (Das, 2010).

Many E-waste products can be reused, refurbished, or recycled. Recuperating treasured metals from E-waste can also offer additional earnings within the disposal technique of end of lifestyles electronics. Consequently, the scrap of electronics should be recycled as an environmental aspect as well as the covering of precious metals (Abhilash et al., 2021). Recycling of E-waste comprises three main steps: (i) collection, (ii) processing, and (iii) valuable metals/materials recovery (Meskers and Hagelüken, 2009).

The accelerated rate of industrialization increases the demand for precious metals, while high quality natural resources are diminished quantitatively, with significant operating costs (Canda et al., 2016). The traditional techniques of recovering precious metals from E-waste are pyrometallurgy and hydrometallurgy. Both have adverse impacts on the environment as well as humans because of the release of toxicants like acidic lixiviates and dioxins (Ahirwar and Tripathi, 2021). Therefore, sustainable and cost-effective solutions should be adopted.

Microbial biotechnology offers a 'natural' way of addressing environmental issues ranging from bioremediation techniques to green bio-hydrometallurgical processes for industrial, agricultural, and municipal effluents. Microbial biotechnology is also a critical component of the 'sustainable development' paradigm, which aims for goals such as waste disposal safety and the recovery of minerals, such as precious metals, that are found in a variety of waste streams from various sources. Using biotechnological approaches, precious metals can potentially be recovered from materials that are not economically beneficial by conventional techniques.

Microbial participation in the management of E-waste is now an emerging area for research. Microbial participation in E-waste management has the potential to make the techniques more economic and eco-friendly, hence greener. This technology can provide a new and emerging area of metallurgy which may facilitate the extraction of metals present in trace quantity from their ores. Microorganisms have the ability to either bind metals to their cell surface, adopt them into the cell for intracellular functions, or chelate metals through generating metabolic ligands (Vakilchap et al., 2020). Precious metals resulted after the recovery processes have the same properties, even after multiple life cycles, therefore recycling allows for (Canda et al., 2016):

- The recovery of valuable material without quality loss.
- Energy saving in comparison with primary production.
- Reducing resulted emissions and reducing greenhouse gas emissions.
- The reduction of mining activities.
- Reducing waste.

11.2 ESTIMATION METHODS OF ELECTRONIC WASTE (E-WASTE)

E-waste is mainly generated in OECD countries (Organization for Economic Cooperation and Development) with highly saturated markets for EEE. To estimate possible global quantities of WEEE, a variety of methodologies have been proposed and applied. It was conducted through the consumption and the use method as illustrated in Lohse and Spiller (1998) and it depends on the average lifetime and average weight of EEE products. On the other hand, this assumption is irrelevant, as it presumes a completely saturated market and comparisons of the studies are difficult (Widmera et al., 2005).

11.3 SUSTAINABLE BIOTECHNOLOGICAL APPROACH FOR E-WASTE RECYCLING

The most commonly recovered precious metals are: Gold from jewellery and electronics; Silver from electronics, radiography, films, photographic emulsions, and industrial applications (catalysts, batteries, glass/mirror); and Platinum group metals from catalytic converters, catalysts for refining crude oil, industrial catalysts, nitric acid manufacturing plants, carbon-based catalysts, and E-waste (Canda et al., 2016; Anandhi et al., 2022; Mahmoud 2022).

Abhilash et al. (2021) used a mixture of *A. ferrooxidans* and *A. thiooxidans* (Bacterial strains) to extract copper (Cu) from shredded printed circuit board (PCB). They could recover 93% of Cu at pH 2 and 308 K, using 8% pulp density in 10 days. Whereas *A. niger* could recover 66% of Cu with the same experimental conditions.

Most literature focuses on the extraction of Cu because more than 75% of which is found in only 11 countries – Chile (23%), Australia (10.2%), Peru (10%), Russia (7%), Mexico (6.1%), USA (5.9%), Indonesia (3.2%), China (3%), Kazakhstan (2.3%), Zambia (2.2%), and the Democratic Republic of Congo (DRC) (2.2%).

11.4 BIOLEACHING: A MICROBIAL PROCESS OF METAL RECOVERY

Microbiological leaching uses the natural ability of microorganisms to transform metals present in the waste in a solid form (in the solid matrix) to a dissolved form. Apart from the possibility of bioleaching of metals in alkaline environment (involving cyan genic bacteria), acidophilus microorganisms and conducting biological process of leaching in an acidic environment play a crucial role in the bio-hydrometallurgical techniques (Willner and Fornalczyk, 2013). The difference between bioleaching and bio-hydrometallurgical is shown in Table 11.2.

TABLE 11.2
Comparison between Bioleaching and Bio-Hydrometallurgical Processes

Bioleaching Process	Bio-Hydrometallurgical Process
• Cheaper and easier to conduct in comparison to conventional techniques. • Its advantage is flexibility microorganisms easily adapt to changing and extreme living conditions.	• Reduces the demand for resources, such as ores, energy, and landfill space • This technology is environmentally friendly (in comparison to chemical method) • Considered a green technology (generates less amount of waste)

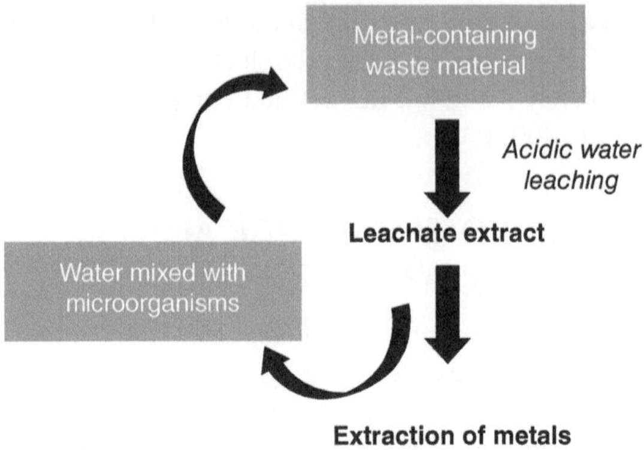

FIGURE 11.2 Microbial leaching process.

Generally, bioleaching refers to the conversion of solid metal values into their water-soluble forms using microorganisms. Bioleaching is a green recycling technology for recovering precious metals. Figure 11.2 shows the microbial leaching process. To achieve microbial leaching, metal-containing waste material is mounded in piles and allows acidic solution to leak through it. Because bacterial oxidation of sulphide ores takes much longer than other biotechnical processes, the leachate is collected and re-circulated throughout the heap (Kour et al., 2021).

Copper sulphide is reduced to copper sulphate by bacteria, and metal values are present in the aqueous phase while the residual solids are eliminated. Microbially metal extraction processes are usually more eco-friendly than physic-chemical processes. When compared to roasting and smelting, they consume less energy and emit no sulphur dioxide or other hazardous pollutants. As a result, this procedure may be compliant with anti-pollution legislation. The majority of naturally occurring bacteria and fungi serve a variety of physiologically significant reactions that enable them to grow and reproduce.

Microbial leaching of uranium follows indirect mechanism. *A. ferrooxidans* responsible for leaching does not interact directly with minerals. Its prime function is to generate Fe^{3+}, the oxidizing agent by oxidation of Fe^{2+} (Kaksonen et al., 2020). Uranium can be successfully recovered by flooding the fractured ores containing uranium with the bacterial community causing the leaching process.

It is worth mentioning that there are two different mechanisms of microbial leaching (direct and indirect mechanisms) (Kour et al., 2021). The direct process includes microorganisms oxidizing metal sulphides through a series of enzymatically catalysed reactions. The electrons required to complete the action are obtained directly from reduced minerals. Direct microbial leaching necessitates a close relationship between the microbial cells and the mineral surface. Adsorption of bacterial cells to mineral particles takes place over a short period of time, in minutes or hours. Indirect process includes the utilization of Fe^{3+} to cause oxidation of reduced metals. In acidic solution, Fe^{3+} possesses a reduction potential of 0.67 V at $pH = 1.5$, making it an oxidizing agent for solubilizing a variety of minerals. Fe^{3+} acts as an oxidant, oxidizing metal sulphides before being reduced to Fe^{2+}. Microorganisms can then oxidize the Fe^{2+} produced, and the cycle continues.

Zn is extracted from sphalerite (ZnS) by *A. ferrooxidans* (Lei et al., 2016). The purpose of bacteria is to restore Fe^{3+} from Fe^{2+} during the entire leaching operation. When the Fe^{2+} concentration is higher than Fe^{3+} concentration, there is an increase in the amount of Zn leaching from sphalerite by *A. ferrooxidans*. The increase is in fact due to the removal of non-porous sulphur layer formed on the surface of sphalerite by chemical oxidation by Fe^{3+} (Schippers et al., 2019).

The biological characteristics of gold (Au) occurrence and extraction from low-grade gold ore have always piqued the interest of academics all over the world. Gold is mined on a huge scale all over the world, with China leading the way, followed by Australia and Russia. Precious gold is continually being thrown as solid trash (i.e., E-waste)/or in streams (primary or secondary gold containing effluents generated during gold ore processing in the form of leachate or spent liquors) and stays unexploited in an era of electronics (Cucchiella et al., 2015; Garlapati, 2016).

The Au content in E-waste is typically of low-grade value, making traditional chemical procedures like cyanidation or chemical leaching difficult to recover. Biological gold biomining is defined as the employment of microbes or their components to extract metal ions from low-grade ores or wastes, according to Rana et al. (2020). It has already been used in industry to process sulphidic and uranium ores, but its promising potential against other metals has only been tested in the lab and has yet to be deployed in industry. Bio-hydrometallurgical techniques, on the other hand, are microbial metabolic agents (oxidants and/or acids)-based metal extraction processes as the primary metal extractors to recover valuable metal ions from low-grade ores or electronic trash. Choi et al. (2020) illustrated the selective separation of Cu and Au from leachates using *Chromobacterium violaceum* associated with recovery of 78.9% Cu and 98.7% Au.

Arab et al. (2020) showed that Luria-Bertani (LB) medium did not provide the highest cyanide production. The maximal cyanide yield of the optimized medium (tryptone and yeast extract = 6 and 5 g/L, respectively) was 1.5 times that of LB medium under ideal culture conditions (25°C, pH 7.5). From 94 bacteria recovered from two E-waste dumps, five efficient indigenous cyanogenic bacterial strains were chosen. For each bacterium, the maximum cyanide concentration was attained by optimizing pH, glycine concentration, and temperature. Copper bioleaching under the optimized circumstances resulted in the range of 96.73% to 31.52% of Cu recovery demonstrating a significant improvement over the results of bioleaching without optimization. Because of their tolerance to metal toxicity, these bacteria are particularly effective at bioleaching other metals such as gold and silver from ores or E-waste. Table 11.3 illustrates the leaching level of various metals from electronic wastes.

Microorganisms and their metabolites are playing a pivotal role for solubilization of metals into aqueous phase from tailings, ores, concentrates, and E-waste. The mobilization of metals from E-waste can be done through the different concentrations of biogenic organic acids such as citric acids $C_6H_8O_7$, Gluconic acid $C_6H_{12}O_7$, Tartaric acid $C_4H_6O_6$, Oxalic acid $C_2H_2O_4$ which are secreted by organotrophs,

TABLE 11.3
Leaching Level Percentage of Various Metals from E-wastes

Microorganisms	Level of Leached Metals	References
Acidithiobacillus ferrooxidans	Cu ~99%	Yang et al. (2009)
Thermosulfidooxidans sulfobacilllus+ *Thermoplasma acidophilum*	Cu ~86%, Zn ~80%, Al ~64%, Ni ~74%	Ilyas et al. (2010)
Chromobacterium violaceum	Au ~11%	Tran et al. (2011)
Thermophilic acidophilic archaea *Acidianus brierley*	Al ~ 35%, Mo ~83%, Ni ~69%	Gerayeli et al. (2013)
Mesophillic Acidithiobacillus thiooxidans	Cu ~98%	Hong and Valix (2014)
Chromobacterium violaceum	Au ~29%	Das et al. (2017)
Pseudomonas balearica	Au ~73%, Ag ~41%	Kumar et al. (2018)
Acidithiobacillus	Cu ~97%	Wei et al. (2020)

bacteria and fungi (Srivastava et al., 2020). For instance, the extraction of copper with the metabolic secreted $C_6H_8O_7$ is illustrated below.

Iron and sulphur oxidizers are playing a large role in metallic extractions from minerals and E-waste. Among those, the properly recognized and studied in element are *Acidithiobacillus ferrooxidans*, *Acidithiobacillus thiooxidans,* and *Leptospirillum ferrooxidans*. However, those are not the most effective iron- and sulphur-oxidizing organisms recognized today which play large role in steel solubilization. Many different genera and species are considered to be gambling lively function in metallic mobilizations. Metal leaching microorganisms are widely disbursed in four phyla particularly Proteobacteria, Nitrospirae, Firmicutes, and Actinobacteria. *Acidithiobacillus, Acidiphilum, Acidiferrobacter,* and *Ferrovum* belongs to Proteobacteria; *Leptospirillum* is a member of *Nitrospirae*; *Alicyclobacillus* and *Sulphobacillus* are classified as Firmicutes; *Ferrimicrobium, Acidimicrobium,* and *Ferrithrix* are Actinobacteria. Those organisms have numerous finest temperatures for their growth and activities which are grouped based on their ideal temperature as mesophiles, slight thermophiles, and thermophiles. However, there aren't any wonderful temperature divisions, for example, *Acidimicrobium ferrooxidans* and *Acidithiobacillus caldus* continue to be active between temperatures 25°C and 55°C, that's the temperature variety of neither mesophiles nor mild thermophiles. Based on the choice of the substrates they are divided into iron oxidizers, sulphur oxidizers, and 1/3 group, which oxidizes both iron and sulphur (Islam et al., 2020).

It is worthy to mention that the cellular membranes of microorganisms have certain adaptations when exposed to metals. Therefore, growth tolerance index (TI) can be measured with time using the following equation (Baniasadi et al., 2019).

$$TI = \frac{\text{Cell count in the presence of metals } \left(\text{cell mL}^{-1}\right)}{\text{Cell count in the absence of metals } \left(\text{cell mL}^{-1}\right)}$$

TABLE 11.4
Factors That Influence the Extraction of Precious Metals from E-wastes (Erüst et al., 2013; Ilyas et al., 2021)

Factors	Effects
• pH	pH of the growth media greatly affects the biotechnological system including the growth rate of microorganisms, metals' speciation and dissolution chemistry.
• Temperature	Significantly influences the rate of reactions in coupled with the microbial growth rate albeit it also depends on the types of microorganisms applied (mesophiles/moderate thermophiles /thermophiles). • Mesophiles: (20°C–40°C)*Acidithiobacillus ferrooxidans, Acidithiobacillus caldusLeptospirillum ferriphilum, Leptospirillum thermoferrooxidans* • Moderate thermophiles (40°C–60°C)*Acidimicrobium ferroxidans, Sulphobacillus thermosulphooxidans, Acidithiobacillus caldus* • Thermophiles (60°C–80°C)*Metallosphaera sedula, Sulphobacillus* sp., *Sulfolobus metallicus*
• Fe^{2+}/Fe^{3+} ratio	Influence the redox potential of a system to drive metals dissolution into the biogenic acid. In biocyanidation, Fe^{2+} forms $Fe(CN)_6^{4-}$ at pH > 8.5, while Fe^{3+} forms $Fe(CN)_6^{3-}$ and CuCN.
• Dissolved oxygen (DO)	DO has two different roles in microbial system: (1) as a respirator for aerobic cells, and (2) as an electron receptor in metal extraction Using *A. ferrooxidans* under the acidic condition, the redox couple conversion of $Fe^{2+} \rightarrow Fe^{3+}$ mainly occurs in the culture medium, Fe^{2+} oxidation greatly influenced by DO of the media.
• Size of feed sample	Can directly be related to the available surface area of contact to the microbial media, thus influencing the progress of extraction process.
• Soluble CO_2	CO_2 is a vital factor as most of the bioleaching activities are performed by autotrophic aerobes. Like O_2, CO_2 is also an essential nutrient for the growth and survival of microorganisms and an adequate supply of these molecules must be ensured for a successful oxidation process.

11.5 FACTORS AFFECTING THE RECYCLING PROCESS

In this section, the possible factors that could influence the recycling process of metals are summarized in Table 11.4.

11.6 CHALLENGES AND PERSPECTIVES OF E-WASTE MANAGEMENT

The major challenge of E-waste management is its massively high volume and complexity. We can get high quality of recycled products when the desired E-wastes are segregated because of the difference in their components (Wang et al., 2017).

Generally, recovery of metals from E-waste is a hard manner. As an example, the restoration charge for cobalt is best at 30%. Metals are critical for laptops,

TABLE 11.5
Summarized Opportunities and Challenges in Developing a Sustainable E-waste Management

Opportunities	Challenges
• E-wastes are rich with precious metals	• High volume • Complexity • Toxicity leaching into water and soil
• Better metal grades in electronics than ores excavated from mines	• Informal sector
• Providing secondary raw materials as alternatives for direct exploitation of natural resources	• Insufficient recycling facilities around the globe
• Reducing E-waste accumulation of E-waste through recycle/reuse	• Ineffective implementation of regulations and frameworks
• Opening additional jobs to support economy	• Lack of knowledge and awareness on E-waste collection

smartphones, and electric-powered vehicle batteries. However, obtaining recycled metals from E-waste is up to 10 times more power green than those from uncooked metallic ores mined (Mudali et al., 2021). Table 11.5 summarizes the opportunities and challenges in developing a sustainable E-waste management.

Advancing the bioleaching processes via developing microbial consortia for improved and efficient leaching of valuable metals from E-waste needs further research. It is hoped that the implementation of these solutions, taken together, should reduce the environmental and health hazards posed by inefficient and improper recycling of new generation of E-waste and should help in effective recovery of the valuable materials from the E-waste (Ahirwar and Tripathi, 2021).

11.7 CONCLUSIONS AND RECOMMENDATIONS

It is expected that the global demand for precious metals will be increased in the future. Therefore, alternative sources for those metals are needed as the natural deposits are finite resources that could be depleted with excessive extraction. Recycling of precious metals by bioleaching is a sustainable process. It is recommended for further research in the extraction of various precious metals using various bacterial strains. As stated in the mentioned literature, the rate of metals recycling especially for Cu is ~90%. Tabelin et al. (2021) expected that the Cu, Au, and Mo reserves will last for 300, 21, and 34 years, respectively. It is highly recommended to create industrial bioleaching plants to develop commercial prospects for the recovery of precious metals and isolate/identify further microorganisms so the percentage recovery of those metals could be improved. Furthermore, technical innovation proposes and uses new materials which could be toxic and no further usage of them. Interdisciplinary or hybrid approaches with advanced biotechnology will facilitate the sustainable recovery of metals.

REFERENCES

Abhilash, Tabassum, S., Ghosh, A., Meshram, P., van Hullebusch, E.D., 2021. Microbial processing of waste shredded PCBs for copper extraction cum separation—comparing the efficacy of bacterial and fungal leaching kinetics and yields. *Metals* 11, 317.

Ahirwar, R., Tripathi, A.K., 2021. E-waste management: A review of recycling process, environmental and occupational health hazards, and potential solutions. *Environmental Nanotechnology, Monitoring & Management* 15, 100409.

Alam, P., Mazhar, M.A., Khan, A.H., Khan, N.A., Mahmoud, A.E.D., 2021. Seasonal characterization of municipal solid waste in the city of Jammu, India, in: *IOP Conference Series: Materials Science and Engineering*. IOP Publishing, p. 012061.

Anandhi, P., Harikrishnan, S., Senthil Kumar, V.J., Lai, W.-C., Mahmoud, A.E.D., 2022. The Enhanced Energy Density of rGO/TiO2 Based Nanocomposite as Electrode Material for Supercapacitor. Electronics 11, 1792.

Arab, B., Hassanpour, F., Arshadi, M., Yaghmaei, S., Hamedi, J., 2020. Optimized bioleaching of copper by indigenous cyanogenic bacteria isolated from the landfill of e-waste. *Journal of Environmental Management* 261, 110124.

Badr, N.B.E., Al-Qahtani, K.M., Mahmoud, A.E.D., 2020. Factorial experimental design for optimizing selenium sorption on *Cyperus laevigatus* biomass and green-synthesized nano-silver. *Alexandria Engineering Journal* 59, 5219–5229.

Baniasadi, M., Vakilchap, F., Bahaloo-Horeh, N., Mousavi, S.M., Farnaud, S., 2019. Advances in bioleaching as a sustainable method for metal recovery from e-waste: A review. *Journal of Industrial and Engineering Chemistry* 76, 75–90.

Belkhir, L., Elmeligi, A., 2018. Assessing ICT global emissions footprint: Trends to 2040 & recommendations. *Journal of Cleaner Production* 177, 448–463.

Canda, L., Heput, T., Ardelean, E., 2016. Methods for recovering precious metals from industrial waste, in: *IOP Conference Series: Materials Science and Engineering*, Vol. 106, p. 012020.

CDA, 2017. Copper Drives Electric Vehicles, https://www.copper.org/publications/pub_list/pdf/A6191-ElectricVehicles-Factsheet.pdf.

Chen, S., Wang, R., Wang, J., Shu, J., Chen, M., Ogunseitan, O.A., 2021. Comparative effectiveness of technical and regulatory innovations to reduce the burden of electronic waste. *Resources, Conservation and Recycling* 167, 105387.

Choi, J.-W., Song, M.-H., Bediako, J.K., Yun, Y.-S., 2020. Sequential recovery of gold and copper from bioleached wastewater using ion exchange resins. *Environmental Pollution* 266, 115167.

Cucchiella, F., D'Adamo, I., Lenny Koh, S.C., Rosa, P., 2015. Recycling of WEEEs: An economic assessment of present and future e-waste streams. *Renewable and Sustainable Energy Reviews* 51, 263–272.

Das, N., 2010. Recovery of precious metals through biosorption — A review. *Hydrometallurgy* 103, 180–189.

Das, S., Natarajan, G., Ting, Y.-P., 2017. Bio-extraction of precious metals from urban solid waste, in: *AIP Conference Proceedings*. AIP Publishing LLC, p. 020004.

Dotaniya, M.L., Meena, V.D., Saha, J.K., Dotaniya, C.K., Mahmoud, A.E.D., Meena, B.L., Meena, M.D., Sanwal, R.C., Meena, R.S., Doutaniya, R.K., Solanki, P., Lata, M., Rai, P.K., 2022. Reuse of poor-quality water for sustainable crop production in the changing scenario of climate. *Environment, Development and Sustainability*, 1–32.

El Din Mahmoud, A., Fawzy, M., 2016. Bio-based methods for wastewater treatment: Green sorbents, in: Ansari, A.A., Gill, S.S., Gill, R., Lanza, G.R., Newman, L. (Eds.), *Phytoremediation: Management of Environmental Contaminants*, Volume 3. Springer International Publishing, Cham, pp. 209–238.

Erüst, C., Akcil, A., Gahan, C.S., Tuncuk, A., Deveci, H., 2013. Biohydrometallurgy of secondary metal resources: A potential alternative approach for metal recovery. *Journal of Chemical Technology and Biotechnology* 88, 2115–2132.

Forti, V., Baldé, C.P., Kuehr, R., Bel, G., 2020. *The Global E-waste Monitor 2020.* United Nations University, International Telecommunication Union International Solid Waste Association, Bonn/Geneva/Rotterdam.

Fungaro, D.A., Silva, K.C., Mahmoud, A.E.D., 2021. Aluminium tertiary industry waste and ashes samples for development of zeolitic material synthesis. *Journal of Applied Materials Technology* 2, 66–73.

Garlapati, V.K., 2016. E-waste in India and developed countries: Management, recycling, business and biotechnological initiatives. *Renewable and Sustainable Energy Reviews* 54, 874–881.

Gerayeli, F., Ghojavand, F., Mousavi, S.M., Yaghmaei, S., Amiri, F., 2013. Screening and optimization of effective parameters in biological extraction of heavy metals from refinery spent catalysts using a thermophilic bacterium. *Separation and Purification Technology* 118, 151–161.

Hong, Y., Valix, M., 2014. Bioleaching of electronic waste using acidophilic sulfur oxidising bacteria. *Journal of Cleaner Production* 65, 465–472.

Ilyas, S., Ruan, C., Bhatti, H.N., Ghauri, M.A., Anwar, M.A., 2010. Column bioleaching of metals from electronic scrap. *Hydrometallurgy* 101, 135–140.

Ilyas, S., Srivastava, R.R., Kim, H., Das, S., Singh, V.K., 2021. Circular bioeconomy and environmental benignness through microbial recycling of e-waste: A case study on copper and gold restoration. *Waste Management* 121, 175–185.

Islam, A., Ahmed, T., Awual, M.R., Rahman, A., Sultana, M., Aziz, A.A., Monir, M.U., Teo, S.H., Hasan, M., 2020. Advances in sustainable approaches to recover metals from e-waste-A review. *Journal of Cleaner Production* 244, 118815.

Kaksonen, A.H., Lakaniemi, A.-M., Tuovinen, O.H., 2020. Acid and ferric sulfate bioleaching of uranium ores: A review. *Journal of Cleaner Production* 264, 121586.

Kiddee, P., Naidu, R., Wong, M.H., 2013. Electronic waste management approaches: An overview. *Waste Management* 33, 1237–1250.

Kour, G., Kothari, R., Mohan Singh, H., Pathania, D., Dhar, S., 2021. Microbial leaching for valuable metals harvesting: versatility for the bioeconomy. *Environmental Sustainability* 4, 215–229.

Kumar, A., Saini, H.S., Kumar, S., 2018. Enhancement of gold and silver recovery from discarded computer printed circuit boards by Pseudomonas balearica SAE1 using response surface methodology (RSM). *3 Biotech* 8, 100.

Lei, Y., Zhang, G., Ai, C., Zhuang, S., 2016. Bioleaching of Sphalerite by the Native Mesophilic Iron-oxidizing Bacteria from a Lead-Zinc Tailing. *Procedia Environmental Sciences* 31, 554–559.

Lohse, G.L., Spiller, P., 1998. Electronic shopping. *Communications of the ACM* 41, 81–87.

Mahmoud, A.E.D., Hosny, M., El-Maghrabi, N., Fawzy, M., 2022. Facile synthesis of reduced graphene oxide by *Tecoma stans* extracts for efficient removal of Ni (II) from water: batch experiments and response surface methodology. *Sustainable Environment Research* 32, 22.

Mahmoud, A.E.D., 2020. Graphene-based nanomaterials for the removal of organic pollutants: Insights into linear versus nonlinear mathematical models. *Journal of Environmental Management* 270, 110911.

Mahmoud, A.E.D., Al-Qahtani, K.M., Alflaij, S.O., Al-Qahtani, S.F., Alsamhan, F.A., 2021a. Green copper oxide nanoparticles for lead, nickel, and cadmium removal from contaminated water. *Scientific Reports* 11, 12547.

Mahmoud, A.E.D., Fawzy, M., 2021. Nanosensors and nanobiosensors for monitoring the environmental pollutants, in: Makhlouf, A.S.H., Ali, G.A.M. (Eds.), *Waste Recycling Technologies for Nanomaterials Manufacturing*. Springer International Publishing, Cham, pp. 229–246.

Mahmoud, A.E.D., Fawzy, M., Hosny, G., Obaid, A., 2020. Equilibrium, kinetic, and diffusion models of chromium(VI) removal using Phragmites australis and Ziziphus spina-christi biomass. *International Journal of Environmental Science and Technology* 18, 2125–2136.

Mahmoud, A.E.D., Umachandran, K., Sawicka, B., Mtewa, T.K., 2021b. 26 - Water resources security and management for sustainable communities, in: Mtewa, A.G., Egbuna, C. (Eds.), *Phytochemistry, the Military and Health*. Elsevier, pp. 509–522.

Mahmoud, A.E.D., 2022. Recent Advances of TiO_2 Nanocomposites for Photocatalytic Degradation of Water Contaminants and Rechargeable Sodium Ion Batteries, in: Shalan, A.E., Hamdy Makhlouf, A.S., Lanceros-Méndez, S. (Eds.), *Advances in Nanocomposite Materials for Environmental and Energy Harvesting Applications*. Springer International Publishing, Cham, pp. 757–770.

Meskers, C., Hagelüken, C., 2009. The impact of different pre-processing routes on the metal recovery from PCs, Resource management and technology for material and energy efficiency, Switserland.

Mudali, U.K., Patil, M., Saravanabhavan, R., Saraswat, V.K., 2021. Review on E-waste recycling: Part I—a prospective urban mining opportunity and challenges. *Transactions of the Indian National Academy of Engineering* 6, 547–568.

Ramesh, A., Hasegawa, H., Sugimoto, W., Maki, T., Ueda, K., 2008. Adsorption of gold(III), platinum(IV) and palladium(II) onto glycine modified crosslinked chitosan resin. *Bioresource Technology* 99, 3801–3809.

Rana, S., Mishra, P., Ab Wahid, Z., Thakur, S., Pant, D., Singh, L., 2020. Microbe-mediated sustainable bio-recovery of gold from low-grade precious solid waste: A microbiological overview. *Journal of Environmental Sciences* 89, 47–64.

Robinson, B.H., 2009. E-waste: An assessment of global production and environmental impacts. *Science of The Total Environment* 408, 183–191.

Schippers, A., Tanne, C., Stummeyer, J., Graupner, T., 2019. Sphalerite bioleaching comparison in shake flasks and percolators. Minerals Engineering 132, 251–257.

Srivastava, R.R., Ilyas, S., Kim, H., Choi, S., Trinh, H.B., Ghauri, M.A., Ilyas, N., 2020. Biotechnological recycling of critical metals from waste printed circuit boards. *Journal of Chemical Technology & Biotechnology* 95, 2796–2810.

Tabelin, C.B., Park, I., Phengsaart, T., Jeon, S., Villacorte-Tabelin, M., Alonzo, D., Yoo, K., Ito, M., Hiroyoshi, N., 2021. Copper and critical metals production from porphyry ores and E-wastes: A review of resource availability, processing/recycling challenges, socio-environmental aspects, and sustainability issues. *Resources, Conservation and Recycling* 170, 105610.

Tran, C.D., Lee, J.-C., Pandey, B.D., Jeong, J., Yoo, K., Huynh, T.H., 2011. Bacterial cyanide generation in presence of metal ions (Na^+, Mg^{2+}, Fe^{2+}, Pb^{2+}) and gold bioleaching from waste PCBs. *Journal of Chemical Engineering of Japan*, 44, 1107120229.

Vakilchap, F., Mousavi, S.M., Baniasadi, M., Farnaud, S., 2020. Development and evolution of biocyanidation in metal recovery from solid waste: a review. *Reviews in Environmental Science and Bio/Technology* 19, 509–530.

Wang, W., Tian, Y., Zhu, Q., Zhong, Y., 2017. Barriers for household e-waste collection in China: Perspectives from formal collecting enterprises in Liaoning Province. *Journal of Cleaner Production* 153, 299–308.

Wei, X., Liu, D., Huang, W., Huang, W., Lei, Z., 2020. Simultaneously enhanced Cu bioleaching from E-wastes and recovered Cu ions by direct current electric field in a bioelectrical reactor. *Bioresource Technology* 298, 122566.

Widmera, R., Oswald-Krapf, H., Sinha-Khetrival, D., 2005. Global perspectives on e-waste. *Environmental Impact Assessment Review*, 25, 436–458.

Willner, J., Fornalczyk, A., 2013. Extraction of metals from electronic waste by bacterial leaching. *Environment Protection Engineering* 39, 197–208.

Xiao, J., Li, J., Xu, Z., 2020. Challenges to future development of spent lithium ion batteries recovery from environmental and technological perspectives. *Environmental Science & Technology* 54, 9–25.

Yang, T., Xu, Z., Wen, J., Yang, L., 2009. Factors influencing bioleaching copper from waste printed circuit boards by Acidithiobacillus ferrooxidans. *Hydrometallurgy* 97, 29–32.

12 Conversion of Organic Waste to Economically Valuable Products

Recent Advancements with Challenges

Shamim Mia, Md. Mehedi Hasan Mithu, Sanjida Aktar, and Ayesa Akter Suhi
Patuakhali Science and Technology University

Ashim Sikdar
Sylhet Agricultural University

Miguel Angel Sanchez-Monedero
CEBAS-CSIC

Tomoyuki Makino
Tohoku University

CONTENTS

DOI: 10.1201/9781003188292-12

12.1 INTRODUCTION

Waste is generated from our daily activities, industrial operations, and agricultural activities. The waste generation is often high reaching out of the capacity of the cities and municipalities to manage them sustainably. Therefore, waste is a serious concern for many countries since it causes multiple problems including environmental pollution, disease dissemination, and greenhouse gas emission if they are not properly managed. For instance, the annual waste generation of major cities of the world is large estimated a ~ 2.1 billion tons in 2016 while it could reach up to 3.42 billion tons in 2050. A large fraction of them remain uncollected (FAO, 2016). This scenario is prevalent in many developing countries listing their cities as the least livable. It is also a problem for developed countries, although there have been significant efforts to manage them.

The waste generation rate is changing with time, most possibly increasing with the betterment of the livelihood of the people. The waste generation rate of developed countries is ~1.0 kg/person/day while it is about 0.5 kg/person/day in the least developed countries (Kaza et al., 2018). Moreover, the population residing in the cities and municipal areas is increasing with time while industrial activities are also increasing. These suggest that the waste generation rate will increase in the future.

Among the waste, a small fraction of waste (i.e., metals, plastic, and wood) is collected and recycled while the largest fraction of waste is organic in nature and remains untreated and disposed of in landfills. The fraction of organic waste can be between 50% and 80% of the municipal waste. This organic or biowaste is basically agriculturally derived product that carries nutrients. These nutrients are harvested from agricultural lands. A continuous harvesting of nutrients from agricultural lands is a serious concern since these lands are getting mined while agricultural production creates large carbon footprint.

Apart from the municipal waste generation, living organisms including human beings also generate a large amount of wastes as urine and feces with a daily individual footprint of ~0.2 and ~0.50 kg, respectively. Moreover, livestock and poultry industry generates large volume of organic waste. When these wastes are combined, the figure becomes quite large with no reliable global estimates. Although sustainable management of animal excreta has been undertaken, similar efforts for managing human excreta have not been noticed. Therefore, this is one of the potential sectors that has not received enough attention for the circular economy.

Waste can be a resource. In the context of circular economy, an economic system should efficiently maintain the value of resources through recycling and reusing them and their products, and conversion of waste to useable products including food, feed, fertilizer, and bioenergy. In this way, waste recycling and reuse can be one of the promising sectors which can help to create new business opportunities while reducing the environmental footprint. In this concept, 4R (reduction, reuse, recycling, and recovery) is usually recommended.

Waste to resources has been considered a new dimension of waste economy. Many processes and techniques are applied to generate useable products from organic wastes. For instance, composting of organic waste has been practiced for hundreds of years. Moreover, harvesting of energy from waste is already been practiced while development of biopolymer, biocomposite, and biosorbents from waste is now starting to be practiced. However, a comprehensive insight into the applicability of these techniques has not been explored since most of the studies focus on the use of a single method. Here, we synthesized the current state of knowledge on the recycling of organic waste to useable products using biological technologies.

12.2 WASTE GENERATE AND ITS COMPOSITION

The daily waste generation varies with the lifestyle and income of the people. The per capita daily waste generation rate is about 2.2 kg for North America while this is about 0.46 kg for sub-Saharan Africa (Table 12.1). In South Asia, the daily per capita waste generation rate is also relatively low, around 0.52 kg. The per capita waste generation is increasing with improving lifestyle, and therefore, it is projected that it would reach 2.50 kg for North America by 2050 while the increment of per capita waste generation rate is expected to be 1.30 kg by 2050 for Latin America. When the per capita generation is multiplied with the population of the country, the amount of waste generation is quite large for East Asia and Pacific countries with estimates of ~1,280 thousand tons per day. Combining all the waste together, the daily global waste generation is about ~5,535 thousand tons per year while it has been estimated to reach ~9,280 thousand tons in the year 2050. The fraction of organic waste also varies across regions with the highest organic fraction in Asia and Africa, and it is also high in the East Asia and Pacific region. The global daily total organic waste generation is about 3,545 thousand tons.

12.3 RECYCLING OPTIONS OF ORGANIC WASTES

Organic waste can be recycled following different processes and a wide range of products can be synthesized (Figure 12.1). The process can be sorting, composting, polymerization, and adsorption while the products can be food for human and feed for animal, fertilizer for agriculture, and bioenergy, biopolymers, and biocomposite

TABLE 12.1
Waste Generation in Different Regions of the World (Kaza et al., 2018)

Region	Population (Million)			Waste Generation Rate (kg/capita/day)			Total Waste Generation (Thousand ton per day)			Fraction of Organic Waste (%)	Organic Waste Generation (Thousand ton per day)
	2016	2030	2050	2016	2030	2050	2016	2030	2050		
Middle East and North Africa	433	539	661	0.81	0.90	1.06	351	485	701	72.0	252.78
Sub-Saharan Africa	985	1400	2118	0.46	0.50	0.63	453	700	1334	53.4	241.89
Latin America and the Caribbean	630	706	762	0.99	1.11	1.30	624	784	991	65.5	408.62
North America	360	391	425	2.21	2.37	2.50	795	926	1063	61.6	489.44
South Asia	1851	2143	2396	0.52	0.62	0.79	962	1328	1893	68.0	654.36
Europe and Central Asia	907	928	923	1.18	1.30	1.45	1070	1207	1338	56.2	601.34
East Asia and Pacific	2286	2424	2420	0.56	0.68	0.81	1280	1648	1960	70.0	896.03
Total	7450.96	8531.17	9704.81	0.96	1.07	1.22	5534.78	7078.67	9279.54	63.81	3544.45

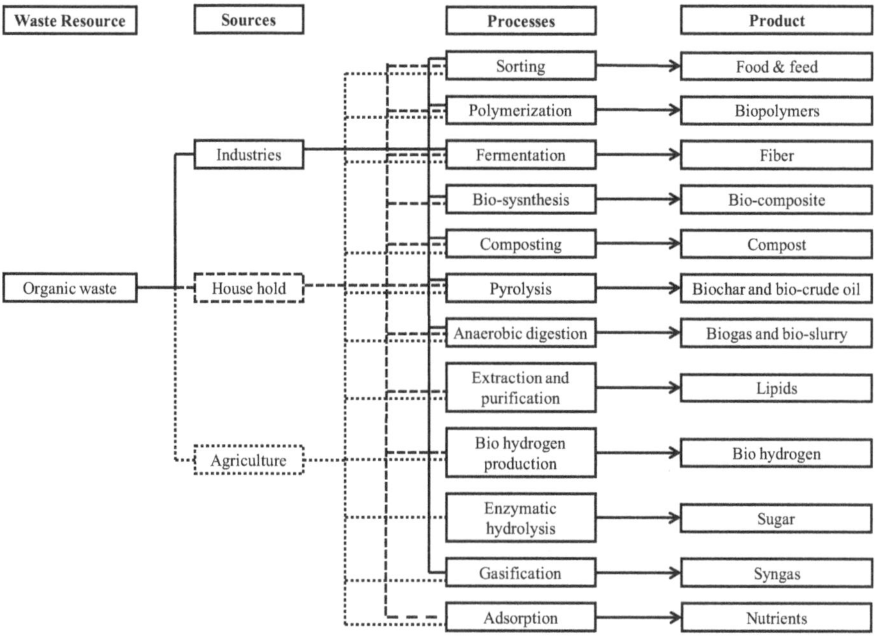

FIGURE 12.1 Potential recycling of organic waste through different processes with their products.

for different uses. The process can be operated singly or in combination with recycling energy and mass from one process to another process allowing synergistic benefits. When waste is collected from households and supermarkets, the high-value products (e.g., food that has not been expired) can be collected separately. In that case, coordinated chain can be developed to collect the food items from household and sale outlets. These foods can then be sterilized to ensure that they do not contain any germs for causing diseases. Also, in many countries and cities, there are food banks where people voluntarily collect food. The collected food can be distributed to meet the food demand of the people. However, as far as we are aware of, such systems have not been adopted largely in either of the cities in the world. Similarly, a fraction of organic waste can be directly used as feed after treating them to ensure there are no germs causing diseases. Moreover, an additional fraction of organic waste can be processed to produce feed for animals. Next, the organic waste can further be sorted into compostable, pyrolyzable, and fiber collecting fractions. Although it is often difficult to mark the boundary between these fractions, easily decomposable waste can be used for composting or anaerobic digestion while a fraction of the waste can be used as feedstock for pyrolysis. Fiber-rich material (e.g., coconut shell) can be used to harvest fiber. Organic waste originated from human excreta can be composted, pyrolyzed, or anaerobically digested while nutrients can also be harvested using different sorbents, e.g., biochar, zeolite. The recent advancement of these processes is discussed in the following subheadings:

12.3.1 Preparation of Food and Feed from Organic Waste

Food preparation, processing, and consumption generate a large fraction of waste estimating up to 33% of the original food item, which is equivalent to 1.3 billion tons (FAO, 2017). On the flipside of this scenario, 820 million people go to bed hungry every day. This is an unequal and unjust fact for the humanity. A large fraction of prepared food can be saved if well organized and coordinated system is followed. For instance, if the prepared food is near to expire its date, these can be sold at lower prices while food left from any events/ceremony or hotels can be collected by a group of people and distributed to people following a model shown in Figure 12.2. Social media or other apps-based operation can ease this system while social awareness is needed to do so. It is also important to change food purchasing habit to reduce food loss as waste.

Food, that is wasted, is usually rich in nutrients and fiber. Therefore, they can potentially be used as animal feed. In many countries, food waste is sorted and used as animal feed either directly or after processing (Table 12.2). The scale of recycling can be from household levels to industrial levels. Depending on the conditions of organic or food waste, several methods are followed, listed below:

- Drying > Grinding > Pelleting
- Pulping > Extruding
- Ensiling
- Chopping > Drying > Grinding > Pelleting
- Fermentation > Filtration
- Fermentation > Filtration > Drying
- Mincing > Drying > Pelleting

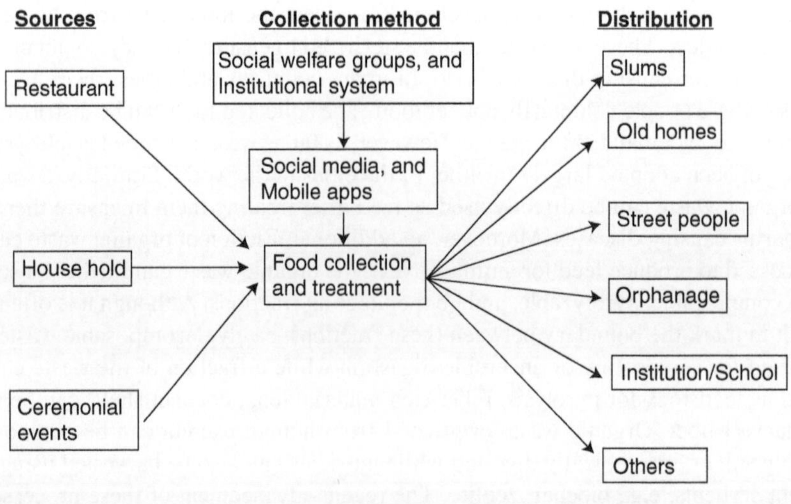

FIGURE 12.2 A proposed model for collection and distribution of food.

TABLE 12.2
Animal Feeding with Food Produced from Different Wastes

Country	Animal	Food Loss/Food Waste	Supply Chain Stage	Processing Method	Optimum Feed Inclusion Level (%)[a]
South Korea, Egypt, US, Nigeria, Brazil, Indonesia, Uganda, Spain, Kingdom of Saudi Arabia, India	Cattle, sheep and goat	Cafeteria food, bakery, biscuit, household/kitchen food, restaurant food, retail food, and vegetable	Market, processing & packaging, handling and storage, consumption	• Grinding-dehydrating • Drying-grinding-pelleting • Grinding-pelleting • Pulping-extruding • Drying-milling • Ensiling	38 (10–100)
China, Japan, Kingdom of Saudi Arabia, Lebanon, Nigeria, Tunisia, Malaysia	Fish feeding- Grass carp Nile tilapia African catfish Common carp	Hotel food, Household/kitchen food, Restaurant food, Retail food	Market-consumption	• Chopping-drying-grinding-pelleting • Drying-grinding-extruding • Drying-milling-pelleting • Pitting-drying-grinding	46 (20–75)
India, South Korea, Japan, Spain, Norway, Mexico, Brazil, Poland, Canada, US	Fig feeding	Cafeteria food, bakery, biscuit, household/kitchen food, hotel/restaurant food	Market-Consumption	• No processing • Fermentation-pelleting-drying • Mincing-drying-pelleting • Milling-pelleting-fluidized bed drying • Grinding-pelleting-drying	39 (4–100)
Egypt, Nigeria, Malaysia, South Korea, Iran, Taiwan, US, Czech Republic, India, Canada, Japan	Poultry feeding	Cafeteria food, bakery, biscuit, household/kitchen food, restaurant food, and retail food	Market-Consumption	• Market-consumption • Grinding-fermentation-drying • Fermentation-drying-grinding • Mixing-grinding-pelleting	29 (5–100)
Kingdom of Saudi Arabia, Brazil, Vietnam, Indonesia	Rabbit feeding	Cafeteria food, bakery, biscuit, household/kitchen food, restaurant food, and retail food	Market-consumption	• No processing • Drying • Drying-grinding	13 (10–15)

Source: Adopted from Rajeh et al. (2021).
[a]Values in the parentheses indicate range.

These food or organic wastes have been shown to be used as animal feed including cattle, poultry, fish, and pig in many countries in the world from developing countries like India to the developed countries the USA. These feeds are usually mixed with regular animal feed with fractions ranging from 5% to 100%. Animals fed to these feeds are shown to perform equally to those that receive a regular feed (Siddiqui et al., 2021). However, the fraction of food or organic waste recycled is still very low. The challenges of these low recycling are collection of waste in a good state to be used as feed and separation of feed from other wastes while processing technologies and negative attitude of the consumer to use this feed for their animal are dominant barriers. The concerns, associated with the dispersion of pathogenic infection with these feeds, are one of the reasons for not using these feeds by the farmers for their animals. Therefore, research is needed to establish a formal system of recycling waste as animal feed in building confidence of the farmer.

12.3.2 Preparation of Biopolymers

Production of biopolymers, macromolecules such as proteins, nucleic acids, lipids, and polysaccharides, can be one of the potential means of reusing organic waste since biopolymers are used in many industries ranging agricultural, food and beverage, and pharmaceutical industry. A range of biomolecules including pectin, dietary fibers, essential oils (matricine, chamazulene, α-bisabolol), and γ-oryzanol have been shown to be produced from biowaste (Lee et al., 2020). Microorganisms are used to synthesize these biopolymers (exopolysaccharides, polyhydroxyalkanoates (PHA) while raw materials (succinic acids, 2,3-butanediol) for biopolymers can be synthesized from lignocellulose-rich biomass (Paul et al., 2021). PHA is considered as a good alternative to synthetic plastic. Bacteria species including *Alcaligenes* spp., *Bacillus* spp., *Pseudomonas* spp., *Azotobacter* spp., *Escherichia coli,* etc. are used to synthesize PHA from a wide range of substrates. Organic waste has been used as substrates for producing PHA while special microbial communities (e.g., recombinant *Bacillus subtilis* 1A304 (105 MU331), *Azotobacter vinelandii* UWD (ATCC 53799), and *C. necator* (*R. eutropha*)) are engineered for accelerating the process (Cho et al., 1997; Ganzeveld et al., 1999; Law et al., 2003). Biopolymers can also be produced during anaerobic digestion processes (discussed in the section below) (Pagliano et al., 2017).

12.3.3 Collection of Fiber

Fiber can be collected from organic waste. For instance, coconut shell has been used to produce ropes and bedding materials. In brief, coconut shell is collected and then, fermented in water. Next, fiber is collected using a crusher and these fibers are then dried for preparing craft items (Figure 12.3). Recently, banana peduncle has been used to collect fiber. After collecting the bananas, the tree is considered agricultural waste. Good-quality fiber or yarn is produced from abandoned banana stem sheaths (Baral et al., 2020). Generally, the sheath is separated from the peduncle of the banana tree. Next, the sheath is then crushed to remove water-dissolved contents while celluse-rich fiber is separated and dried. The collected fibers are then prepared

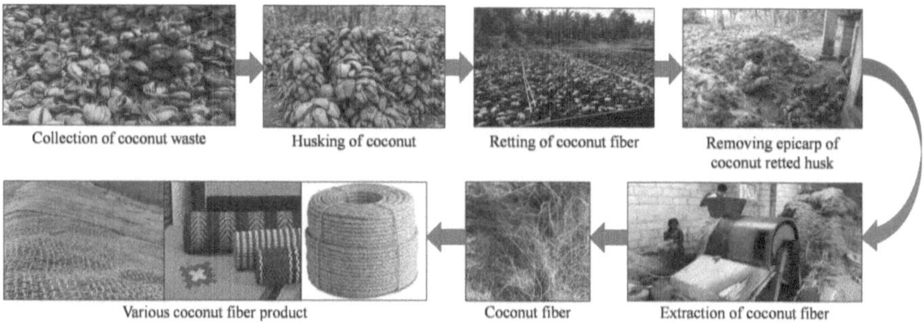
Collection of coconut waste
Husking of coconut
Retting of coconut fiber
Removing epicarp of coconut retted husk
Various coconut fiber product
Coconut fiber
Extraction of coconut fiber

FIGURE 12.3 Preparation of fiber and craft items from coconut shell.

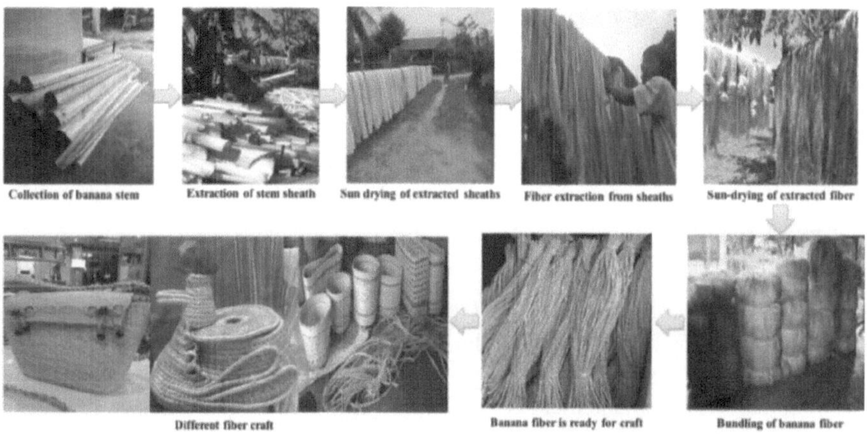
Collection of banana stem
Extraction of stem sheath
Sun drying of extracted sheaths
Fiber extraction from sheaths
Sun-drying of extracted fiber
Different fiber craft
Banana fiber is ready for craft
Bundling of banana fiber

FIGURE 12.4 Extracting banana fiber from waste banana stems. (The photos are taken from a social media post, link: https://www.facebook.com/photo/?fbid=6150399608365984&set=pcb.6150401791699099.)

for marketing in bundle form. These fibers were later used for preparing many different handicrafts (Figure 12.4).

The world generates 2.01 billion tons of waste every year, 18% of which comes from paper and cardboard (Kaza et al., 2018). Therefore, there is urgent need to find means to recycle waste to resources. Recently, preparation of paper or cellulose-based boards has been receiving increased attention. Pulp is produced from paper and then paper or cellulose-based materials are prepared (Figure 12.5). Paper preparation is in practice in small scale to industrial scales (Alam et al., 2016).

12.3.4 Development of Biocomposite

Biocomposite is a mixture of distinct materials while organic matter can be used as raw material for producing biocomposites including hard board, plywood, thermal insulator, etc. For instance, biowaste (e.g., cereal husk, wood, coir, and textile fiber)

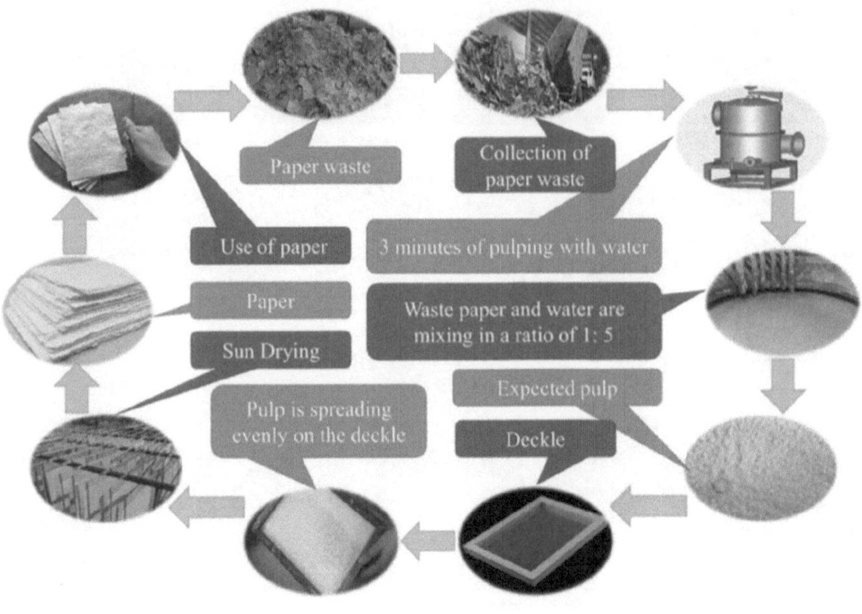

FIGURE 12.5 Preparation of paper from recycled paper (small-scale business).

is used to prepare thermal insulator (Figure 12.6). Muthuraj et al. (2019) prepared thermal insulator by blending drying the rice/wheat husks with a bioresin (Ecovio®).

Moreover, biocomposite can also be produced from materials developed from waste biomass. Thermochemical technologies (e.g., pyrolysis) have been receiving increased attention for managing organic wastes through converting waste to value-added products (e.g., biochar). These biochars can be used to produce biocomposite. Biochar-based biocomposite can be produced through methods followed for natural fibers. These are extrusion, injection molding, and hot pressing. In the biochar-based composite a range of polymers can be used including thermoplastic (polyethylene, polypropylene, polystyrene) and thermoset (phenol formaldehyde resin, urea formaldehyde resin) polymers. However, the use of thermoset polymers is limited since their formability and fluidity. In addition, reactive carbon (activated carbon) can be produced from biochar and these activated carbons have been shown to be used for different industrial uses including for preparing composite fertilizers, biosorbents, and drugs.

12.3.5 Composting

Composting is a decomposition process that converts organic matter into more stable organic substances through microbial processes that are regulated by physicochemical conditions of the composting chamber (moisture, temperature, and aeration) (Figure 12.7). Traditionally, composting has been used for the preparation of manure from agricultural wastes while reducing the volume and water content of wastes. Moreover, during the composting process, the harmful pathogens are destroyed

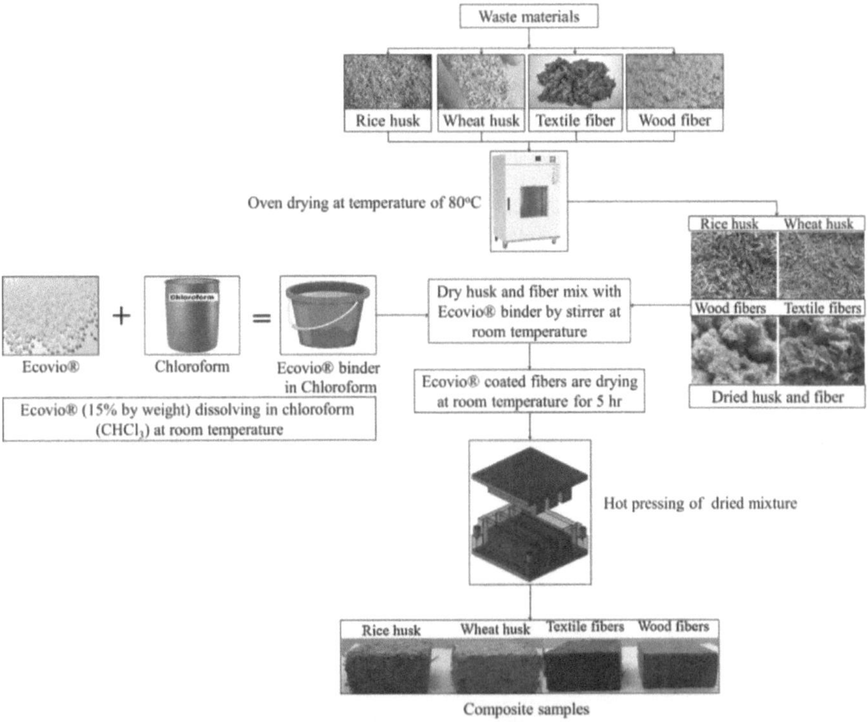

FIGURE 12.6 Preparation of thermal insulation biocomposites from different waste materials. (Adopted from Muthuraj et al., 2019.)

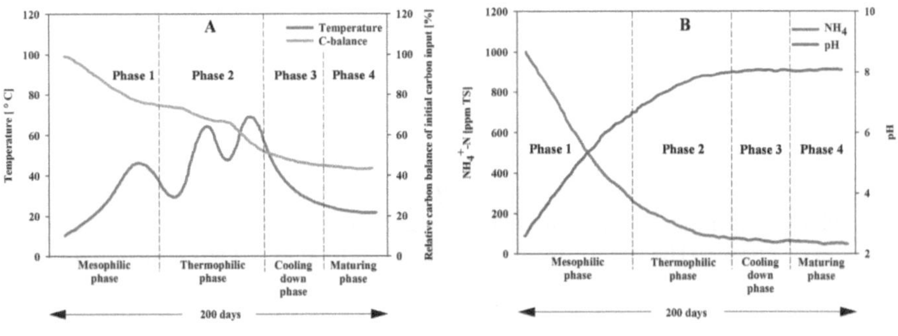

FIGURE 12.7 Composting processes with changes in nutrients and mass of biomass along with time. (Adopted from Fischer & Glaser 2012.)

while the odor is reduced. In recent decades, composting has widely been established as an eco-friendly management approach to manage the organic fraction of municipal solid wastes (MSW) and industrial wastes (Sallwey et al., 2017). For instance, there has been an increasing trend to prepare useful products including compost from waste in many countries including in Europe since the landfilling with waste has been discouraged (EU, 2008; European Union, 1999). As an alternative to landfilling, composting provides multiple benefits including efficient management of organic waste, avoidance of environmental hazards associated with traditional treatment, recycling of nutrients to soils, sanitation, and active involvement in the economic process (Park et al., 2004).

12.3.5.1 Composting Process

The composting process is carried out by a diverse population of microorganisms that regulate several biochemical transformations. The composting process involves four main phases. In each of the phases, different communities of microorganisms predominate the composting process (Bünemann et al., 2006). These phases include:

a. **Mesophilic**: Microorganisms such as fungi, bacteria, and actinomycetes decompose fresh biomass at relatively low temperatures ranging between 15°C and 40°C (Sundberg et al., 2004). Due to high microbial activities, i.e., respiration, the temperature of composting pile starts to increase. During this phase, the ammonium concentration is relatively higher than in other phases while the pH of the composting pile starts to increase.
b. **Thermophilic**: At this stage, the microbial activities reach the maximum leading to a higher temperature ranging between 40°C and 70°C (Sundberg et al., 2004). A large fraction of substrate is degraded during this time (Novinscak et al., 2008). As a result, the labile organic matter is exhausted rapidly. The substrate is reduced due to the degradation of sugar and proteins and thus, the temperature of the composting pile started to reduce (25°C and 45°C) at the end of the process with consequences for shifting of microbial communities from thermophiles to mesophiles (Novinscak et al., 2008; Zeng et al., 2011).
c. **Cooling phase**: As the supply of high-energy compounds becomes exhausted, more heat is lost from the pile than it is generated. During this phase, the pH starts to get stabilized.
d. **Compost maturation**: Soil macro and meso fauna are primarily active at this stage while the temperature reaches almost close to ambient temperature. The C:N ratio of the composting pile is much narrower at the starting phase ranging between 15 and 20 since the carbon has been lost in the previous phases. The pH is also stabilized around 8.0–8.5. One of the characteristics of this stage is the production of sufficient humic materials (Hsu & Lo, 1999).

12.3.5.2 Factors Affecting the Composting Process

Many factors can affect composting processes, including temperature, moisture, gas flow, and many other physical, chemical, and biological variables (Figure 12.2) (Ekinci, 2001; Ljung & Glad, 1994). Oxygen, moisture, porosity, C/N ratio, and temperature of the compost pile are the major determinants (Haug, 2018; Ruggieri et al., 2009; Sánchez, 2007; Tiquia et al., 2002). Microorganisms are the key players in converting biomass to compost while their occurrence and multiplication depend on feedstock, nutrient supply, and composting conditions. Bacteria, actinomycetes, and fungi of mesophilic and thermophilic groups are mainly responsible for biological degradation in composting. The common actinomycetes in compost are *Streptomyces* sp. and *Micromonospora* sp. while the latter is more prevalent. The common fungi in compost are *Thermonomyces* sp., *Penicillium dupontii,* and *Asperigallus fumigatus.* Besides, inoculation of *Phanerochaete chrysosporium* might improve humification and maturity as well as reduce the metal load of Cd, Pb, and Cu (Chen et al., 2018). The amount and quality of carbon is an important factor for composting since carbon is required for supplying the energy to microorganisms while nitrogen helps to grow and reproduce more organisms to oxidize the carbon. Therefore, a low C:N ratio (25–30) is good for composting (Ros et al., 2006). Oxygen is needed for oxidizing the carbon (Gao et al., 2010) while water is required in the right amount to maintain microbial activities without creating the anaerobic condition (Cooperband, 2000; Mata-Alvarez et al., 2000). An optimum temperature favors composting process while low temperature may lengthen the composting duration since microbial growth is low. Moreover, sufficient high temperature is required to destroy weed seeds, pathogens, and fly larvae. The influencing factors and their optimum conditions are stated in Table 12.3.

12.3.5.3 Composting Systems or Methods

Several composting methods can be applied, and the selection of the method is dependent on the capital cost, labor cost, time, the availability of land, etc. The main methods include windrow composting, static aerated static pile composting, in-vessel composting, and vermicomposting.

12.3.5.4 Composting Technologies

A range of composting technologies is available. A few of them are highlighted below.

12.3.5.4.1 Open Windrows

This is the least sophisticated technique which involves placing a mixture of organic waste materials into long, narrow piles approximately 6 feet high by 12 feet wide and as long as it is necessary. Enough ventilation facilities are kept for gas exchange while piles are turned over for mixing of wastes.

12.3.5.4.2 Covered Windrow

The covered window is synonymous to controlled microbial composting that involves the production of compost in covered windrows (1.2 m width × 1.8 m height and any length) over a 6–8 weeks period (Diver, 2004). The feedstocks are carefully chosen to include a balance of well-structured materials and should have a C/N ratio of around 30. They are mixed, water is added if necessary and covered with a waterproof, breathable membrane. The windrows are monitored daily for CO_2, moisture levels and temperature, and the windrows are turned with a purpose-built compost turner every time the temperature exceeds 60°C. This often means that the windrows are turned daily at the start of the process. Compost maturity is estimated by measuring temperature and CO_2 emission from the windrows.

TABLE 12.3
Factors Influencing Composting Process and Their Optimal Conditions

Influencing Factor	Explanation	Optimum Condition	Reference(s)
Microorganisms	The breakdown of proteins and other readily biodegradable organic matter is occurred by thermophilic bacteria whereas fungi and actinomycetes are mainly responsible for the decomposition of cellulose and lignin.	Mesophiles are organisms that grow optimally at temperatures from 20°C to 35°C while thermophiles prefer to grow between 50°C and 60°C.	Birkett and Lester (1999); Henis (1987)
Moisture	Decomposing microorganisms need water to continue microbial activity.	A moisture of 50%–60% is considered good for microbial growth.	Gaur (1997)
Temperature	Changes in temperature are essential to create suitable environment for the microbes in different phases of composting.	Optimal temperature varies with phases. However, a higher temperature >60°C accelerates the composting.	Gaur (1997)
C/N ratio	Nitrogen is required for decomposition of substrate while a higher N could accelerate the N loss through volitization.	A C/N ratio between 25 and 30 is usually considered as the optimum ratio for composting. It is necessary to maintain an initial C/N ratio of 30:1.	Awasthi et al. (2014)
Aeration	Sufficient aeration is essential to supply O_2 required for microbial process in aerobic composting.	Optimal oxygen concentration is between 15% and 20%.	Bernal et al. (2009)
pH	Slightly acidic to neutral pH is suitable for microbial activities. Highly acidic or alkaline conditions affect the composting process.	For composting the optimum pH is 6–8.	Smårs (2002)
Particle size	Small particles carry larger surface area and thus, increase the chances for microbial reproduction by providing larger space.	A particle size of 5–10 mm size is suitable for composting.	Gaur (1997)

12.3.5.4.3 Aerated Static Pile

This system involves supply of ambient air through mechanical means and requires no turning of the organic mixture once the pile is formed. By controlling air mechanically, this process allows the use of larger piles. For composting under this method, an air plenum is constructed and the organic mixture is placed in piles on top of the air plenum. Piles are built as high as the equipment allows, normally it is kept eight to twelve feet high. Aerated static piles can be constructed individually or in extended piles. Individual piles, constructed all at once, allow the composting to occur in batches. Extended piles consist of a series of cells created over the course of many days and stacked against each other to form one long rectangular pile. A temperature sensor placed within the pile works in conjunction with the blower to control temperature and oxygen concentration within the pile.

12.3.5.4.4 *In-vessel Composting*

It involves confining the composting process into a variety of containers or vessels. These systems usually include provisions for aeration, mixing, temperature control, and containment of odors.

12.3.5.4.5 *Vermicomposting*

Vermicomposting is produced with the combined activity of microorganisms and earthworms. Earthworms break down sewage sludge and other organic wastes (Neuhauser et al., 1980). A range of earthworm including *Eisenia foetida* has been shown to use while they can grow in a wide range of wastes including pig and cattle solid and slurries, horse manure, and potato waste (Edwards et al., 1985). Worms are useful in converting agricultural wastes into useful soil conditioners, but also the worms can be harvested and processed into a nutritious protein feed supplement for fish, poultry, and pigs. *E. foetida* prefers a pH of 5, and temperatures <35°C. Composting may require a large area for preparing vermicompost (Reddy & Galab, 1998; Sannigrahi & Chakrabortty, 2002).

12.3.5.5 Advances in Organic Waste Composting

12.3.5.5.1 *Technologies to Improve Composting Processes*

One of the important aspects of adopting composting techniques for organic waste recycling would be the technological advancement suited for both small (household) and large-scale (industrial) operations. A model composting unit should be equipped with facilities to control the factors (temperature and aeration) that affect composting processes and compost quality (Figure 12.8). For instance, composting processes can be divided based into four sections (i.e., phases) with assignment of specific environments for each of the phases to accelerate the processes. It can be done through movement of composting piles from one chamber to the next or by changing conditions with time. The first process can be followed in the industries while the next process can be followed for household composting units (Figure 12.9).

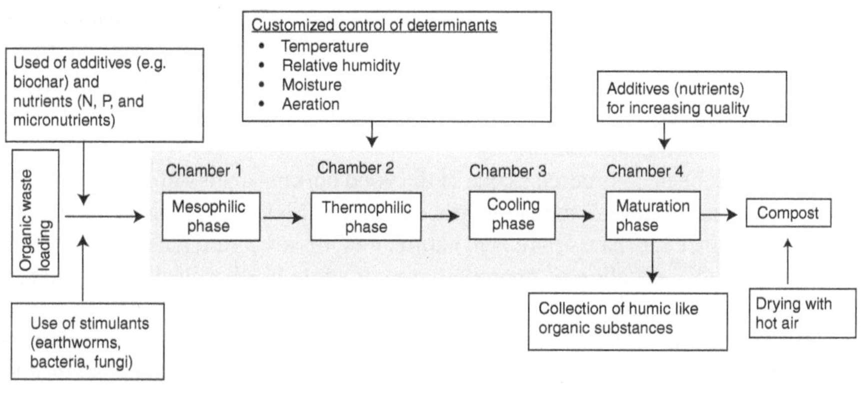

FIGURE 12.8 A model composting unit with control of composting conditions.

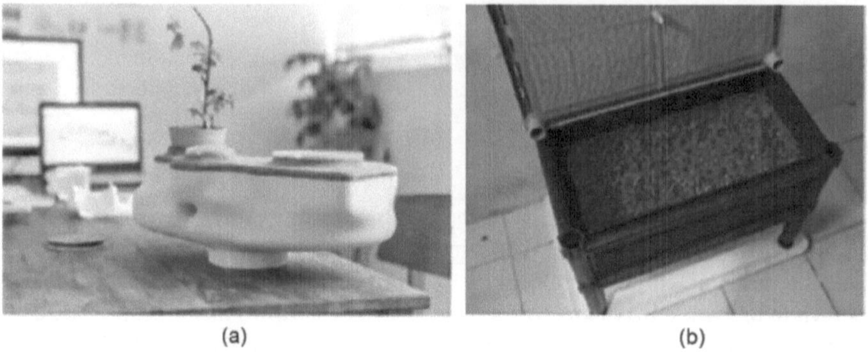

FIGURE 12.9 Household ornamental composting unit (adopted from Peng et al., 2020.).

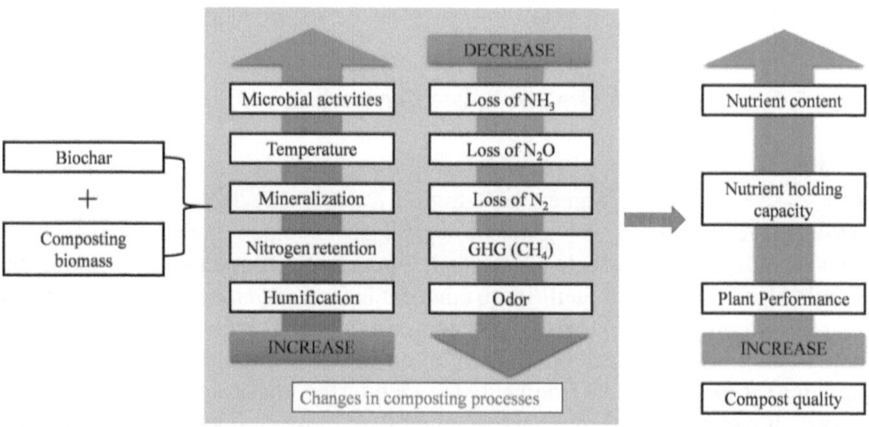

FIGURE 12.10 Changes in composting process and compost quality after biochar amendment (Guo et al., 2020; Mia et al., 2018; Sánchez-Monedero et al., 2021.).

12.3.5.5.2 Use of Additives to Composting Biomass

The composting process can be accelerated using several additives including (1) bulking agents such as rice husk, biochar, sawdust, or any other materials that increase space inside the pile, (2) use of microbes (e.g., earthworms, bacteria, fungi), (3) addition supplementary nutrients (N, P, and micronutrients), and (4) adsorbents (Zeolite) (Andraskar et al., 2021; Rastogi et al., 2020; Sanchez-Monedero et al., 2018; Sánchez-Monedero et al., 2021).

Biochar has been considered as one of the good bulking agents to composting biomass since it can change composting processes in multiple ways (Figure 12.10) (Mia et al., 2018). Since biochar is porous in nature, it increases aeration in the composting pile leading to acceleration of microbial growth while biochar itself hosts microorganisms. As a result, the temperature of the composting pile increases and composting processes is accelerated (i.e., composting duration is shortened). Biochar can adsorb mineralizing nitrogen that increases its concentration in composting piles.

An increase in nitrogen concentration can further accelerate microbial activities and thus, composting processes. Nitrogen retention reduces its losses as NH_3 volatilization, N_2O, and N_2 emission while greenhouse gas emission can also be reduced since an increase in aeration can reduce methane production (Guo et al., 2020). During composting process, the quality of biochar (i.e., surface functionalization) is also enhanced through microbial actions with implications for increased cation exchange capacity. Therefore, use of biochar in composting is considered as a win-win scenario (Sánchez-Monedero et al., 2021).

Microorganisms are the key players in converting biomass to compost, and therefore, the use of suitable microorganisms could accelerate the composting process and improve compost quality. A range of microbial cultures has been shown to be effective in composting.

These are mixed culture (*Nitrobacter* and *Thiobacillus*, lignin decomposition composite, and fungi), cellulolytic thermophilic actinomycetes, cellulolytic microbial inoculum (*Phanerochaete chrysosporium*, *Trichoderma viride, Trichoderma reesei*), *Bacillus subtilis* and *Pseudomonas*, *Aspergillus niger* and *Aspergillus flavus* (Modderman, 2020; Rastogi et al., 2020).

12.3.6 Bioenergy Generation and Biochar Production

Generation of power in the form of heat or electricity from organic waste is one of the possible means of generation bioenergy generation through different processes including pyrolysis and fermentation (Kant Bhatia et al., 2021). There are several options for pyrolysis and the most common are:

a. **Pyrolysis**: Heating at relatively low temperature (300°C–800°C) biomass in absence or limited oxygen. Heat is generated while biochar is produced as a by-product of the pyrolysis process. Syngas (a mixture of H_2, CH_4, CO, and CO_2) can also be harvested and recycled for electricity generation. Pyrolysis can be of two types depending on the operation conditions. Slow pyrolysis is carried out at a relatively low heating rate (0.1°C–1°C/s) at 300°C–800°C while the heating period lasts for long ranging from several hours to days. In contrast, the feedstock is at relatively high heating rate (>500°C) for short time for a few minutes. Pyrolysis has been carried out using a range of designs suited for small to industrial-scale production. For instance, biochar can be produced in small retort meant for cooking while large industrial setup has been practiced (e.g., Black is green in Australia). In addition, pyrolysis reactor varies (such as fixed bed, free-fall, rotary, auger, and fluidizied) (Gabhane et al., 2020; Gholizadeh et al., 2020; Sakhiya et al., 2020). Given the large diversity of pyrolysis designs and kilns/retort, the efficiency of energy recovery and biochar production from different methods are not available. However, the main basic principle of pyrolysis is that the biomass is initially heated with external energy until the pyrolyzing biomass starts to generate heat for carrying out the process. Once the pyrolyzing biomass starts producing heat and syngas, these are then used for carrying

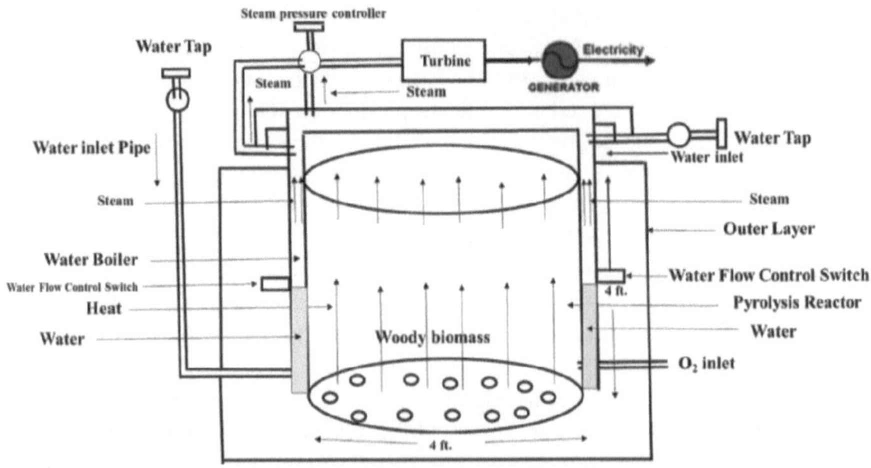

FIGURE 12.11 A model slow pyrolysis kiln for converting heating energy to electricity.

out pyrolysis while a part of the heat energy can be used to convert energy type (i.e., heat to electricity) (Figure 12.11).

There are several factors (feedstock, temperature, oxygen flow rate, residence time) that control the pyrolysis efficiency.

b. **Gasification**: Biomass is heated at a relatively higher temperature (500°C–1,400°C) for decomposition mainly to gases (H_2, CO, CH_4, etc.) under oxygen-limited conditions. The decomposition process can be accelerated using catalysts including steam, and CO_2.
c. **Hydrothermal carbonization**: In this process, wet biomass is heated at a relatively low temperature (150°C–350°C) under high pressure for a longer duration.
d. **Hydrothermal liquefaction**: Conversion of biomass into liquid fractions (e.g., biocrude) with compressed reactive water (374°C, 22.0MPa) through hydrolysis, depolymerization, and self-condensation.

12.3.7 Valorization and Bioethanol Production from Waste

Waste biomass rich in carbohydrates (i.e., cellulose and hemicellulose) can be hydrolyzed and fermented by enzymatic actions to produce ethanol that can be used as fuel directly or after mixing with gasoline (Cheng & Brewer, 2021). Carbohydrate-rich waste biomass including straw of cereals is usually selected as feedstock for valorization. The biomass undergoes several processes to produce bioethanol. First, the inorganic acids and enzymes break down the ether bonds, which link the monomers, resulting in the release of monomers glucose, galactose, xylose, mannose, etc. through the hydrolysis process. Next, these monomers are converted to bioethanol through the fermentation process. During ethanol production additives (e.g., acid or alkali), saccharification enzymes, yeast for accelerating the fermentation process are used while the production conditions (46°C–60°C and 24–168 h for saccharification, 28°C–37°C and 24–168 h for fermentation) are also optimized to harvest maximum bioethanol (Uddin et al., 2021). In a recent review, a description of bioethanol production has been presented with the synthesis of data on production conditions and catalysts (Table 12.4) (Cheng & Brewer, 2021).

12.3.8 Biogas Generation and Bio-Slurry Production

The energy demand is increasing with time due to rapid industrialization, growth of population, and changing the lifestyle of people (Ncube et al., 2021; *UN DESA*, 2019). A large fraction of the power is generated using non-renewable resources, e.g., coal, crude oil, natural gas, and lignite, with consequences for greenhouse gas emissions (Sawyerr et al., 2020). Moreover, there are deep concerns about the exhaustion of non-renewable resources placing the people in challenge to meet their future energy needs. The share of current renewable power generation (13.8%) has to increase by 65% by 2050 for ensuring access of population to power (Kapoor et al., 2018). As an alternative, generation of power from renewable sources including biomass and solar can lessen the pressure on fossil fuels while reducing carbon footprint. Through effective management of these important bio-resources, we can cut global greenhouse gas (GHG) emissions by 10% which is equivalent to 3,290–4,360 Mt CO_2 by 2030. Moreover, the global biogas market is fast-growing and has doubled to $33.1 billion in 2022 from $17.3 billion in 2012 (Yousuf et al., 2017).

Biogas is basically a mixture of different gases (e.g., methane (CH_4), carbon dioxide (CO_2), water (H_2O), hydrogen sulfide (H_2S), and ammonia (NH_3)) generated by anaerobic digestion (Budiyono et al., 2018). The typical methane percentage from anaerobic digestion (AD) usually ranges between 50% and 70% (Bharathiraja et al., 2018). AD is a biological process and is generally composed of four major stages: hydrolysis, acidogenesis, acetogenesis, and methanogenesis (Figures 12.12 and 12.13). During the whole process, microorganisms convert the hydrogen and acetic acid to methane gas and carbon dioxide where the bacteria responsible for this conversion, known as methanogens, work under strictly anaerobic conditions. During the first step—hydrolysis, the hydrolytic enzymes excreted by bacteria break down insoluble polymers, carbohydrates, lipids, and protein into soluble mono- and oligomers and become available to microorganisms directly. In acidogenesis (the second step), simple sugars, fatty acids, and amino acids are further degraded into carbon dioxide, acetate, hydrogen, and volatile fatty acids and alcohols, while in third step, acetogenesis, volatile fatty acids and alcohols are further degraded into H_2, CO_2, and acetic acid. Finally, methanogenic bacteria transform the mixture of CO_2, H_2, methanol, formate, and acetate into the final product methane (Kasinath et al., 2021).

The gas mixtures generated during the AD process are of good value and can be used for many different purposes from cooking to running generators or buses. It is important to note that methane creates a large carbon footprint, the methane gas itself is one of the greenhouse gases, and if they are not trapped, they are used with consequences for global warming. Moreover, the biogas slurry contains about 2.10% nitrogen, 2.20% potassium, and 0.046% phosphorous and thus is a good source of plant nutrients that might have also been an un-trapped resource (Ding et al., 2014;

TABLE 12.4
Production of Ethanol from Different Organic Waste with Their Efficacies

Feedstock	Dry Matter (%)	Pretreatment Agent	Pretreatment Temperature (°C)	Pretreatment Duration (min)	Enzyme Type	Yeast	Hydrolysis Temperature (°C)	Hydrolysis Time (h)	Fermentation Temperature (°C)	Fermentation Time (h)	Ethanol Yield (%)[a]
Wheat straw	20	HT	195	18.5	Cellic CTec 2	*S. cerevisiae*			34	168	86.32
Wheat straw	30	HT	195	18.5	Cellic CTec 2 + PEG3000	*S. cerevisiae*	50	24	34	144	89.07
Wheat straw	20	HT	195	18.5	Cellulcast:Novozym 188 = 5:1	*S. cerevisiae*			34	168	66.34
Wheat straw	10	H_2SO_4 (0.5%)	160	10	Advanced, Novozymes and Genencor	*S. cerevisiae*			38	72	78
Wheat straw	5	AFEX	220	2.5	NS50013 and NS50010	*S. cerevisiae*			35	72	63.4
Wheat straw	10	HT	205	6	Celluclast 1.5 FG: Novozym 188	Rehydrated Thermosacc Dry	50	24	37	144	92
Energy cane bagasse	10	HT	160	60	Spezyme CP	*S. cerevisiae* D5A	55	24	30	48	21
Energy cane bagasse	10	AFEX	160	60	Spezyme CP	*S. cerevisiae* D5A	55	24	30	48	64
Rape seed stover	14.1	H_3PO_4 (85%)	50	60	Celluclast 1.5L	*S. cerevisiae* D5A			38	96	97.3
Corn stover	10	H_2SO_4 (0.05%)	195	15	Celluclast 1.5L: Novozym 188	*S. cerevisiae*	50	24	30	120	89.3
Corn stover	20	H_2SO_4 (0.5%)	150	25	Accellerase 1500	*S. cerevisiae* D5A			37	48	90.5

(Continued)

TABLE 12.4 (*Continued*)
Production of Ethanol from Different Organic Waste with Their Efficacies

Feedstock	Dry Matter (%)	Pretreatment Agent	Pretreatment Temperature (°C)	Pretreatment Duration (min)	Enzyme Type	Yeast	Hydrolysis Temperature (°C)	Hydrolysis Time (h)	Fermentation Temperature (°C)	Fermentation Time (h)	Ethanol Yield (%)[a]
Corn cob	13.4	H_2SO_4 (1.38%)	165	8.3	P. decumbens JUA10-1	*S. cerevisiae*			30	117.5	88.8
Agricultural waste	0.02	NA			Cellulase and endo-1,4- xylanase enzymes	*S. cerevisiae*			37	72	48
Cashew apple bagasse	10	H_2SO_4 (0.6 m)	120	15	Celluclast 1.5 L	*Kluyveromyces marxianus* ATCC36907	40	12	40	32	93
Barley straw	10	Steam explosion	210	5	NS50013 and NS50010	*Kluyveromyces marxianus* CECT 10875			42	72	67.3
Barley straw	10	H_2SO_4 steam explosion	180	3.5	Celluclast and 15 Novozyme 188	*S. cerevisiae*			35	72	56.9
Barley straw	10	H_2SO_4 steam explosion	180	3.5	Celluclast and 15 Novozyme 188	*S. cerevisiae*			35	72	78.4
Blue Agave tequilana bagasse	10	Ethanol and H_2SO_4	160	10	CTec2 and HTec2	*Escherichia coli* strain MS04	50	18	37	48	85.3
Miscanthus	10	H_2SO_4 (0.45)	150	30	Spezyme cellulose cocktail and Novozyme 188	*S. cerevisiae* DA2416			30	48	63

(*Continued*)

TABLE 12.4 (*Continued*)
Production of Ethanol from Different Organic Waste with Their Efficacies

		Pretreatment					Hydrolysis		Fermentation		
Feedstock	Dry Matter (%)	Agent	Temperature (°C)	Duration (min)	Enzyme Type	Yeast	Temperature (°C)	Time (h)	Temperature (°C)	Time (h)	Ethanol Yield (%)[a]
Miscanthus	10	H_2SO_4 (0.6)	150	30	Spezyme cellulose cocktail and Novozyme 188	*S. cerevisiae* DA2416			30	48	62
Bermuda grass	13.8	H_3PO_4 (85%)	50	60	Celluclast 1.5 L	*S. cerevisiae* ATCC			38	96	93
Common Reeds	22.1	H_3PO_4 (85%)	50	60	Celluclast 1.5 L	*S. cerevisiae* ATCC			38	96	98.7
Switchgrass	20	NA			CTec2 + HTec2	*S. cerevisiae* strain BY4741	50	18	37	72	83.3
Kan low switchgrass		HT	200	10	Fibrilase	*S. cerevisiae* D5A			37	168	92.3
Napiergrass	10	H_2SO_4 (1.5%)	121	60	NS50013 and NS50010	*S. cerevisiae*			37	176	52
Wet Distiller's Grain cellulose	15	HT	160	20	Spezyme CP and Novozyme 188	*S. cerevisiae* D5A			28	72	78.4
Wet Distiller's Grain cellulose	15	AFEX	90	5	Spezyme CP and Novozyme 188	*S. cerevisiae* D5A			28	72	79
Whole stillage fiber	15	H_2SO_4 (1.5%)	100	270	Cellic Ctec2	Neurospora intermedia CBS 131.92	45	72	35	96	91

(*Continued*)

TABLE 12.4 (*Continued*)
Production of Ethanol from Different Organic Waste with Their Efficacies

Feedstock	Dry Matter (%)	Pretreatment			Enzyme Type	Yeast	Hydrolysis		Fermentation		Ethanol Yield (%)[a]
		Agent	Temperature (°C)	Duration (min)			Temperature (°C)	Time (h)	Temperature (°C)	Time (h)	
Brewery spent Grains	15	H_3PO_4 (2%)	155		Cellic CTec3 and Novozyme 50010	*Escherichia coli* SL100			40	72	78
Digestate	0.02	NA			Cellulase and endo-1,4- xylanase enzymes	*S. cerevisiae*			37	72	33
Shea Tree Sawdust	10	H_2O_2 (1%)	120	30	Trichoderma reesei, and β-glucosidase	*S. cerevisiae*			30	72	24.53
Spent Sawdust Matrix	10	HT	121	20	Celluclast 1.5 L and Novozyme 188	*S. cerevisiae* IR-2			30	168	75
Primary wastewater solids	0.1	NA			Trichoderma reesei QM9414 (ATCC 26921)	*S. cerevisiae*			40	24	32.3
Palm kernel press cake	35	NA			45 endomannanase +15 β-mannosidase + 1.5 cellulase	*S. cerevisiae*	50	48	32	168	70
Eruca sativa seedcake (solvent extracted)	0.02	NaOH (8%)	100	60	Celluclast 1.5 L and Novozyme 188	*S. cerevisiae*			37	48	58.8

Source: After Cheng & Brewer, (2021).
[a]Indicates percentage of theoretical maximum.

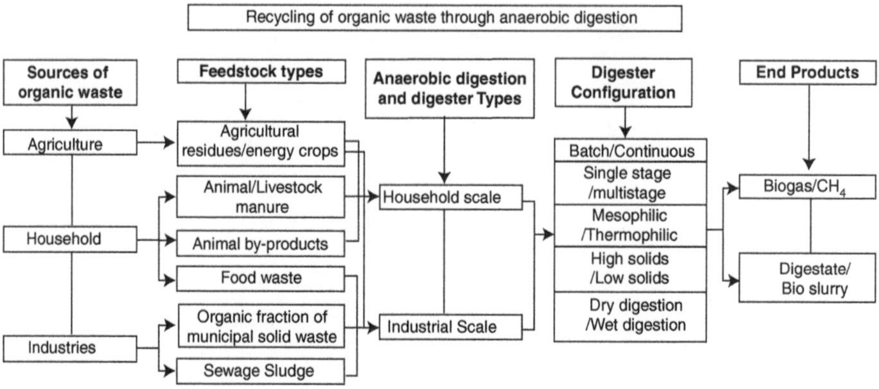

FIGURE 12.12 Anaerobic digestion processes of organic waste from diverse sources.

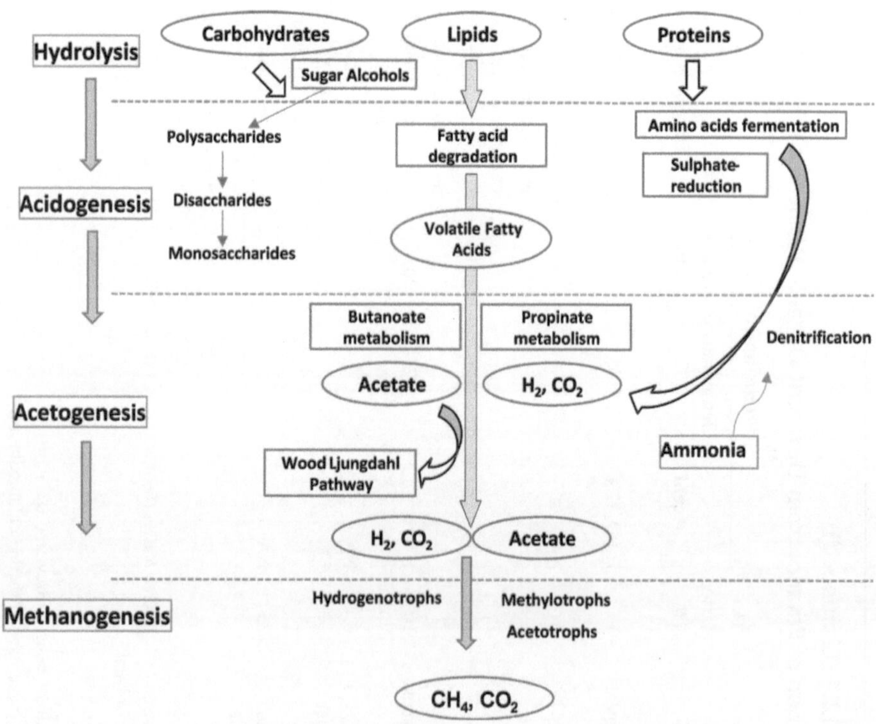

FIGURE 12.13 Schematic pathways of microbial decomposition of organic substances to methane (redrawn from Kougias & Angelidaki, 2018.).

Drosg et al., 2015; Rajendran et al., 2012). Altogether, anaerobic can be referred to as a net zero-waste process due to the creation of energy from biogas and utilization of digested material (digestate) as an organic fertilizer (Atelge et al., 2020). Although significant effort has been made to promote AD installation plants with a growth rate of 11.2%, a large scope remains un-trapped (Wainaina et al., 2020).

12.3.8.1 Factors Affecting Anaerobic Digestion Process

There are several factors that affect the performance of the AD process. For instance, biogas composition depends upon the substrate composition along with the conditions in the anaerobic digester (temperature, pH, substrate concentration, digestion kinetics, and digester retention time) (Anukam et al., 2019). Among the factors temperature, pH, hydraulic retention time, loading rate, and C:N ratio are relatively more influential in methane production. Although the optimal conditions for these factors may vary with digester types, feedstock, and ambient environment, the optimal conditions for AD are listed in Table 12.5.

12.3.8.2 Anaerobic Digestion Technologies

Biogas production through the AD techniques varies from household to industrial scales while it also varies with the income and technological know-how of the population. The most common anaerobic technologies are: (1) floating dome digester, (2) fixed dome digester and Balloon Plants/Plug Flow Digesters. A comparative description of the major technologies is listed in Table 12.6.

12.3.8.2.1 Recent Advancements for Accelerating Anaerobic Digestion Processes

12.3.8.2.1.1 Use of Additives AD in a specific digester depends on the complex enzymatic reactions of microorganisms. Many of these enzymes require co-factors for accelerating enzymes. So, the yield of biogas can be enhanced through various additives. By adding these materials, enhanced enzymatic activity and desirable conditions for bacteria could be provided (Abanades et al., 2021a). Additives can be in the form of biochar, trace metals, nanoparticles, catalysts, chlorides, and activated carbon while biological additives are added for optimizing AD (Abanades et al., 2021b). For instance, the application of essential elements (N, P, Fe, and Ni) has been shown to promote AD (Qin et al., 2017). Moreover, the application of biochar could effectively enhance AD performance by increasing the buffering capacity of the system and accelerating the transformation of macromolecular substances to dissolved substrates (Dudek et al., 2019; Pan et al., 2019). Studies indicated that the addition of biochar proceeds methanogenic conversion up to five times higher rate than the control (Cruz Viggi et al., 2017) while biochar application has been shown to reduce lag phase (Fagbohungbe et al., 2016). Biochar application reduces inhibitory products such as ammonia and volatile fatty acids, establishes bioelectrical connections for microbial colonies, reinforces buffer capacity, and improves the degradation of lignocellulosic biomass (Pan et al., 2019; Yu et al., 2021). Additionally, activated carbon is treated as an effective additive by promoting electron transfer between microorganisms, discouraging the selection of resistant bacteria, reducing the horizontal transfer

TABLE 12.5
Factors Controlling Anaerobic Digestion

Factors	Optimal Conditions	References
pH	A pH of 6.8–7.2 can accelerate anaerobic digestion process.	Náthia-Neves et al. (2018); Mamun and Torii (2015)
Temperature	Mesophilic temperatures: 20°C–45°C with optimum at 32°C–35°C and in thermophilic temperatures (50°C–65°C) pathogen destruction and CO_2 increase occur	Náthia-Neves et al. (2018)
Hydraulic retention time (HRT)	HRT is 30–50 days in tropical countries and up to 100 days in temperate climate as it depends on temperature and can be calculated by HRT=>V/Q, V = Volume (m^3) and Q = daily flow (m^3/day)	Lohani and Havukainen (2018)
Organic loading rate (OLR)	0.5–3 kg VS/m^3/day and can be calculated by QLR= $\frac{Q*VS}{V}$ V = volume (m^3), Q = daily flow (kg/day), and VS = volatile solids (kg kg^{-1})	Náthia-Neves et al. (2018); Mamun and Torii (2015)
C: N:P ratio	C: N: P ratio of 100:3:1	Lohani and Havukainen (2018)
Feedstock types	High biodegradability such as fats, sugars, proteins, and starch-based compounds	and Rupf et al. (2016)
Solid content	5%–9%	Saraswat et al. (2019)
Seeding of biogas plant	Seeding bacteria into the digester from sludge	Open access
Stirring/mixing	Gas production increase due to intimate contact between microorganisms and substrate through stirring	Rupf et al. (2016)
Particle size	Smaller particle size as (1.02–2.14 mm) yield more gas	Lohani and Havukainen (2018)
Moisture	Moisture-60%–80%	Lohani and Havukainen (2018)

of antibiotic resistance genes, and aiding in the hydrolysis of DNA. Granular activated carbon and carbon cloth help to increase the growth of some specific populations, can withstand low temperatures, and increase methanogenic activity (Paritosh et al., 2020). Besides, a wide variety of chemical additives like NaOH, $Ca(OH)_2$, NH_4OH, H_3PO_4, etc., can improve the associated biogas production yield. Biological additives can also be a better option for increasing methane yield (Abanades et al., 2021b). Microbial augmentation (anaerobic bacteria as *Methanobacterium* and fungi Neocallimastigomycota) is widely used to directly introduce specific microorganisms into biogas digesters for improving the performance of the AD process. For

TABLE 12.6
Comparison of Different Anaerobic Digestion Technology

Name of AD Technology	Main Features	Structural Design	Advantages	Disadvantages	References
Fixed dome digester	a) A Chinese or hydraulic in nature b) Constructed underground with variable sizes (6–8 m^3). c) Built with the locally available materials like stones, bricks, cement, plastic or reinforced fiber	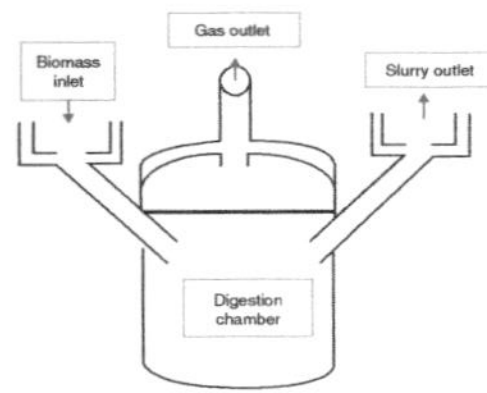	a) Low initial cost b) Long useful lifespan (20 years) c) No rusting d) Less land space required if built underground e) Less maintenance required	a) High technical skills is required for gas-tight construction b) Repair is difficult in case of leakage c) Gas is not visually visible d) Incarnate fluctuation in gas pressure	Rajendran et al. (2012); Pilloni and Hamed (2021); Kechrist et al. (2020); Mang et al. (2013)
Floating dome digester	a) An Indian type digester b) Built partially underground with bricks and concrete c) Drum is made of metal or steel	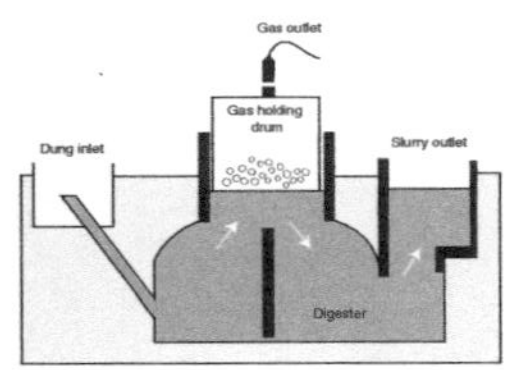	a) A simple digester with easy operation b) Gas volume is visible c) Gas pressure is constant d) Construction is relatively easy	a) High installation cost b) Difficult to maintain and manage c) Clogging is encountered due to scum d) A short lifespan because of steel drum corrosion	Mang et al. (2013)
Balloon Plants/Plug Flow Digesters	a) Portable digester with a size of 2.4 to 7.5 m^3 b) Placed inclined to the ground c) Feeding ratio manure: water 1:1 or 1:3	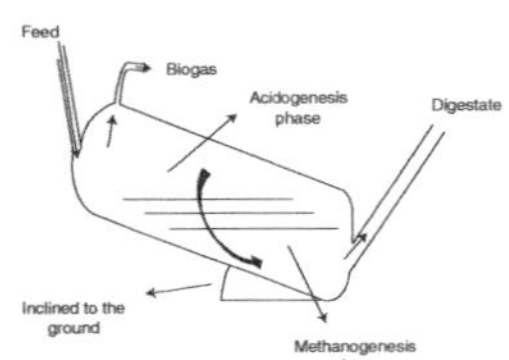	a) Low cost b) Easy to install c) Easy to transport d) Uncomplicated and affordable maintenance	a) Short life span (2–5 years) b) Leak identification is tedious c) High susceptibility to damage d) Gas pressure is low e) Not eco-friendly	Surendra et al. (2014); Mishra et al. (2015); Pilloni and Hamed (2021); Mang et al., (2013)

(Continued)

TABLE 12.6 (*Continued*)
Comparison of Different Anaerobic Digestion Technology

Name of AD Technology	Main Features	Structural Design	Advantages	Disadvantages	References
Prefabricated biogas digesters/Bag digesters	a) A Taiwan type plastic digester b) As known as balloon digesters, tube digesters, ball-type digester and bladder digesters c) Installed in temperature countries	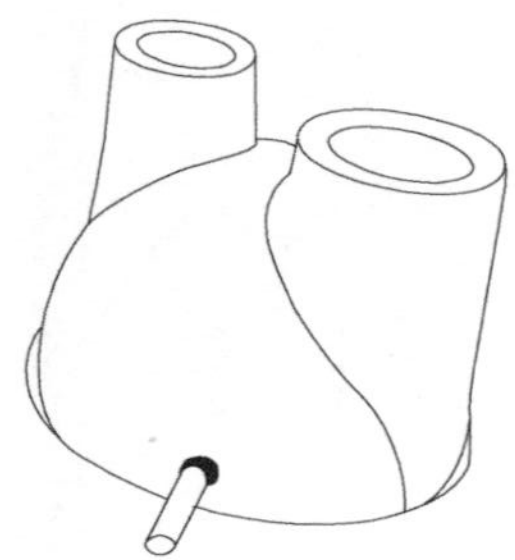	a) Suitable for remote and/or mountainous areas b) Low cost and easy to operate c) Easy to transport and install d) Easy to agitate the slurry	a) A short life span b) Prone to damaged c) Large sedimentation and difficult to remove d) Difficult to maintain temperature	Mang et al. (2013)
Prefabricated biogas digesters/ Composite material digester (CMD)	a) A China type b) Made of polyester, gel-coated resin	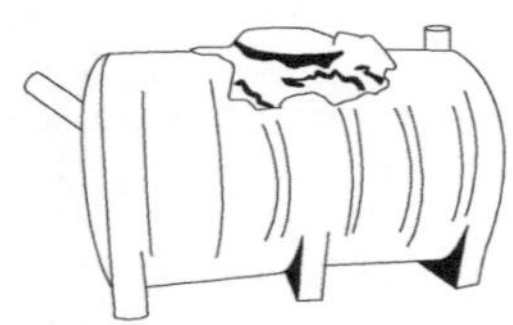	a) Easy to install b) Water and gas tight c) No leakage of gas	a) a high initial investment b) Customized digested is not available	Mang et al. (2013)
Ferro-cement digester	a) A vessel type digester with 6 m^3 b) Made of ferro-cement	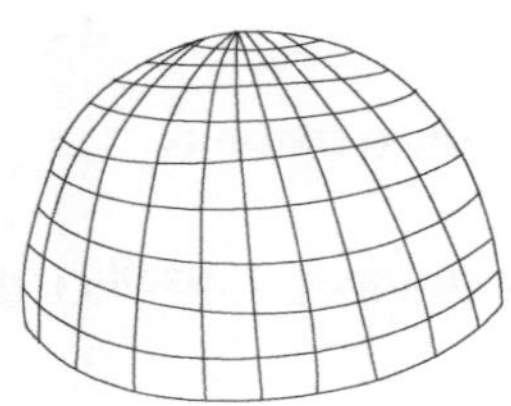	Low cost	High-quality cement is required	Mang et al. (2013)

example, *Enterobacter cloacae* bacteria can influence the microbial composition and maintain stable cell numbers in the AD system whereas anaerobic fungi attack plant structures and yields great potential for enhancement of the AD process (Liu et al., 2021).

12.3.8.3 Co-digestion

Co-digestion is the simultaneous digestion of two or more organic waste. The co-digestion process usually improves the biogas yields from anaerobic conditions by dint of synergisms established in the digestion medium and also the supply of missing nutrients by the co-substrates. Co-digestion can be in the form of mixing of kitchen waste with sewage sludge, activated sludge and organic MSW, pig manure, municipal and agricultural waste with dairy cow manure, cheese whey with cattle manure, co-substrate of goat manure and crop residues, and co-digestion of food waste and human excreta (Phill et al., 2020).

12.3.8.4 Pretreatment

Pretreatment techniques are employed to make the organic matter more accessible to anaerobic microorganisms. This process improves the overall digestion efficiency, reducing retention time and increasing the degree of digestion and methane production rates. Different pretreatment techniques such as thermal, chemical, mechanical, and biological and their combinations are employed significantly (Phill et al, 2020). Thermal pretreatment through heat supply breaks the chemical bonds of the cell wall and thus makes the protein content easily accessible for biological digestion which can be conducted at high temperature >100°C and also low temperature <100°C (Phill et al, 2020). Moreover, pretreatment with acid (HCl, H_2SO_4, H_3PO_4, and HNO_3) alkali (KOH, $Mg(OH)_2$, and $Ca(OH)_2$) has been used for accelerating the AD process. Recently, pretreatment with ozone and ultrasound has also been practiced (Baredar et al., 2016).

12.3.8.5 Biogas Production Potential and Biomethane Production

Globally, the amount of biogas generation capacity of the existing plants is about 19.5 GW (Abanades et al., 2021a). Biogas plants can be small units suitable for household uses and top industrial units for commercial production. The small biogas plants are is usually installed in developing countries in Asia and Africa while large units are usually established in European countries (Ding et al., 2014). In Europe, the primary biogas producers are Finland, Austria, Denmark, and Germany (Piekutin et al., 2021) while similar efforts have been taken in the USA, China, and Turkey.

Production of biomethane, purified methane up to 90%, from biogas is receiving increased attention globally since biomethane can be included in the grid and used as an alternative to natural gas (Kapoor et al., 2018). The removal of harmful and/or toxic compounds (such as H_2S, moisture, siloxanes, volatile organic compounds (VOCs), and NH_3) is often challenging and requires several technologies including adsorption and precipitation that are outlined in Figure 12.14 (Kapoor et al., 2018).

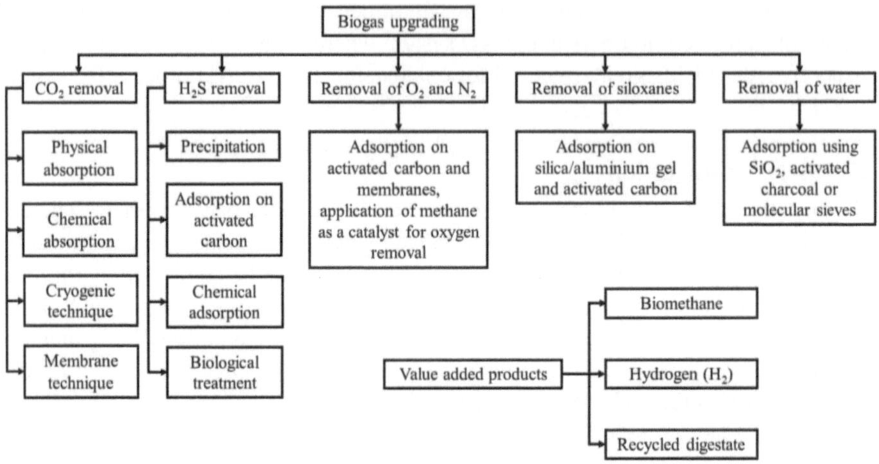

FIGURE 12.14 Production of biomethane and hydrogen gas from biogas.

12.3.9 Solid-State Fermentation

Solid-state fermentation (SSF) is carried out in the absence or near the absence of water. A range of products including different biomolecules (e.g., enzymes) can be obtained from SSF of waste materials. These products are used in agro and food industries. Different bioreactors are traditionally used for SSF while significant development has been achieved in recent years in the manufacturing of bioreactor for SSF. During the operation of SSF, several factors need to be considered: (1) selection of substrate, (2) use of suitable microorganisms, (3) optimization of process parameters, and (4) separation and purification of the products (Pandey, 2003). Although fungi and yeast are considered suitable microorganisms for SSF, several bacteria have also been found to be effective in carrying out the SSF successfully. Moreover, particle size, initial moisture, and pH of the pile during fermentation play important role in producing quality products.

12.3.10 Nutrient Harvesting through Combined Pyrolysis and Composting Techniques

Organic waste and human excreta carry a considerable amount of nutrients (Tables 12.7 and 12.8). Our estimate showed that the daily global carbon, nitrogen, phosphorus, and potassium loading from organic waste are ~1,600, 63, 24, and 65 thousand tons while these figures are 252, 673, 52, and 370 thousand tons from human excreta (feces and urine combined). These nutrients are basically lost since organic waste and human excreta were not recycled. Recycling of organic waste and human excreta can be done with the simultaneous application of several methods. For instance, combined pyrolysis and composting of organic waste to be a sustainable means of recycling organic waste (Mia et al., 2018). Similarly, human excreta can also be pyrolyzed and the produced biochar can be used for trapping nutrients from urine or other nutrient-loaded water flows (Figure 12.15). Using the estimate of Mia et al. (2020), the potential

TABLE 12.7
Nutrient Loading from Municipal Organic Waste at Different Regions

Region	Population (Million)	Waste Generation Rate (kg/capita/day)	Fraction of Organic Waste (%)	Organic Waste Generation (Thousand ton per day)	Nutrient Loading (Thousand ton per day)			
					C	N	P	K
MENA	433.43	0.81	72.00	252.78	113.75	4.47	1.72	4.63
SSA	984.73	0.46	53.40	241.89	108.85	4.28	1.64	4.43
LAC	630.14	0.99	65.50	408.62	183.88	7.23	2.78	7.48
NA	359.52	2.21	61.60	489.44	220.25	8.66	3.33	8.96
SA	1850.57	0.52	68.00	654.36	294.46	11.58	4.45	11.97
ECA	906.77	1.18	56.20	601.34	270.60	10.64	4.09	11.00
EAP	2285.79	0.56	70.00	896.03	403.21	15.86	6.09	16.40
Global total	7450.96	0.96	63.81	3544.45	1595	62.74	24.10	64.86

Source: Carbon (C), nitrogen (N), phosphorus (P) and potassium (K) concentration in dry organic waste was considered as 45%, 1.77%, 0.68% and 1.83% respectively. These figures were adopted from a recent review article that used average value of literature data (Mia et al., 2018).

EAP, East Asia and Pacific; ECA, Europe and Central Asia; LAC, Latin America and the Caribbean; MENA, Middle East and North Africa; NA, North America; SA, South Asia; SSA, Sub-Saharan Africa.

TABLE 12.8
Nutrient Loading from Human Excreta at Different Regions

Region	Human Excreta Generation (Thousand ton per day)[a]		Nutrient loading (Thousand ton per day)[b]			
	Feces	Urine	C	N	P	K
MENA	21.67	73.80	14.70	39.16	3.02	21.45
SSA	49.24	167.68	33.39	88.97	6.86	48.73
LAC	31.51	107.30	21.37	56.93	4.39	31.18
NA	17.98	61.22	12.19	32.48	2.50	17.79
SA	92.53	315.11	62.75	167.19	12.89	91.57
ECA	45.34	154.41	30.75	81.92	6.32	44.87
EAP	114.29	389.22	77.51	206.51	15.92	113.11
Global Total	372.55	1268.75	252.65	673.17	51.90	368.69

EAP, East Asia and Pacific; ECA, Europe and Central Asia; LAC, Latin America and the Caribbean; MENA, Middle East and North Africa; NA, North America; SA, South Asia; SSA, Sub-Saharan Africa.

Feces and urine generation rates were considered as 0.050 kg dry feces/day and 0.17 kg moisture free urine kg/day (Mia et al., 2020; Schouw et al., 2002).

[b]Carbon, nitrogen, phosphorus and potassium concentration in feces and urine were considered as 45%, 3.16%, 1.84%, 2.28% and 6.7%, 52.13%, 3.55%, 28.39%, respectively (Mia et al., 2020).

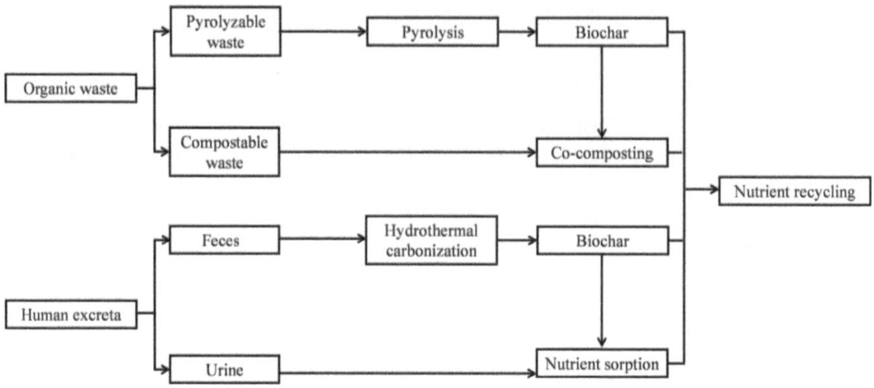

FIGURE 12.15 A proposed model for simultaneous adoption of different methods for harvesting nutrients.

harvestable nutrients in the world are estimated at 720, 81, 52, and 48 thousand tons of C, N, P, and K, respectively, per day (Table 12.9). The amount of potential N, P, and K recovery is equivalent to 351 thousand tons of urea fertilizer, 517 thousand tons of triple superphosphate, and 159 thousand tons per day of muriate of potash.

12.4 CHALLENGES OF WASTE RECYCLING

Recycling of organic waste and preparation of waste products carry several challenges. These include:

12.4.1 Waste Sorting

One of the most dominant challenges of waste recycling is the non-compliance of the citizens to sort waste according to their nature. Most often, wastes are mixed with many different types of by-products and used leftover materials. When wastes are collected and combined, it is very difficult to sort them according to nature. In developed countries, mechanical separators are used to separate waste while in developing countries it is mostly carried out by human labor. In using a mechanical separator, it is difficult to completely separate the waste according to the nature while human labor is costly. Health hazard associated with laborers is also a problem. Therefore, the most feasible way of getting waste sorted can be the classification of waste at the source and citizens' compliance with the waste sorting rules.

12.4.2 Technologies

Although a significant effort has been made to reduce the environmental footprint of waste, it is still not enough for putting the policy into practice. Therefore, most wastes are currently used in landfills. Both technological development and government policies for implementing these technologies are required to have a waste based-economy.

TABLE 12.9
Nutrient Recovery with Proposed Model

Region	Total Organic Waste Generation (Thousand ton per day)[a]	Nutrient Recovery (Thousand ton per day)[b]			
		C	N	P	K
MENA	348.25	50.09	4.80	3.22	2.87
SSA	458.81	55.47	10.26	5.78	5.85
LAC	547.43	80.05	7.06	4.87	4.25
NA	568.64	90.65	4.53	3.97	2.94
SA	1062.00	139.31	19.67	11.79	11.39
ECA	801.08	117.53	10.18	7.08	6.15
EAP	1399.54	187.48	24.46	14.97	14.25
Global Total	5185.75	720.59	80.95	51.68	47.69

EAP, East Asia and Pacific; ECA, Europe and Central Asia; LAC, Latin America and the Caribbean; MENA, Middle East and North Africa; NA, North America; SA, South Asia; SSA, Sub-Saharan Africa.
[a]Total organic waste generation = Organic waste generation + Human excreta generation.
[b]Carbon, nitrogen, phosphorus, and potassium concentration in total organic waste generation was considered as 39%, 11%, 68%, and 11%, respectively (Mia et al., 2020).

REFERENCES

Abanades, S., Abbaspour, H., Ahmadi, A., Das, B., Ehyaei, M. A., Esmaeilion, F., El Haj Assad, M., Hajilounezhad, T., Jamali, D. H., Hmida, A., Ozgoli, H. A., Safari, S., AlShabi, M., & Bani-Hani, E. H. (2021a). A critical review of biogas production and usage with legislations framework across the globe. *International Journal of Environmental Science and Technology*. https://doi.org/10.1007/s13762-021-03301-6

Abanades, S., Rodat, S., & Boujjat, H. (2021b). Solar thermochemical green fuels production: A review of biomass pyro-gasification, solar reactor concepts and modelling methods. *Energies*, *14*(5), 1494. https://doi.org/10.3390/en14051494

Alam, M., Rikta, S. Y., Hasnine, T., & Ahmed, F. (2016). Production of Eco-friendly Handmade Paper from The Waste Paper Generated Production of Eco-friendly Handmade Paper from The Waste Paper Generated in Municipalities of Dhaka City, Bangladesh. May.

Andraskar, J., Yadav, S., & Kapley, A. (2021). Challenges and control strategies of odor emission from composting operation. *Applied Biochemistry and Biotechnology*, *193*(7), 2331–2356. https://doi.org/10.1007/s12010-021-03490-3

Anukam, A., Mohammadi, A., Naqvi, M., & Granström, K. (2019). A review of the chemistry of anaerobic digestion: methods of accelerating and optimizing process efficiency. *Processes*, *7*(8), 504. https://doi.org/10.3390/pr7080504

Atelge, M. R., Krisa, D., Kumar, G., Eskicioglu, C., Nguyen, D. D., Chang, S. W., Atabani, A. E., Al-Muhtaseb, A. H., & Unalan, S. (2020). Biogas production from organic waste: recent progress and perspectives. *Waste and Biomass Valorization*, *11*(3), 1019–1040. https://doi.org/10.1007/s12649-018-00546-0

Awasthi, R., Kaushal, N., Vadez, V., Turner, N. C., Berger, J., Siddique, K. H. M., & Nayyar, H. (2014). Individual and combined effects of transient drought and heat stress on carbon assimilation and seed filling in chickpea. *Functional Plant Biology*, *41*(11), 1148. https://doi.org/10.1071/FP13340

Baral, P. B., Divyadarshan, C. S., & Lija, M. G. (2020). Banana Fiber Craft - Ernakulam, Kerala.

Baredar, P., Suresh, S., Kumar, A., & Krishnakumar, P. (2016). A review on enhancement of biogas yield by pre-treatment and addition of additives. In: *MATEC Web of Conferences*. Vol. 62. https://doi.org/10.1051/matecconf/20166206002

Bernal, M. P., Alburquerque, J. A., & Moral, R. (2009). Composting of animal manures and chemical criteria for compost maturity assessment. A review. *Bioresource Technology, 100*(22), 5444–5453. https://doi.org/10.1016/j.biortech.2008.11.027

Bharathiraja, B., Sudharsana, T., Jayamuthunagai, J., Praveenkumar, R., Chozhavendhan, S., & Iyyappan, J. (2018). Retraction notice to "Biogas production -A review on composition, fuel properties, feed stock and principles of anaerobic digestion" [*Renew. Sustain. Energy Rev.*, 90(2018) 570–82]. *Renewable and Sustainable Energy Reviews, 94*, 1229. https://doi.org/10.1016/j.rser.2018.08.010

Birkett, J., & Lester, J. (1999). *Microbiology and Chemistry for Environmental Scientists and Engineers*. CRC Press. https://doi.org/10.4324/9780203477397

Budiyono, A. P., Ardhannari, L., Matin, H., & Sumardiono, S. (2018). Study of biogas roduction rom cassava industrial waste by anaerobic process. In: *MATEC Web Conference on 2018*, p. 156.

Bünemann, E. K., Schwenke, G. D., & Van Zwieten, L. (2006). Impact of agricultural inputs on soil organisms—a review. *Soil Research, 44*(4), 379. https://doi.org/10.1071/SR05125

Chen, X., Zeng, D., Xu, Y., & Fan, X. (2018). Perceptions, risk attitude and organic fertilizer investment: Evidence from rice and banana farmers in Guangxi, China. *Sustainability, 10*(10), 3715. https://doi.org/10.3390/su10103715

Cheng, F., & Brewer, C. E. (2021). Conversion of protein-rich lignocellulosic wastes to bioenergy: Review and recommendations for hydrolysis + fermentation and anaerobic digestion. *Renewable and Sustainable Energy Reviews, 146*(July), 111167. https://doi.org/10.1016/j.rser.2021.111167

Cho, K. S., Ryu, H. W., Park, C. H., & Goodrich, P. R. (1997). Poly(hydroxybutyrate-co-hydroxyvalerate) from swine waste liquor by Azotobacter vinelandii UWD. *Biotechnology Letters, 19*(1), 7–10. https://doi.org/10.1023/A:1018342332141

Cooperband, L. R. (2000). Composting: Art and science of organic waste conversion to a valuable soil resource. *Laboratory Medicine, 31*(5), 283–290. https://doi.org/10.1309/W286-LQF1-R2M2-1WNT

Cruz Viggi, C., Simonetti, S., Palma, E., Pagliaccia, P., Braguglia, C., Fazi, S., Baronti, S., Navarra, M. A., Pettiti, I., Koch, C., Harnisch, F., & Aulenta, F. (2017). Enhancing methane production from food waste fermentate using biochar: The added value of electrochemical testing in pre-selecting the most effective type of biochar. *Biotechnology for Biofuels, 10*(1), 303. https://doi.org/10.1186/s13068-017-0994-7

Ding, W., Wang, L., Chen, B., Xu, L., & Li, H. (2014). Impacts of renewable energy on gender in rural communities of north-west China. *Renewable Energy, 69*, 180–189. https://doi.org/10.1016/j.renene.2014.03.027

Diver, S. (2004). *Controlled Microbial Composting and Humus Management: Luebke Compost*, pp. 1–23. http://www.ibiblio.org/steved/Luebke/Luebke-compost2.html

Drosg, B., Fuchs, W., Al Seadi, T., Madsen, M., & Linke, B. (2015). Nutrient recovery by biogas digestate processing. In: *Integrated Sustainable Urban Water, Energy, and Solids Management*. https://doi.org/10.1002/9781119593683.ch9

Dudek, M., Świechowski, K., Manczarski, P., Koziel, J. A., & Białowiec, A. (2019). The Effect of biochar addition on the biogas production kinetics from the anaerobic digestion of brewers' spent grain. *Energies, 12*(8), 1518. https://doi.org/10.3390/en12081518

Edwards, C. A., Burrows, I., Fletcher, K. E., & Jones, B.A. (1985). The use of earthworms for composting farm wastes. In: J. K. R. Gasser, ed. *Composting Agricultural and Other Wastes*. Elsevier Applied Science Publishers, London, pp. 229–241.

Ekinci, K. (2001). *Theoretical and experimental studies on the effects of aeration strategies on the composting process.* Ph.D. Dissertation, the Ohio State University, Columbus, USA.

EU. (2008). Directive 2008/104/EC of the European Parliament and of the Council of 19 November 2008 on temporary agency work. *Official Journal of the European Union, 51*(L–327), 9–14. http://eur-lex.europa.eu/LexUriServ/LexUriServ.do?uri=OJ:L:2008:327:0009:0014:EN:PDF

European Union. (1999). Council Directive 1999/31/EC on the landfill. *Official Journal of the European Communities, 10*, L182/1-19. https://doi.org/10.1039/ap9842100196

Fagbohungbe, M. O., Herbert, B. M. J., Hurst, L., Li, H., Usmani, S. Q., & Semple, K. T. (2016). Impact of biochar on the anaerobic digestion of citrus peel waste. *Bioresource Technology, 216*, 142–149. https://doi.org/10.1016/j.biortech.2016.04.106

FAO. (2016). The state of food and agriculture, 2016. In *The Eugenics Review* (Vol. 59, Issue 2).

FAO. (2017). *The Future of Food and Agriculture Trends and Challenges.*

Fischer, D., & Glaser, B. (2012). Synergisms between compost and biochar for sustainable soil amelioration. In *Management of Organic Waste.* InTech. https://doi.org/10.5772/31200

Gabhane, J. W., Bhange, V. P., Patil, P. D., Bankar, S. T., & Kumar, S. (2020). Recent trends in biochar production methods and its application as a soil health conditioner: a review. *SN Applied Sciences, 2*(7), 1–21. https://doi.org/10.1007/s42452-020-3121-5

Ganzeveld, K. J., Van Hagen, A., Van Agteren, M. H., De Koning, W., & Uiterkamp, A. J. M. S. (1999). Upgrading of organic waste: Production of the copolymer poly-3-hydroxybutyrate-co-valerate by *Ralstonia eutrophus* with organic waste as sole carbon source. *Journal of Cleaner Production, 7*(6), 413–419. https://doi.org/10.1016/s0959-6526(99)00159-6

Gao, M., Li, B., Yu, A., Liang, F., Yang, L., & Sun, Y. (2010). The effect of aeration rate on forced-aeration composting of chicken manure and sawdust. *Bioresource Technology, 101*(6), 1899–1903. https://doi.org/10.1016/j.biortech.2009.10.027

Gaur, A. C. (1997). Bulky organic manures and crop residues. In: Tandon H.L.S., Ed., *Fertilizers, Organic Manures. Recyclable Wastes and Biofertilizers*, FDCO, New Delhi, India, pp. 37–51.

Gholizadeh, M., Li, C., Zhang, S., Wang, Y., Niu, S., Li, Y., & Hu, X. (2020). Progress of the development of reactors for pyrolysis of municipal waste. *Sustainable Energy and Fuels, 4*(12), 5885–5915. https://doi.org/10.1039/d0se01122c

Guo, X.X, Liu, H.T., & Zhang, J. (2020). The role of biochar in organic waste composting and soil improvement: A review. *Waste Management, 102*, 884–899. https://doi.org/10.1016/j.wasman.2019.12.003

Haug, R. T. (2018). *The Practical Handbook of Compost Engineering.* Routledge. https://doi.org/10.1201/9780203736234

Henis, Y. (1987). Survival and dormancy of bacteria. In: *Survival and Dormancy of Microorganisms* (Y. Henis, Ed.). John Wiley and Sons, Inc., New York, pp. 1–108.

Hsu, J. H., & Lo, S. L. (1999). Chemical and spectroscopic analysis of organic matter transformations during composting of pig manure. *Environmental Pollution, 104*(2), 189–196. https://doi.org/10.1016/S0269-7491(98)00193-6

Kant Bhatia, S., Palai, A. K., Kumar, A., Kant Bhatia, R., Kumar Patel, A., Kumar Thakur, V., & Yang, Y. H. (2021). Trends in renewable energy production employing biomass-based biochar. *Bioresource Technology, 340*(June), 125644. https://doi.org/10.1016/j.biortech.2021.125644

Kapoor, R., Gupta, R., Son, L. H., Jha, S., & Kumar, R. (2018). Boosting performance of power quality event identification with KL Divergence measure and standard deviation. *Measurement, 126*, 134–142. https://doi.org/10.1016/j.measurement.2018.05.053

Kasinath, A., Fudala-Ksiazek, S., Szopinska, M., Bylinski, H., Artichowicz, W., Remiszewska-Skwarek, A., & Luczkiewicz, A. (2021). Biomass in biogas production: Pretreatment and codigestion. *Renewable and Sustainable Energy Reviews, 150*, 111509. https://doi.org/10.1016/j.rser.2021.111509

Kaza, S., Yao, L., Bhada-Tata, P., & Van Woerden, F. (2018). *What a Waste 2.0: A Global Snapshot of Solid Waste Management to 2050* (Vol. 148).

Kechrist, O., Mamphweli, N. S., Meyer, E. L., Makaka, G., Nwokolo, N., & Onyeaka, H. (2020). Comparative Study on the Performance of Aboveground and Underground Fixed- Dome Biogas Digesters. *Chemical Engineering & Technology, 43*(1), 68–74.

Kougias, P. G., & Angelidaki, I. (2018). Biogas and its opportunities—A review. *Frontiers of Environmental Science and Engineering, 12*(3). https://doi.org/10.1007/s11783-018-1037-8

Law, K. H., Cheng, Y. C., Leung, Y. C., Lo, W. H., Chua, H., & Yu, H. F. (2003). Construction of recombinant *Bacillus subtilis* strains for polyhydroxyalkanoates synthesis. *Biochemical Engineering Journal, 16*(2), 203–208. https://doi.org/10.1016/S1369-703X(03)00039-1

Lee, J. K., Patel, S. K. S., Sung, B. H., & Kalia, V. C. (2020). Biomolecules from municipal and food industry wastes: An overview. *Bioresource Technology, 298*(September), 122346. https://doi.org/10.1016/j.biortech.2019.122346

Liu, M., Wei, Y., & Leng, X. (2021). Improving biogas production using additives in anaerobic digestion: A review. *Journal of Cleaner Production, 297*, 126666. https://doi.org/10.1016/j.jclepro.2021.126666

Ljung, L., & Glad, T. (1994). Modeling of dynamic systems. *Control Engineering Practice, 3*(6), 897–898. https://doi.org/10.1016/0967-0661(95)90022-5

Lohani, S. P., & Havukainen, J. (2018). Anaerobic digestion: Factors affecting anaerobic digestion process. *Energy, Environment, and Sustainability*, 343–359. https://doi.org/10.1007/978-981-10-7413-4_18

Mamun, M. R. Al, & Torii, S. (2015). Removal of hydrogen sulfide (H_2S) from biogas using zero-valent iron. *Journal of Clean Energy Technologies, 3*(6), 428–432. https://doi.org/10.7763/JOCET.2015.V3.236

Mang, H.-P., Li, Z., Porres Lebofa, M. M., Huba, E.-M., Schwarz, D., Schnell, R., Luong, N. G., Kellner, C., & Selke, J. (2013). Biogas production developing country biogas production, developing countries biogas production developing countries. In: *Renewable Energy Systems.* Springer, New York, pp. 218–246. https://doi.org/10.1007/978-1-4614-5820-3_250

Mata-Alvarez, J., Macé, S., & Llabrés, P. (2000). Anaerobic digestion of organic solid wastes. An overview of research achievements and perspectives. *Bioresource Technology, 74*(1), 3–16. https://doi.org/10.1016/S0960-8524(00)00023-7

Mia, S., Alam, M. R., Sattar, M. A., & Dijkstra, F. A. (2020). Nutrient loading in the river systems around major cities in Bangladesh: A quantitative estimate with consequences and potential recycling options. *Statistics for Data Science and Policy Analysis*, 111–128. https://doi.org/10.1007/978-981-15-1735-8_9

Mia, S., Uddin, M. E., Kader, M. A., Ahsan, A., Mannan, M. A., Hossain, M. M., & Solaiman, Z. M. (2018). Pyrolysis and co-composting of municipal organic waste in Bangladesh: A quantitative estimate of recyclable nutrients, greenhouse gas emissions, and economic benefits. *Waste Management, 75*, 503–513. https://doi.org/10.1016/j.wasman.2018.01.038

Mishra, S., Tenneti, S., & Mishra, S. (2015). Design of domestic scale bio-digester assembly, experimentation for biogas production and comparison of results with conventional digester. *Jurnal Teknologi, 75*(11), 51–59. https://doi.org/10.11113/jt.v75.5332

Modderman, C. (2020). Composting with or without additives. *Animal Manure: Production, Characteristics, Environmental Concerns, and Management*, 245–254. https://doi.org/10.2134/asaspecpub67.c19

Muthuraj, R., Lacoste, C., Lacroix, P., & Bergeret, A. (2019). Industrial crops & products sustainable thermal insulation biocomposites from rice husk, wheat husk, wood fibers and textile waste fibers : Elaboration and performances evaluation. *Industrial Crops & Products*, *135*(April), 238–245. https://doi.org/10.1016/j.indcrop.2019.04.053

Náthia-Neves, G., Berni, M., Dragone, G., Mussatto, S. I., & Forster-Carneiro, T. (2018). Anaerobic digestion process: technological aspects and recent developments. *International Journal of Environmental Science and Technology*, *15*(9), 2033–2046. https://doi.org/10.1007/s13762-018-1682-2

Ncube, A., Fiorentino, G., Colella, M., & Ulgiati, S. (2021). Upgrading wineries to biorefineries within a circular economy perspective: An Italian case study. *Science of The Total Environment*, *775*, 145809. https://doi.org/10.1016/j.scitotenv.2021.145809

Neuhauser, E. F., Kaplan, D. L., Malecki, M. R., & Hartenstein, R. (1980). Materials supporting weight gain by the earthworm Eisenia foetida in waste conversion systems. *Agricultural Wastes*, *2*(1), 43–60. https://doi.org/10.1016/0141-4607(80)90046-3

Novinscak, A., Surette, C., Allain, C., & Filion, M. (2008). Application of molecular technologies to monitor the microbial content of biosolids and composted biosolids. *Water Science and Technology*, *57*(4), 471–477. https://doi.org/10.2166/wst.2008.019

Pagliano, G., Ventorino, V., Panico, A., & Pepe, O. (2017). Integrated systems for biopolymers and bioenergy production from organic waste and by-products: A review of microbial processes. *Biotechnology for Biofuels*, *10*(1), 1–24. https://doi.org/10.1186/s13068-017-0802-4

Pandey A. (2003). Solid state fermentation. *Biochemical Engineering Journal*, *13*, 81–84.

Pan, J., Ma, J., Liu, X., Zhai, L., Ouyang, X., & Liu, H. (2019). Effects of different types of biochar on the anaerobic digestion of chicken manure. *Bioresource Technology*, *275*(010), 258–265. https://doi.org/10.1016/j.biortech.2018.12.068

Paritosh, K., Balan, V., Vijay, V. K., & Vivekanand, V. (2020). Simultaneous alkaline treatment of pearl millet straw for enhanced solid state anaerobic digestion: Experimental investigation and energy analysis. *Journal of Cleaner Production*, *252*, 119798. https://doi.org/10.1016/j.jclepro.2019.119798

Park, M., Singvilay, O., Shin, W., Kim, E., Chung, J., & Sa, T. (2004). Effects of long-term compost and fertilizer application on soil phosphorus status under paddy cropping system. *Communications in Soil Science and Plant Analysis*, *35*(11–12), 1635–1644. https://doi.org/10.1081/CSS-120038559

Paul, E., Bessière, Y., Dumas, C., & Girbal-Neuhauser, E. (2021). Biopolymers production from wastes and wastewaters by mixed microbial cultures: strategies for microbial selection. *Waste and Biomass Valorization*, *12*(8), 4213–4237. https://doi.org/10.1007/s12649-020-01252-6

Peng, L., Zheng, P., & Siswanto, I. (2020). Good earthworm-kitchen waste decomposition device. *Journal of Physics: Conference Series*, *1456*(1). https://doi.org/10.1088/1742-6596/1456/1/012029

Piekutin, J., Puchlik, M., Haczykowski, M., & Dyczewska, K. (2021). The efficiency of the biogas plant operation depending on the substrate used. *Energies*, *14*(11), 3157. https://doi.org/10.3390/en14113157

Pilloni, M., & Hamed, T. A. (2021). Small-size biogas technology applications for rural areas in the context of developing countries. *Anaerobic Digestion in Natural and Built Environments*. https://doi.org/10.5772/intechopen.96857

Qin, Y., Pan, X., Kubicek, C., Druzhinina, I., Chenthamara, K., Labbé, J., & Yuan, Z. (2017). Diverse plant-associated pleosporalean fungi from saline areas: Ecological tolerance and nitrogen-status dependent effects on plant growth. *Frontiers in Microbiology*, *8*. https://doi.org/10.3389/fmicb.2017.00158

Rajeh, C., Saoud, I. P., Kharroubi, S., Naalbandian, S., & Abiad, M. G. (2021). Food loss and food waste recovery as animal feed: a systematic review. *Journal of Material Cycles and Waste Management*, *23*(1), 1–17. https://doi.org/10.1007/s10163-020-01102-6

Rajendran, K., Aslanzadeh, S., & Taherzadeh, M. J. (2012). Household biogas digesters—A review. *Energies*, *5*(8), 2911–2942. https://doi.org/10.3390/en5082911

Rastogi, M., Nandal, M., & Khosla, B. (2020). Microbes as vital additives for solid waste composting. *Heliyon*, *6*(2), e03343. https://doi.org/10.1016/j.heliyon.2020.e03343

Reddy, S., & Galab, S. (1998). *An Integrated Economic and Environmental Assessment of Solid Waste Management in India – the Case of Hyderabad, India.* A report, Centre for Economic and Social Studies, Andhra Pradesh, India.

Ros, M., Klammer, S., Knapp, B., Aichberger, K., & Insam, H. (2006). Long-term effects of compost amendment of soil on functional and structural diversity and microbial activity. *Soil Use and Management*, *22*(2), 209–218. https://doi.org/10.1111/j.1475-2743.2006.00027.x

Ruggieri, L., Gea, T., Artola, A., & Sánchez, A. (2009). Air filled porosity measurements by air pycnometry in the composting process: A review and a correlation analysis. *Bioresource Technology*, *100*(10), 2655–2666. https://doi.org/10.1016/j.biortech.2008.12.049

Rupf, G. V., Bahri, P. A., de Boer, K., & McHenry, M. P. (2016). Broadening the potential of biogas in Sub-Saharan Africa: An assessment of feasible technologies and feedstocks. *Renewable and Sustainable Energy Reviews*, *61*, 556–571. https://doi.org/10.1016/j.rser.2016.04.023

Sakhiya, A. K., Anand, A., & Kaushal, P. (2020). Production, activation, and applications of biochar in recent times. *Biochar*, *2*(3). https://doi.org/10.1007/s42773-020-00047-1

Sallwey, J., Hettiarachchi, H., & Hülsmann, S. (2017). Challenges and opportunities in municipal solid waste management in Mozambique: a review in the light of nexus thinking. *AIMS Environmental Science*, *4*(5), 621–639. https://doi.org/10.3934/environsci.2017.5.621

Sanchez-Monedero, M. A., Cayuela, M. L., Roig, A., Jindo, K., Mondini, C., & Bolan, N. (2018). Role of biochar as an additive in organic waste composting. *Bioresource Technology*, *247*(July), 1155–1164. https://doi.org/10.1016/j.biortech.2017.09.193

Sánchez-Monedero, M. A., Sánchez-Garcıá, M., Castejón-Del Pino, R., Fornes, F., Belda, R. M., Lidón, A., & Cayuela, M. L. (2021). Biochar as an additive in composting: impact on process performance and on the agronomical quality of the end product. *Acta Horticulturae*, *1317*, 175–187. https://doi.org/10.17660/ActaHortic.2021.1317.21

Sánchez, A. (2007). A kinetic analysis of solid waste composting at optimal conditions. *Waste Management*, *27*(6), 854–855. https://doi.org/10.1016/j.wasman.2006.07.003

Sannigrahi, A. K., & Chakrabortty, S. (2002). Beneficial management of organic wastes by vermi composting. *Indian Journal of Environmental Protection*, *22*(4), 405–408.

Saraswat, M., Dixit, A., Goel, A., & Ram Chauhan, N. (2019). Performance and emission evaluation of butanol blends in SI engine. *IOP Conference Series: Materials Science and Engineering*, *691*, 012081. https://doi.org/10.1088/1757-899X/691/1/012081

Sawyerr, N., Trois, C., Workneh, T. S., Oyebode, O., & Babatunde, O. M. (2020). Design of a household biogas digester using co-digested cassava, vegetable and fruit waste. *Energy Reports*, *6*, 1476–1482. https://doi.org/10.1016/j.egyr.2020.10.067

Schouw, N. L., Danteravanich, S., Mosbaek, H., & Tjell, J. C. (2002). Composition of human excreta - A case study from Southern Thailand. *Science of the Total Environment*, *286*(1–3), 155–166. https://doi.org/10.1016/S0048-9697(01)00973-1

Siddiqui, Z., Hagare, D., Jayasena, V., Swick, R., Rahman, M. M., Boyle, N., & Ghodrat, M. (2021). Recycling of food waste to produce chicken feed and liquid fertiliser. *Waste Management*, *131*(July), 386–393. https://doi.org/10.1016/j.wasman.2021.06.016

Smårs, S. (2002). Improvement of the composting time for household waste during an initial low pH phase by mesophilic temperature control. *Bioresource Technology*, *84*(3), 237–241. https://doi.org/10.1016/S0960-8524(02)00056-1

Sundberg, C., Smårs, S., & Jönsson, H. (2004). Low pH as an inhibiting factor in the transition from mesophilic to thermophilic phase in composting. *Bioresource Technology*, *95*(2), 145–150. https://doi.org/10.1016/j.biortech.2004.01.016

Surendra, K. C., Takara, D., Hashimoto, A. G., & Khanal, S. K. (2014). Biogas as a sustainable energy source for developing countries: Opportunities and challenges. *Renewable and Sustainable Energy Reviews*, *31*, 846–859. https://doi.org/10.1016/j.rser.2013.12.015

Tiquia, S. M., Richard, T. L., & Honeyman, M. S. (2002). Carbon, nutrient, and mass loss during composting. *Nutrient Cycling in Agroecosystems*, *62*(1), 15–24. https://doi.org/10.1023/A:1015137922816

Uddin, M. N., Siddiki, S. Y. A., Mofijur, M., Djavanroodi, F., Hazrat, M. A., Show, P. L., Ahmed, S. F., & Chu, Y. M. (2021). Prospects of bioenergy production from organic waste using anaerobic digestion technology: A mini review. *Frontiers in Energy Research*, *9*(March). https://doi.org/10.3389/fenrg.2021.627093

United Nations, Department of Economic and Social Affairs (UN DESA). (2019). In *The United Nations, Department of Economic and Social Affairs-Highlights 2018-2019*. Accessed at https://www.un.org/development/desa/en/wp-content/uploads/2019/12/Anual_Report_1211.pdf on 26 July, 2022.

Wainaina, S., Awasthi, M. K., Sarsaiya, S., Chen, H., Singh, E., Kumar, A., Ravindran, B., Awasthi, S. K., Liu, T., Duan, Y., Kumar, S., Zhang, Z., & Taherzadeh, M. J. (2020). Resource recovery and circular economy from organic solid waste using aerobic and anaerobic digestion technologies. *Bioresource Technology*, *301*, 122778. https://doi.org/10.1016/j.biortech.2020.122778

Yousuf, A., Sultana, S., Monir, M. U., Karim, A., & Rahmaddulla, S. R. B. (2017). Social business models for empowering the biogas technology. *Energy Sources, Part B: Economics, Planning, and Policy*, *12*(2), 99–109. https://doi.org/10.1080/15567249.2016.1255677

Yu, Q., Liu, S., Yu, L., Xiao, Y., Zhang, S., Wang, X., Xu, Y., Yu, H., Li, Y., Yang, J., Tang, J., Duan, H.-C., Wei, L.-H., Zhang, H., Wei, J., Tang, Q., Wang, C., Zhang, W., Wang, Y., … Jia, G. (2021). RNA demethylation increases the yield and biomass of rice and potato plants in field trials. *Nature Biotechnology*. https://doi.org/10.1038/s41587-021-00982-9

Zeng, J., Singh, D., & Chen, S. (2011). Thermal decomposition kinetics of wheat straw treated by Phanerochaete chrysosporium. *International Biodeterioration & Biodegradation*, *65*(3), 410–414. https://doi.org/10.1016/j.ibiod.2011.01.004

Index

Note: **Bold** page numbers refer to tables; *Italic* page numbers refer to figures.